Th. Rabe · B. Runnebaum

Fertility Control – update and trends

Springer
Berlin
Heidelberg
New York
Barcelona
Budapest
Hong Kong
London
Milan
Paris
Singapore
Tokyo

Thomas Rabe · Benno Runnebaum

Fertility Control – Update and Trends

With 54 Figures, some in Color, and 29 Tables

Springer

Thomas Rabe, Prof. Dr. med., Dr. h.c. mult.
Division of Gynecology and Reproductive Medicine
WHO Collaborating Centre for Research in Gynaecological
Endocrinology and Reproducative Medicine
University Women's Hospital
Voßstrasse 9
69115 Heidelberg
Germany

Benno Runnebaum, Prof. Dr. med., Dr. h.c. mult.
Division of Gynecology and Reproductive Medicine
WHO Collaborating Centre for Research in Gynaecological
Endocrinology and Reproducative Medicine
University Women's Hospital
Voßstrasse 9
69115 Heidelberg
Germany

Library of Congress Cataloging-in-Publication Data.

Fertility control / [edited by] Thomas Rabe.
p. cm.
Includes bibliographical references and index.

ISBN 978-3-642-86698-2 ISBN 978-3-642-86696-8(eBook)
DOI 10.1007/978-3-642-86696-8

1. Contraception-Congress. I. Rabe, T. (Thomas), 1951-
RG136.A2F48 1999
613.9'4-dc21

98-33842
CIP

Softcover reprint of the hardcover 1st edition 1999

Cover design: E. Kirchner, Heidelberg

Typesetting: Goldener Schnitt, Sinzheim

SPIN: 10484727 13/3135 5 4 3 2 1 0 – Printed on acid-free paper

Preface

Dedication to Professor Dr. med. Dr. h.c. mult. Benno Runnebaum on his 65th Anniversary

The name of Benno Runnebaum is closely tied to the status of gynaecological endocrinology and reproductive medicine. Therefore, we would like to dedicate this conference book entitled "Fertility Control" to him in recognition of his achievements.

Who is Benno Runnebaum?

Benno Runnebaum was born on 22 July, 1933, in Rüschendorf, Germany. After taking his A-levels, he studied medicine in Münster, Bonn and Cologne. He graduated from Cologne University in 1961 and then prepared his doctoral thesis on the "Identification and quantification of progesterone, 20α-dihydroprogesterone, 20β-dihydroprogesterone and 17α-hydroxyprogesterone in the plasma of human placental blood". This

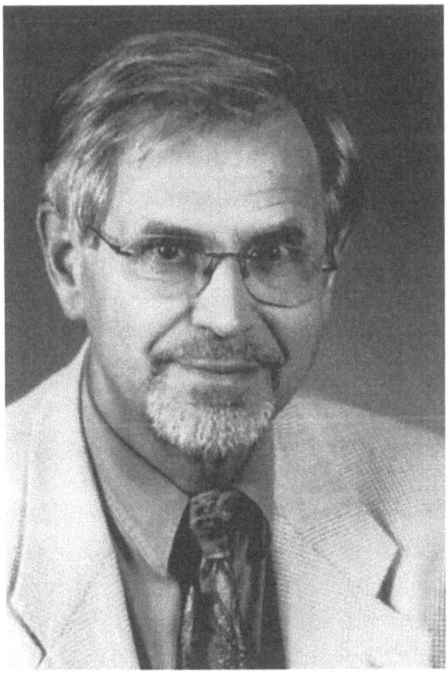

Benno Runnebaum

publication was the first to describe the progestin cycle in the feto-placental unit. His thesis was supported by Professor Dr. med. Dr. h.c. Josef Zander. It was graded "summa cum laude" and won him a scholarship from the National Institute of Health for training in steroid biochemistry at the Biochemical Institute in Salt Lake City (Professor Samuels) in 1962 and 1963. After his return to Germany he worked at the University Women's Hospital of Cologne. He received his further specialist training in 1964 at the Heidelberg Women's Hospital, under the chairmanship of his teacher, Professor Zander. In 1969, Benno Runnebaum wrote his professorial thesis on the "Identification and quantification of progesterone and 20α-dihydroprogesterone in the human uterine muscle during pregnancy". In the same year, he became a "Facharzt" for Gynaecology and Obstetrics. In early 1970, he joined the 1st University Women's Hospital in Munich together with Professor Zander to work there as a university lecturer and consultant. In 1971, he was appointed Head of Department for Gynaecological Endocrinology at the University Women's Hospital in Heidelberg. Since 1975, he has been the Medical Director of the Department for Gynaecological Endocrinology and Fertility Disorders.

Professor Runnebaum has investigated various aspects of gynaecological endocrinology and reproductive medicine. From his first experimental studies, he has analysed the close endocrine link between the child, the placenta and the mother and made substantial contributions with respect to endocrine regulation and maintenance of pregnancy. He has also dealt with the control of hormonal processes involving the brain stem, the pituitary and the ovaries and made a number of new findings of great relevance for special therapies, e.g. of women with cyclic disorders, myomata and endometriosis. He has also taken an interest in research of direct clinical relevance and translated new findings quickly into patient treatment. A number of clinical sections ("Spezialsprechstunden") were set up in his divisions to look at special issues, such as hormones and infertility, virilism and hair loss, in vitro fertilisation, endometriosis, the menopause, environmental influences and fertility disorders.

He has organised three international symposia in Heidelberg on "Future aspects of contraception". In this context, new ideas have emerged, advancing the development of contraceptive methods.

Apart from his membership in many national professional associations and his activities on the boards of several scientific societies (Deutsche Gesellschaft für Gynäkologie und Geburtshilfe, Deutsche Gesellschaft für Endokrinologie, Deutsche Menopausegesellschaft, Deutsche Gesellschaft zum Studium für Fertilität und Sterilität), he was the co-founder of a number of scientific societies and journals; in recent years, he has been a corresponding editor for the American Journal of Obstetrics and Gynecology. As spokesman of the Working Group for Gynaecological Endocrinology and Reproductive Medicine (AGGEF) since 1992, he has managed to bring together a heterogeneous group of gynaecological endocrinologists, experts on reproductive medicine and microsurgeons to form a strong voice for gynaecological endocrinology and reproductive medicine.

His team has always been open to international scientific exchange, especially with visiting doctors from Greece, Hungary, Rumania, Saudi-Arabia, Chile, China, Venezuela, Turkey and Poland. The most recent exchange programme started 1 year ago with the women's hospitals of Ho Chi Minh City and Hanoi/Vietnam as a partner programme with the WHO (HRP).

His clinical and research work is reflected in more than 450 original scientific publications. In 1987, he edited a textbook on gynaecological endocrinology. The second edition was published in 1994 as two volumes: Gynaecological Endocrinology and Reproductive Medicine. Altogether, he has published a total of 12 books and written 87 book articles.

On account of his achievements in gynaecological endocrinology and reproductive medicine, he received the "Bundesverdienstkreuz" (Federal Order of Merit) in 1994. In the same year, his department was declared WHO Collaborating Centre for Research in Gynaecological Endocrinology and Reproductive Medicine. This implies a great honour since there are only 52 WHO collaborating centres for human reproduction in the world. It is an important acknowledgement, not just to his Division at the Women's Hospital, but also to the University of Heidelberg.

As mentioned above, many young scientists and doctors from home and abroad have received their further clinical and scientific training in his department. In 1991, Benno Runnebaum was awarded the honorary doctorate of the Semmelweis University, Budapest and, in 1998, the honorary doctorate of the University of Cluj, Rumania, in recognition of his co-operation and his achievements in the field of gynaecological endocrinology and reproductive medicine.

All along, he has worked to establish the discipline of gynaecological endocrinology and reproductive medicine at many German University Women's Hospitals and other large outpatient clinics to provide the best diagnostic and therapeutic care available to many women and couples with hormone and fertility problems.

Despite all efforts of Professor Runnebaum to establish new departments for gynecological endocrinology and reproductive medicine at German universities, no new independent departments for gynaecological endocrinology and reproductive medicine have been founded there so far; the number of existing departments or divisions has steadily been reduced.

However, due to the enormous growth in knowledge, the importance of gynaecological endocrinology and reproductive medicine has increased world-wide and certainly in Germany; most patients have been treated in large, well-equipped and well-staffed out-patient clinics. Unfortunately, German universities have experienced an exodus of qualified doctors and scientists because of lack of employment prospects. Calls for more basic research in molecular biology and molecular genetics as a prerequisite for catching up with the international standard are big but empty words, without an adequate structure at the women's hospitals. Best wishes of all of us!

Finally, I would like to thank Professor Runnebaum as a mentor and friend for his achievements in the field of gynaecological endocrinology and reproductive medicine, also on behalf of the Working Group on Gynaecological Endocrinology and Reproductive Medicine (AGGEF).

Together with the staff of the University Women's Hospital, research workers, his patients and many former colleagues and friends at home and abroad, I would like to wish Professor Benno Runnebaum good health, creativity and continued success in the future to fulfil all his wishes in family life, lifestyle and art, and also in science – and please don't forget the Chinese proverb:

If we radiate goodness,
we will receive goodness in return.

Thomas Rabe, Heidelberg, den 22.6.1998

Contents

List of Contributers

d'Arcangues, Catherine, Dr.
Special Programme of Research, Development and Research,
Training in Human Reproduction
World Health Organization
12211 Geneva 27, Switzerland

Baulieu, Etienne, Emile, Prof.
Collége de France, INSERM U 33
80 rue du Général Leclerc, F-94276 Le Kremlin-Bicetre Cedex, France

Benagiano, Giuseppe P., Prof.
Direcor General, Istituto Superiore Di Sanitá
Viale Regina Elena 299, I-00161 Roma, Italy

Bydgdeman, Marc, Prof., MD, PhD
Department of OB/GYN, Karolinska Hospital
S-17176 Stockholm, Sweden

Danielsson, Kristina Gemzell, MD, PhD
Department of OB/GYN, Karolinska Hospital
S-17176 Stockholm, Sweden

Diszfalusy, Egon, Prof. Dr. Dr. h.c. mult.
Rönningevägen 21, S-14461 Rönninge, Sweden

Eckardstein, Sigrid von, Dr. med.
Westfälische Wilhelms-Universität
Zentrum für Frauenheilkunde
Institut für Reproduktionsmedizin
WHO Kollaborationszentrum
Domagkstraße 11, 48129 Münster, Germany

Filshie, Marcus, Prof.
Reader/Consultant in OB/GYN, Queen's Medical Centre
University Hospital Nottingham, Nottingham NG7 2 UH, United Kingdom

Freundl, Günter, Prof. Dr. med.
Chefarzt Frauenklinik D-Benrath
Urdenbacher Allee 83, 40593 Düsseldorf, Germany

Garbe, Edeltraut, Dr. med.
ZEG - Zentrum für Epidemiologie
Schönerlinder Straße 11-12
16341 Zepernick, Germany

Heinemann, Lothar A.J., Prof. Dr. med.
ZEG-Zentrum für Epidemiologie
Schönerlinder Straße 11-12, 16341 Zepernick, Germany

Lähteenmäki, Pekka, Prof.
Vice President, Research & Development

Newton, John R., Prof.
Head of Reproductive Medicine
Director of the West Midlands Laser Endoscopy Centre
Birmingham Women's Hospital, Edgbaston, Birmingham B 15 2 TG, United Kingdom

Marions, Lena, MD
Department of OB/GYN, Karolinska Hospital
S-17176 Stockholm, Sweden

Nieschlag, Eberhard, Prof. Dr. med.
Westfälische Wilhelms-Universität
Zentrum für Frauenheilkunde
Institut für Reproduktionsmedizin
WHO Kollaborationszentrum
Domagkstraße 11, 48129 Münster, Germany

Pera, Alessandra
Istituto Superiore Di Sanita
Viale Regina Elena 299, I-00161 Roma, Italy

Rabe, Thomas, Prof. Dr. med., Dr. h.c.mult.
Univ.-Frauenklinik, Gynäkologische Endokrinologie und Fertilitätsstörungen, Abt. 4.2
WHO Collaborating Centre for Research in Gynaecological Endocrinology and Reproductive Medizine
Voßstraße 9, 69115 Heidelberg, Germany

Runnebaum, Benno, Prof. Dr. med, Dr. h.c.mult.
Univ.-Frauenklinik, Gynäkologische Endokrinologie und Fertilitätsstörungen, Abt. 4.2
WHO Collaborating Centre for Research in Gynaecological Endocrinology and Reproductive Medizine
Voßstraße 9, 69115 Heidelberg, Germany

Snow, Rachel, Prof. Dr. med.
Hygiene-Institut Heidelberg
Im Neuenheimer Feld 324, 69120 Heidelberg, Germany

Swahn, Marja-Liisa, MD, PhD
Department of OB/GYN, Huddinge Hospital
S-14146 Huddinge, Sweden

Vladescu, Elena, Dr. med.
Bega-Clinic Timisoara
BD. Victor Babes. 12, 1900 Timisoara, Rumänien

Wagner, Horst, Prof. Dr. med.
Chefarzt der Abt. für Gynäkologie
Zweckverband Stadt- und Kreiskrankenhaus Klinikum Minden
Friedrichstraße 17, 32427 Minden, Germany

1 The Contraceptive Revolution: Its Past and Future "History"*

Egon Diczfalusy

Do I contradict myself?
Very well then, I contradict myself;
(I am large – I contain multitudes.)
WALT WHITMAN, 1855.

The Brave New World of Doublethink

"Every truth has its sect and every sect its truth" says an old Chinese proverb, and even those of us who are gathered here today from many countries, from almost all continents of the world, to celebrate the 25th anniversary of the World Health Organization's (WHO's) Human Reproduction Programme, belong to a particular sect of scientists, who believe profoundly in a bright future for the United Nations, in general, and for WHO in particular. Perhaps we have more in common in terms of fundamental values than with people within our own societies – or even within our own families. Still, except for our strong commitment to our common ideals and to the Special Programme during the past quarter of a century, we are rather different from each other and represent a multitude of views and a variety of approaches to life.

I myself represent the future. Yes, you heard it right, I said the future. I represent the future of the past. As Paul Valéry puts it : "Are you not the future of all memories stored within you? The future of the past." [1]. Indeed, my memories cover many, many years; a substantial part of the 20th century. During those years I have seen many changes, some of them fundamental, a few of them almost incredible. Times are changing, very rapidly and often irreversibly.

All of us, who studied Latin know very well the saying: "Tempora mutantur, nos et mutamur in illis"; times change and we change with them, but perhaps not too many classical students know its origin. No wonder, since it is misty and very uncertain. Matthias Borbonius [2] attributes it bravely and bluntly – indeed without any good evidence – to Emperor Lothar I. (795-855 A.D.) who was involved in very bitter twists and wars with his two younger brothers, the subject of the controversy being – needless to say – power. At any rate, the above quote doesn't seem to originate from the great thinkers of the Roman Empire; it is quoted much later in the literature, perhaps for the first time by A. Gartner in 1566 [3]. But why is this quotation of such an interest to us? – because of its next two lines: "Quomodo? Fit semper tempore peior homo"; How? Man will be worse with time.

Reprinted with permission from: L. Kovács and B.A. Resch (eds): Research on Human Reproduction. Albert Szent-Györgyi Medical University Press, Szeged (1998).

Well, well, is this indeed true? Some 160 years ago, Giacomo Leopardi remarks that "Each generation believes, on the one hand, that the ancients were better than the moderns and, on the other hand, that the human race is continually progressing and improving" [4]. Voilá!

Our next stop on this somewhat philosophical journey is George Orwell's Nineteen eighty-four [5], in which a modern inquisitor of our time, O'Brian, is brainwashing his victim, poor Winston: "Doublethink means the power of holding two contradictory beliefs in one's mind simultaneously, and accepting both of them". On first reading, I was smiling at all this; nowadays, I don't smile any longer, simply because even I became a "doublethinker", who believes that fundamental truths are recognized by the fact, that the opposite proposition is also a fundamental truth. Is this a new philosophy? Certainly not; already Aristotle stated that "the knowledge of the opposites is one" and I am just one of those late followers, like the poet Palinurus [6]: "I believe in two-faced truth, the Either, the Or and the Holy Both".

To me, this philosophy is a prerequisite for accepting – in an optimistic mood – our world full of paradoxes, a world that today is more integrated and fragmented than ever (just to mention one of those paradoxes). Other "doublethinkers" who still find it disturbing to accept that intrinsic contradiction is almost the quintessence of the human condition, might find some comfort in learning that, indeed, many of our favourite and often paradoxical modern slogans "require us to hold two or more contradictory propositions in our minds at the same time. The capacity to do that, I seem to recall" remarks Harlan Cleveland – was Sigmund Freud's definition of maturity [33].

The Power of Nonsensus

"Nonsensus" is one of my favourites, a special subgroup of consensus, defined by J. W. Webber in a letter to the editor of the Financial Times (1 November 1997) as "the fervent possession by a group of a belief or a set of beliefs which to an intelligent and dispassionate observer is clearly untrue", and I agree with Mr. Webber that nonsensus is one of the powerful instruments shaping our history, but hopefully not human destiny. Let me give a "politically sensitive" example, the issue of witch processes, something that was greatly appreciated by Homo sapiens during its history.

With an exceptional wisdom and vision, the young Hungarian King, Kálmán the Learned (1095-1116) issued a royal decree almost 900 years ago, stating that "De stregiis, quae non sunt, nulla mentio fiat"; Witches don't exist and should not be mentioned. Well, that was then the end, wasn't it? Certainly not; rather it was the beginning.

Almost 400 years thereafter, two fanatic monks, Jacob Spreger and Heinrich Krämer persuade the new Pope Innocentius VIII that witches represent an utmost danger to true Christianity, if not to entire human species; the Pope issues a Papal Bull, Summis desiderantes affectibus (1484) and gives full pouvoir to the two inquisitors for the persecution of the evil forces, and they do it very well, indeed. Of course, Spreger and Krämer are profoundly convinced of the fundamental solidity of their case and describe how to reveal, persecute and punish witches in a book entitled "Malleus maleficarum" (Strassbourg, 1490), the hammer of witches. What follows then, during a couple of centuries, are tens of thousands of witch processes, in which a very large number of "witches" are executed on the basis of "convincing and reliable testimonies", not infrequently by children. In Sweden, the last execution took place in 1704 and the last (and rather prolonged) witch process during the years 1757-1763. What did Friedrich Nietzsche say? "Convictions are more dangerous enemies of truth than lies." [7].

Of course, this couldn't happen in our day. Couldn't it? I myself have witnessed the history of the 20th century, in which some 200 million human beings were killed frequently in a systematic, carefully organised fashion – by other human beings on the orders of "deeply and honestly convinced" policy makers. And that time in history, there was no longer any need for witch processes, or child witnesses; many children also became witches.

The Power of Progress

I think it was Alexander Pope (1735) who felt, that "there must be shadows, if there should be light" and I have also seen an incredible amount of light. In my lifetime, I have seen more progress in science than all scientists of all preceding periods put together since the dawn of history, a progress that resulted in a major improvement of the human condition. It was observed already by Friedrich Engels that "science progresses in proportion to the mass of knowledge that is left to it by preceding generations, that is, under the most ordinary circumstances, in geometrical proportion" [8].

Indeed, I have also been part of the first age since the dawn of civilization, which dared to think it not only desirable, but also practicable, to make the benefits of progress available to the entire human race. I have been part of a generation that dared to establish the United Nations with all its important specialised agencies, such as WHO, a generation which – for the first time in history – felt it both feasible and mandatory to provide large-scale assistance jointly in any corner of the world to those stricken by famine or other natural catastrophes.

It was our generation, that – for the first time in history – acquired a truly holistic view of the world and a global consciousness. Do you doubt it? Just look around this room and consider the number of countries represented by us and our joint commitment to improve the human condition. Nothing of this sort existed during the previous centuries of our common past.

Indeed, history is much more than just an account of how people are double-crossing and killing each other; it is also an account of major intellectual revolutions, true progress, the gradual improvement of the human condition and the development of new ideas. My generation was a most privileged one, witnessing what I called the nine revolutions of the 20th century, the demographic, scientific, technological and environmental ones, together with those in communication, global identity, contraception, reproductive health and gender equity [9]. Many of us here today were and are part of the three last-mentioned ones, the three major intellectual, social revolutions of our time [10], and the contraceptive revolution is supposed to be the topic of this chapter, as suggested by its title, but perhaps not by this prolonged introduction.

The Contraceptive Revolution

How strong can an idea be, when it really corresponds to the exigency of the epoch? Very strong; the contraceptive revolution provides a good example. The year was 1952, when the government of India – for the first time in history – established a national family-planning programme. They did it at a time, when no oral contraceptives (OCs), or intrauterine devices were as yet available! The Indian example was followed – at first hesitatantly, later enthusiastically – by other governments. Today, some 150 governments support family-planning programmes, directly or indirectly.

The concept of the contraceptive revolution is intimately associated with the introduction of steroidal contraception, which was indeed a major revolution, scientifically, medically and socially, and which then resulted in another two powerful revolutions, those in reproductive health and gender equity [11]. It may be worth looking back at it with the wisdom of hindsight, particularly, since I was "present at the creation" [12] (for a review of the early history of " the pill", see references [13-15]).

In 1955, Professor Axel Westman, my chief at the Karolinska Hospital and the Editor-in-Chief of Acta Endocrinologica, brought back with him a few manuscripts from the Congress of the International Planned Parenthood Federation in Tokyo, and asked me to review them. One of those papers was presented by Gregory Pincus with the not too glamorous title: "Some effects of progesterone and related compounds upon reproduction and early development in mammals". The paper dealt with the results of various animal experiments, but it mentioned – in a rather cursory fashion – that huge doses (several hundred milligrams) of orally administered progesterone also inhibit ovulation in women [16]. What we didn't know in Stockholm at that time, was that Pincus and co-workers (among others Edris Rice-Wray and Celso Garcia) already had far-advanced clinical studies underway in Puerto Rico, using relatively small doses of orally active progestogens, norethisterone [17] and norethynodrel [18].

I was also "present at the creation" the following year, in 1956, witnessing the "birth of the pill" at the Laurentian Hormone Conference in Mont Tremblant. The triumvirate, John Rock, Celso Garcia and "Goody" Pincus, presented a paper on the effects of synthetic progestins in women [19], which were effective in far-smaller doses than natural progesterone in inhibiting ovulation. However, because of the aggressively hostile "public opinion" at the time (isn't it always against innovations?), it was unthinkable to John Rock (a devoute Bostonian catholic) to present such a revolutionary new concept: oral contraception. No, the idea had to be presented with plenty of sugar coating and the name of the game was: the rebound phenomenon. The objective of the studies was – the authors emphasized – to treat infertility and induce ovulation by means of a rebound effect. The synthetic progestins administered inhibit the disturbed pituitary secretion of gonadotrophins. This then constitutes a powerful stimulus for a rebound, the release of gonadotrophins in amounts sufficient to induce ovulation. But what about ovulation inhibition? Well, of course, ovulation is inhibited temporarily and in a reversible fashion during the therapeutic administration of the progestins, but this is a very reasonable price to pay for the return of normal ovulation and fertility, isn't it?

"What is amusing now had to be taken in desperate earnest once" wrote Virginia Woolf [20] and, of course, this applies equally to "bad news" and "good news" of times past. At any rate, the argument of "Goody" was so convincing, that the following year, in

1957, the Food and Drug Administration (FDA) of the United States approved two synthetic progestin preparations, norethynodrel and norethisterone, for "menstrual regulation". Did they really regulate menstruation? That's a very good question. What those menstrual regulators did in reality, was to introduce irregular intermenstrual bleedings, unless they were supplemented with small amounts of a synthetic estrogen. And what was a complete impossibility in 1957, became a matter-of-fact reality in 1959: the FDA approved the first (estrogen–progestin) combined oral contraceptive, Enovid. This was followed by regulatory action in Berlin: the Bundesgesundheitsamt approved Anovlar in 1961 and then the FDA approved Ortho Novum in 1962 [14]. The contraceptive revolution arrived in order to stay. Why? Because the modern methods of contraception enabled humankind, for the first time, to move contraception "out of the bathroom".

And the intrauterine devices? To insert an intrauterine device was a criminal offence in many countries as late as in the 1950s. Then, within a few years, things and perceptions changed, rather dramatically. The Margulies spiral was launched in 1960, Lippes loop in 1962 and the ice was definitely broken at an international Conference sponsored by the Population Council in New York, in 1962, which was followed by renewed research efforts in the field resulting in a new generation of medicated devices, Zipper's Copper-T (1974), the Progestasert (1976) and the Levonorgestrel device (1982) (for a review [21]). By the 1980s and 1990s, intrauterine devices were used by a couple of hundred million women around the world [22].

Revolution, or Way of Life?

In 1960, the number of contraceptive users in the developing world was around 30 million; by 1990 their number exceeded 380 million [23]. The United Nations estimate that around 1990, some 900 million couples used contraceptives [24]; the percentage of users was lowest in Africa (18%) and highest in Eastern Asia (79%); in fact, higher than in the developed regions of the world (72%) (Table 1).

Table 1. Contraceptive use – around 1990

Region	Couples (millions)	Users %
World	900	57
Africa	97	18
Asia	545	58
(Eastern Asia)	236	79
Latin America	67	58
Developed R.	186	72

United Nations, 1995 [24]

It is projected that by the year 2000, more than half a billion people of the developing world will use modern methods of contraception [22], as indicated by the data of Table 2.

In a world with some 900 million contraceptive users, a fundamental question is: when does a revolution cease to be a revolution and become simply a way of life? How many acceptors are needed for it and how do we measure its success in numerical

Table 2. Contraception in 2000

Method	Million users
Tubectomy	207
Vasectomy	47
Oral contraceptives	75
Injectables	21
Intrauterine devices	125
Condom	35
Traditional methods	57

Source: Shah I. H., 1994 [22]

terms? And how long should contraception be referred to as "controversial", just because a few religious and political leaders (but certainly not the many millions of their followers) are unwilling to accept a new idea? A "new idea" that is no longer new and no longer an idea, but rather a widely accepted fact of life?

The Changing Nature of Unmet Need

In the euphoric atmosphere of the "golden years" of the 1960s and 1970s, with a seemingly unlimited public and government support for research, the prospects for developing a large variety of methods for fertility regulation appeared to be rosy [25], and many of us were requested to indulge in futurology and speculate on the future need for methods and on methods that would probably be developed during the next few decades.

With the wisdom of hindsight, it may be of some interest to review here and now the "futurology of the past". Twenty years ago, I suggested six areas in which major development should take place:

a) worldwide epidemiological studies on "pill safety";
b) improved methods of ovulation prediction;
c) orally active prostaglandins;
d) methods for interfering with sperm maturation and motility;
e) improved methods for sterilization; and
f) better toxicological methods for the assessment of safety [26].

Ten years later, in 1989, Carl Djerassi also suggested six areas:

a) a spermicidal antiviral agent for local use;
b) a "menses inducer";
c) a reliable ovulation predictor;
d) reversible male sterilization; and
e) a male contraceptive pill and
f) a "male" and "female" antifertility vaccine [27].

Then just 3 years ago, on the initiative of Mahmoud Fathalla [28], the Rockefeller Foundation launched the Second Contraceptive Technology Revolution, with a women-centred agenda. The development of three types of methods is considered to be of top priority:

a) self-administered, "local" contraceptives that also offer protection against sexually transmitted diseases, including HIV;
b) various types of "menses inducers" and/or monthly methods; and
c) new contraceptives for men.

The women-centred agenda also addresses two fundamental concerns women have:
1. concern for control over their own bodies and
2. concern for equity in terms of physical safety and wellbeing.

The Rockefeller programme is the logical consequence of what has happened and what has not happened during the past two decades. There is still an "unmet need", estimated around 120 million couples, because of non-use, or misuse of contraceptives; 28% of all pregnancies (some 52 million) are still interrupted; too many women opt for surgical sterilisation (at least 200 million worldwide) instead of reversible methods; no reliably reversible methods can be offered as yet to the male population of the world, and there is a rapidly increasing global burden of sexually transmitted diseases, with more than 330 million new cases annually [29, 30].

Past and Present Obstacles

It is, by now, a truism that the development of new fertility-regulating agents is very time consuming and very costly. Looking into the future, in 1979, I tried to define the obstacles interfering with the development of a greatly needed wide variety of contraceptives and identified seven major causes:
a) gaps in fundamental knowledge;
b) animal models of doubtful predictive value;
c) shortage in qualified investigators;
d) a long lead time;
e) high developmental costs;
f) hesitation of industry; and
g) absence of political support [26].

Is the situation basically different today? Hardly. Latest estimates by the representatives of the Pharmaceutical Industry put the development time (including phase-III studies, but not those beyond phase III) to approximately 10 years, and the cost of bringing to the market a new chemical entity over 200 million US dollars; spin-off products cost perhaps half of this amount [31].

Future Users and their Future

Paul Valéry remarks somewhere that "the magic of history is the most dangerous poison to the human intellect" and I feel that he has a point, also in the context of the history of contraception, and that we have to look a bit more into its future "history", as suggested the title of this chapter. Some 200 years ago, Edmund Burke warned that "you can never plan the future by the past" [32], but our entire political system in its

Table 3. *Tempora mutantur.* Regional distribution of the global population (%)

Region	Year 1950	2000	2050
Africa	9	14	22
Asia	56	61	58
Latin America	7	9	9
North America	7	5	4
Europe	22	12	7

United Nations, 1995 [24]

Table 4. Female population aged 15-49 (millions)

Region	Year 2000	2020	2040
Africa	194	339	514
Asia	963	1194	1292
Latin America	139	176	188
North America	78	79	82
Europe	183	158	136

United Nations, 1995 [24]

present organisation with relatively short periods of time between elections does not entice policy makers to invest a great deal of time and effort into long-term planning instead of re-election campaigns.

What are the likely projections for our future "history"? The United Nations (1995) project that, between 1950 and 2050, the global population will increase from 2.5 billion to some 10 billion people [24]. Major geopolitical changes are also projected, as indicated by the data of Table 3.

In 1950, the population of Africa constituted 9% of the global population and that of Europe 22%; by the year 2050, Africa will represent 22% of the world population and Europe only 7%. The regional distribution of the population in the fertile age will - logically - follow the same pattern; the projected changes in the female population aged 15-49 years, between the years 2000 and 2040, are shown in Table 4.

Today it is estimated that 50%, or perhaps even more, of the contraceptive market is in Northern America; however, between 2000 and 2040, the number of consumers of contraceptives will hardly increase there, whereas it will markedly decline in Europe; by 2040, 90% of the fertile female population will live in Africa, Asia and Latin America [24].That's where the market of the future will be, provided they, or the international community, will be able and willing to pay for those future contraceptives.

In an attempt to put all this into an economic perspective of our present decade, the gross national product (GNP) of different economic areas of the world (in 1993) is presented in Table 5 [29]. We all agree that contraception is an indispensable ingredient of reproductive health and, as such, it is not only a fundamental human right for all, but also a social and economic imperative [34]. We also agree, that there still is a major need worldwide for safe, effective and acceptable methods of fertility regulation; but what are we going to do in order to make them affordable? In the Chairman's Foreword to the Report of the World Commission on Environment and Development [35], Mme. Gro Harlem Brundtland remarked that "Since the answers to fundamental and serious concerns are not at hand, there is no alternative but to keep on trying to

Table 5. Some basic indicators (1995)

	POPULATION (Millions)	GNP (US$)
World	5701	4229
Market economies	823	23262
Economy in transition	391	1992
Developing countries	3898	1043
Least developed countries	589	200

WHO, 1996 [29]

find them". It would appear, therefore, that a great deal more research, development and advocacy will still be needed when humankind enters the third millennium.

Changing the Past and Inventing the Future

More than 100 years ago, Samuel Butler remarked "It has been said that although God cannot alter the past, historians can; it is perhaps because they can be useful to Him in this respect that He tolerates their existence" [36]. Then, one of the great physicists of our century, a former Hungarian, Leo Szilárd, emphasized that "the most important facet of the future is that it is inherently different from past and present. Furthermore, it is impossible to know in what way the future will be different. Hence the most illogical premise of all was the belief most economists held, that by observing the past and present they would find clues to the future." [37]. Eliminating in this way, all historians and economists from our consideration of the future, we have to rely (like so many times before!) on poets. They are more likely to help, as observed in the early 1930s by Frederic Wood-Jones: "Whoever wins to a great scientific truth, will find a poet before him in the quest". So, I found somewhere Gabriel Garcia Marqués saying that "Como no es posible predecir el futuro, hay que inventarlo". Since it is not possible to predict the future, we have to invent it. So, permit me to re-invent the future by converting the "here and now" into Our Common Future and the Great Beyond, hoping that posterity will not be upset too much. After all, why should it be? As Heywood Broun pointed out, "posterity is as likely to be wrong as anybody else" [38] and this includes, of course, our forefathers as much as our grandchildren.

The National Historical Memorial Park at Opusztaszer – with the world famous cyclorama of Árpád Feszty – is in the vicinity of Szeged, perhaps 15 miles away. The cyclorama presents the Hungarian conquest from 11 centuries ago; it was painted by Feszty between 1892 and 1894 with the support of several of his colleagues. Thus, the famous horse-battle scene can be attributed to Pál Vágó. It conveys masterfully to the observer the very special – almost symbiotic – relationship of Hungarians to their horses; no doubt, a nation of legendary horsemen! However, not even the very best Hungarian huszár would be able to ride the horse shown in Figure 1, which shows the famous statue by Salvador Dali, the horse of destiny; only time represented by Dali's speciality, a soft clock – but no human being – can ride this horse, and the fateful horse of destiny is well on its way into the third millennium. Homo sapiens tries to follow him, with uncertain and hesitant steps, as depicted by A. Penck in his impressive painting, entitled "Der Übergang"; transition (1963) (Fig. 2).

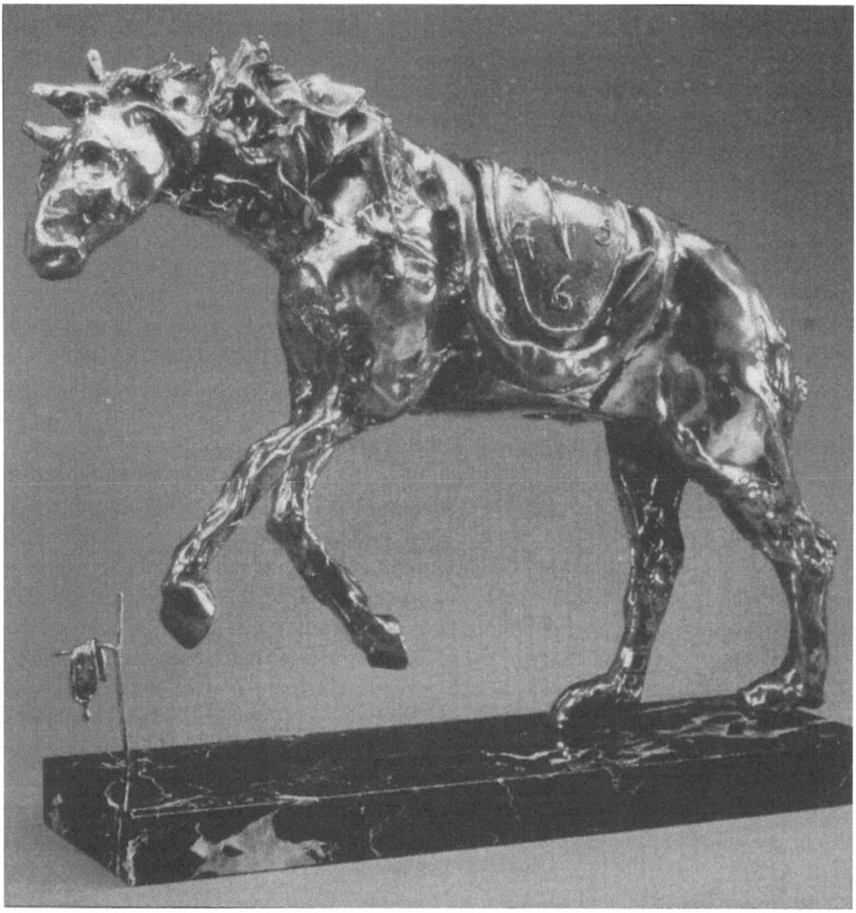

Fig. 1. Salvador Dali. Le Cheval avec la montre molle. © 1981, Original Sculptures Ltd. – D 513

Although the painting is most expressive, I find that something is missing, since homo sapiens doesn't travel empty handed. He carries with him several things into the third millennium, like the seven obstacles on our "golden road to Samarkand" (Table 6).

Homo sapiens also carries with him many diseases, among those an insufficiently observed one of critical importance for our future, described by Feodor Dostoyevsky

Table 6. Seven obstacles on humankind's "golden road to samarkand"

Population growth
Ageing of populations
Environmental degradation
Global unemployment
Poor health
Persistent poverty
Intra-species aggression

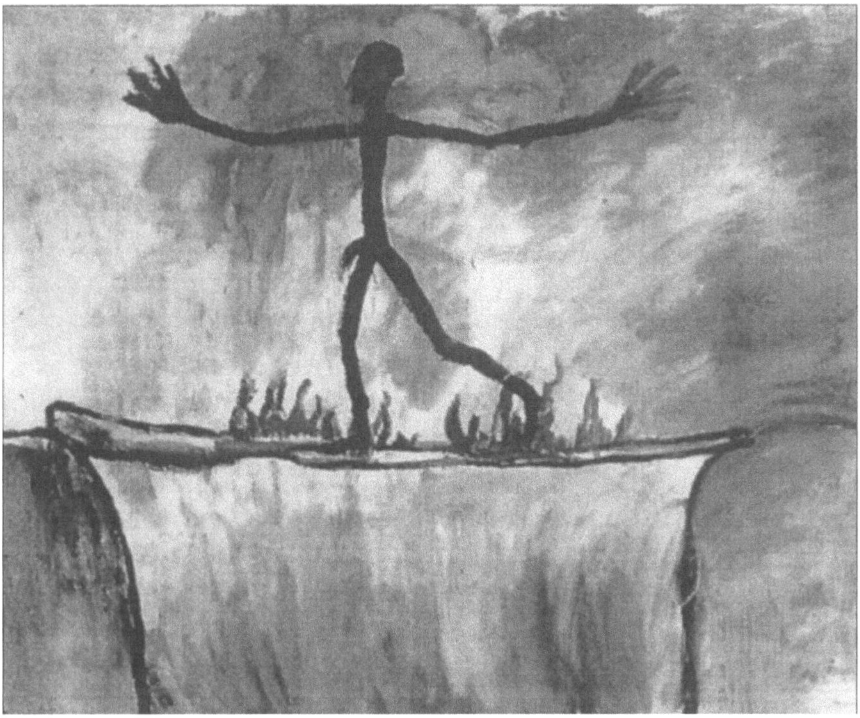

Fig. 2. A.R. Penck. Der Übergang - 1963

as the "Don Quijote disease"; a passionate search for reality. In this search, I could identify at least nine approaches: the scientific, cultural, religious, ethical, economical, ecological, sociocritical, philosophical and political [9]; when these approaches converge, they can create a confluence of spiritual influences of different character, resulting in a flourishing culture and amazingly rapid scientific progress. If they don't, then the world becomes a vast temple of discord, with the political approach assuming a controlling role [10].

It is very important to remember that each of the above approaches can enormously enrich human existence. However, it is equally important to bear in mind that their impact on the wellbeing of humankind is not equal and that - as P. C. Snow [39] observed, "The scientific revolution is the only method by which people can gain the primal things (years of life, freedom from hunger, survival for children)." Indeed, it can't be overemphasised that "the acquisition and systematisation of positive knowledge is the only human activity that is truly cumulative and progressive" [40].

Indeed, science has a unique self-correcting propensity and its "track record" in improving the human condition is unparallelled by any other human activity. Of course, all human knowledge is imperfect and will remain imperfect forever; however, it is indefinitely perfectible. Homo sapiens doesn't travel empty handed, since never before has humankind had so many resources, so much knowledge and such powerful technologies at its disposal. And - most importantly - homo sapiens carries with him into the third millennium – what I called – the infinite wisdom of hope, a robust hope in the ultimate success of the human race in its struggle to eventually establish on this Earth "the empire of human dignity", a world in which every human being has sufficient food, potable water, shelter, sanitation, health services, a healthy environment, education, employment and personal security [41]. This will be the greatest of all social revolutions ever; a universal search for human dignity. All this can happen, if we let it happen! Why don't we try? I like to quote in this context the Roman philosopher, Publilius Syrus: "Nobody knows what he can do till he tries" [42], and an impressive writer, a son of Bánnát, Danilo Kis : "Beware of cynicism, even your own". However, in the final analysis, as a "take-home" message from Hungary, the timeless words of Imre Madách reflect best the fundamentals of the human condition: "Mondottam ember: küzdj és bizva bizzál"; Oh Man, strive on, strive on; have faith and trust! [43].

References

1. Valéry P (1942) Mauvaises pensées at autres, 8th edn, Gallimard, Paris
2. Matthias Borbonius, Delitiae poetarum Germanorum. J. Gruber (ed) 1612-/685
3. Gartner A. (1566) Proverbialia dicteria 16; fol. C4
4. Leopardi G (1824-1832) "Sayings of Filippo Ottonieri". In: Essays and Dialogues
5. Orwell G (1944) Nineteen eighty-four. Seeker & Warburg, London
6. Palinurus (1945) The Unquiet Grave. Hamish Hamilton, London
7. Nietzsche F (1878-1886) Human, All Too Human
8. Engels F (1963) In: Karpov M.M (ed) Osnovyyie zakonomernosti razvitiya estestvoznaniya, Rostov State University; Quoted by Ebison M. (ed) (1977) Scientific Quotations: the Harvest of a Quiet Eye, p 54. Crane, Russak and Co., New York
9. Diczfalusy E (1998) Farewell to the 20th century and reproductive ill health. Eur J Obstet Gynecol Reprod Biol 77: 1-9
10. Diczfalusy E (1997). In search of human dignity: gender equity, reproductive health and healthy ageing. Int J Gynecol Obstet 59: 159-206.
11. Diczfalusy E (1997) The contraceptive revolution. An era of scientific and social development. Casterton Hall, Parthenon
12. Acheson D (1969) Present at the creation. My years in the State Department. Washington DC
13. Diczfalusy E (1978) Gregory Pincus and steroidal contraception: a new departure in the history of mankind. J Steroid Biochem 11:3-11
14. Diczfalusy E (1989) The history of steroidal contraception: what is past and what is present? In: Michal F (ed) Safety requirements for contraceptive steroids. Cambridge University Press, Cambridge pp 1-18
15. Djerassi C (1979) The politics of contraception. Stanford Alumni Association, Stanford, California
16. Pincus G (1956) Some effects of progesterone and related compounds upon reproduction and early development in mammals. Acta Endocrinol (Kbh) [Suppl 28] 18
17. Djerassi C, Miramontes L & Rosenkranz G (1952) Steroids. 19-nor-ethynyltestosterone and 19-nor-methyltestosterone. Paper presented at the Milwaukee, Wisconsin, Meeting of the American Chemical Society, April, 1952. Division of Medicinal Chemistry, Abstract 18J
18. Colton F.B (1955) 13-methyl-17ethynyl-17-hydroxy-1,2,3,4,6,7,8,9,11,12,13,14,16,17-tetradecahydro-15H-cyclo-penta(alpha)phenanthren-3-one and its preparation. U.S. Patent No. 2,725,389
19. Rock J, Garcia CR & Pincus G (1957) Synthetic progestins in the normal human menstrual cycle. Rec Progr Hormone Res 13:323-346
20. Woolf V (1929) A room of one's own. London
21. Rowe PJ (1987) Intrauterine contraception: advances and future prospects. In: Matsumoto S (ed) Recent advances in fertility control. Excerpta Medica, Amsterdam, pp 22-55
22. Shah IH (1994) The advance of the contraceptive revolution. World Health Stat.Q. 47:9-15
23. United Nations Department of International Economic and Social Affairs (1989) Levels and trends of contraceptive use as assessed in 1988. UN Publication Sales No. E89, X11. 1989, New York, pp 4

24. United Nations Department for Economic and Social Information and Policy Analysis, Population Division (1995) World population prospects: the 1994 revision. Document ST/ESA/SER/A/145. United Nations, New York.
25. Harper MJK (1983) Birth control technologies. William Heinemann Medical Books Ltd., London
26. Diczfalusy E (1979) Future methods of fertility regulation. Int J Gynaecol Obstet 16:571-578
27. Djerassi C (1989) The biller pill. Science 245:354-361
28. Fathalla M (1994) Fertility control technology: a woman-centered approach to research. In: Chen L, Germain A & Sen G (eds) Population policies reconsidered: health, empowerment and rights. Harvard University Press, Cambridge, Mass
29. World Health Organization (1996) The World health report 1996. Fighting disease, fostering development. World Health Organization, Geneva
30. Harrison PF, Rosenfield A (eds) (1996) Contraceptive research and development. Looking to the future. National Academy Press, Washington DC
31. Rockefeller Foundation (1997). Public/private sector collaboration in contraceptive research and development. A new partnership. Report of a Bellagio meeting, March 10-14
32. Burke E (1953) Letter to a member of the National Assembly. Quoted by the Oxford Dictionary of Quotations. Oxford University Press, London, pp 102: 6
33. Cleveland H (1997) Leadership and the information revolution. World Academy of Art and Science, Minneapolis MN
34. World Health Organization (1994). Health, population and development. WHO position paper for the international conference on population and development, Cairo, 1994. WHO/FHE/94. World Health Organization, Geneva
35. The World Commission on Environment and Development (1987) Our Common Future. Oxford University Press, Oxford
36. Butler S (1953) Erewhon, ch 14 Quoted by the Oxford Dictionary of Quotations. Oxford University Press, London, pp 111:28
37. Lanouette W (1992) Genius in the shadows. A biography of Leo Sziáird, the man behind the bomb. The University of Chicago Press, Chicago, pp 44
38. Broun H (1924) Sitting on the world. Quoted by Gross J. The Oxford Book of Aphorisms (1983) Oxford University Press, Oxford, pp 322
39. Snow CP (1963) The two cultures: a second look. Cambridge University Press, London
40. Sarton GAL (1957) The study of the history of science. Dover, New York
41. Diczfalusy E (1995) From population policy to reproductive health: numbers, rates or human beings? In: Elstein M (ed) From contraception to reproductive health care. Parthenon, New York, pp 16-38
42. Publilius Syrus (circa 42 BC) Maxim 786. Quoted in: Bartlett J. (ed) Familiar Quotations, Mac Millan, London, pp 46
43. Madách I (1860) The tragedy of man. Corvina, Budapest (1964), p.196

2 Decreasing Abortion: The Potential and the Constraints

Giuseppe Benagiano, Alessandra Pera

In the whole field of health there is no topic that has, throughout history, created more controversy than the voluntary interruption of an already-established pregnancy. Already centuries before Christ, the issue was debated and Hippocrates, the great Greek Physician of the 5th Centrury B.C., placed in his oath the prohibition to induce an abortion in a pregnant woman.

This fact alone is sufficient to explain why voluntary abortion has been the source of bitter disagreement even among gynaecologists. Indeed, the ethical considerations brought forward in favor or against abortion are so opposing that nothing one can say will ever create unanimity.

For this reason, it is probable that each reader of this paper will find some reason for disagreement; the truth of the matter here is that everything said about voluntary abortion borders on philosophy. It is important, therefore, to state that we are convinced that the termination of a pregnancy entails the termination of a human life and is something that, intrinsically, should be avoided; at the same time, we believe that voluntary abortion should not be criminalized, because – as physicians – we have to recognize that abortion, when performed, must be safe. We therefore find that the position held by President Clinton, that "abortion must be safe, legal and rare" [1], deserves consideration.

Under the circumstances, we wonder whether it is possible to establish a dialogue – any dialogue – between those who consider abortion an evil to be fought at all costs and those who believe that women have a right to terminate an early pregnancy.

The answer we propose is a daring "yes" and the reason for an optimism so unwarranted by the reality we see around the world, is that we know that there is a sufficiently large portion of the international community which would easily agree with the idea that our main goal is to minimize the need to recur to the voluntary termination of pregnancy. Therefore, to make an alliance based on this fundamental premise seems – in theory – possible, although it will be necessary to keep the two extremes out of the effort, because no dialogue seems possible with those who consider abortion such an abominable crime to warrant bombing abortion clinics or, at the other end of the spectrum, with those who advocate abortion as a method of family planning, and therefore wish to see more – not fewer – women utilizing it.

The creation of a minimum common ground, however implies decreasing the need for abortion by increasing contraceptive prevalence – a fact, unfortunately, not accepted by everyone.

The best way to start this discussion is to explain why restrictive legislation might have been good to appease the conscience of policy makers and a part of the public, but definitely has never deterred women from terminating a pregnancy when they felt strongly they could not afford it, nor has it - per se - moved women to prevent unwanted pregnancies.

In a conversation held almost 3 years ago in London, the President of IPPF's Central Council, François Ekam of Togo, a businessman, explained that his interest in family planning dated back to when he was a student at the Sorbonne in Paris more than 30 years ago. He was then a member of the board of the student health insurance plan, and this insurance group was chronically in the red; being an economics student, he started investigating the reasons for the deficit and found out that female students purchased large quantities of antibiotics. He then discovered that this was a consequence of the fairly large number of clandestine abortions among these students, which - of course - carried complications necessitating treatment. Therefore, the criminalization of abortion and the lack of access to contraception simply made termination of pregnancy a health hazard, rather than a procedure that young French women would not utilize.

Legalizing abortion does not entail, per se, a more widespread utilization of the procedure, and may - on the contrary - help decrease its incidence, provided decriminalization is linked to a series of other public health measures. The situation is however very complex; to prove this complexity, we have three examples - all from Europe - of the consequences of legislation liberalizing voluntary pregnancy termination.

The first is the United Kingdom. As shown in Figure 1, following legalization in England, both the number of legal abortions and the ratio of abortion to live births continued to increase [2]. Several observations can be made about these statistics: first of all, looking at the incredibly low numbers and rates in the 1970s, it is easy to suspect that, in fact, what we observe here is a gross underreporting in the early days. In addition, all pill scares in Europe originated from the United Kingdom; each involved a steep surge in the number of abortions performed, thereby nullifying the positive effects of contraception.

The impact - locally and internationally - of the latest pill scare, caused by action taken by the U.K. Committee on Safety of Medicines at the end of 1995, has been analyzed in detail by the British Birth Control Trust. They have calculated that some 3000 extra abortions took place because of the sudden abandonment of contraception by women worried about their health [3].

The second example is France where, historically, the situation has been different from England. There, as shown in Figure 2, a decrease could be observed between 1973 and 1993 both in the absolute number of abortions, in the ratio of abortions to term pregnancies (which is today approximately 0.3) and in the number of abortions per woman (which is approximately 0.5). France has today one of the lowest abortion rates in the world; however, it has to be stressed that, although it legalized contraception quite late in 1968, the country has made good progress in its utilization [4].

The third example is Italy, where, following legalization, abortions decreased from about 235,000 in 1984 to some 150,000 in 1993. Also, the ratio of abortion to live birth decreased from 38% to 27%. Finally, abortion rates among women of reproductive age decreased from 17 to a very low 10.5 per thousand. The downtrend continues to this day [5].

As can be imagined, there are many factors contributing to this very positive trend; the first is that, in Italy, a voluntary abortion is taken very seriously from an ethical

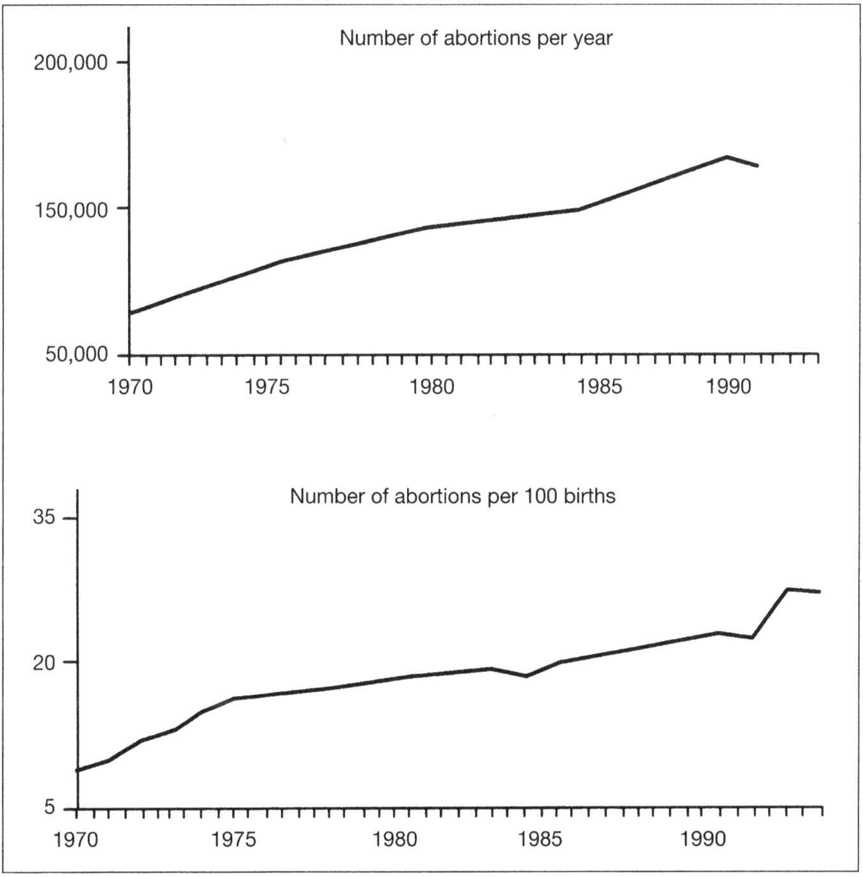

Fig. 1. Evolution of voluntary pregnancy termination in the United Kingdom [2]

point of view. Women would recur to it if they felt there was no other alternative, but they would also make every effort to avoid being in the situation to need an abortion. The second reason is that in order for contraception to successfully decrease the need for abortion, there has to be active promotion; this has been the case in Italy.

Recently, the Ministry of Health launched a very good initiative called "Women's Welfare"[6]. Consider Figure 4. The text under the centre picture says: "this woman is happy not because she found the ideal shampoo against dandruff, but because (right picture) she now knows that she will be able to avoid abortion with a contraceptive adapted to her needs". Thus, we can conclude that in Italy, it is family planning that has created the conditions for a major reduction in the need to resort to abortion.

A counterexample of the inverse relationship between abortion and the use of modern contraceptives is provided by the diagram in Figure 5, showing that, as abortion decreased, oral contraceptive use increased [7]. It is interesting to note that, given motivation and education, this reduction in abortion can occur with just about any contraceptive mix.

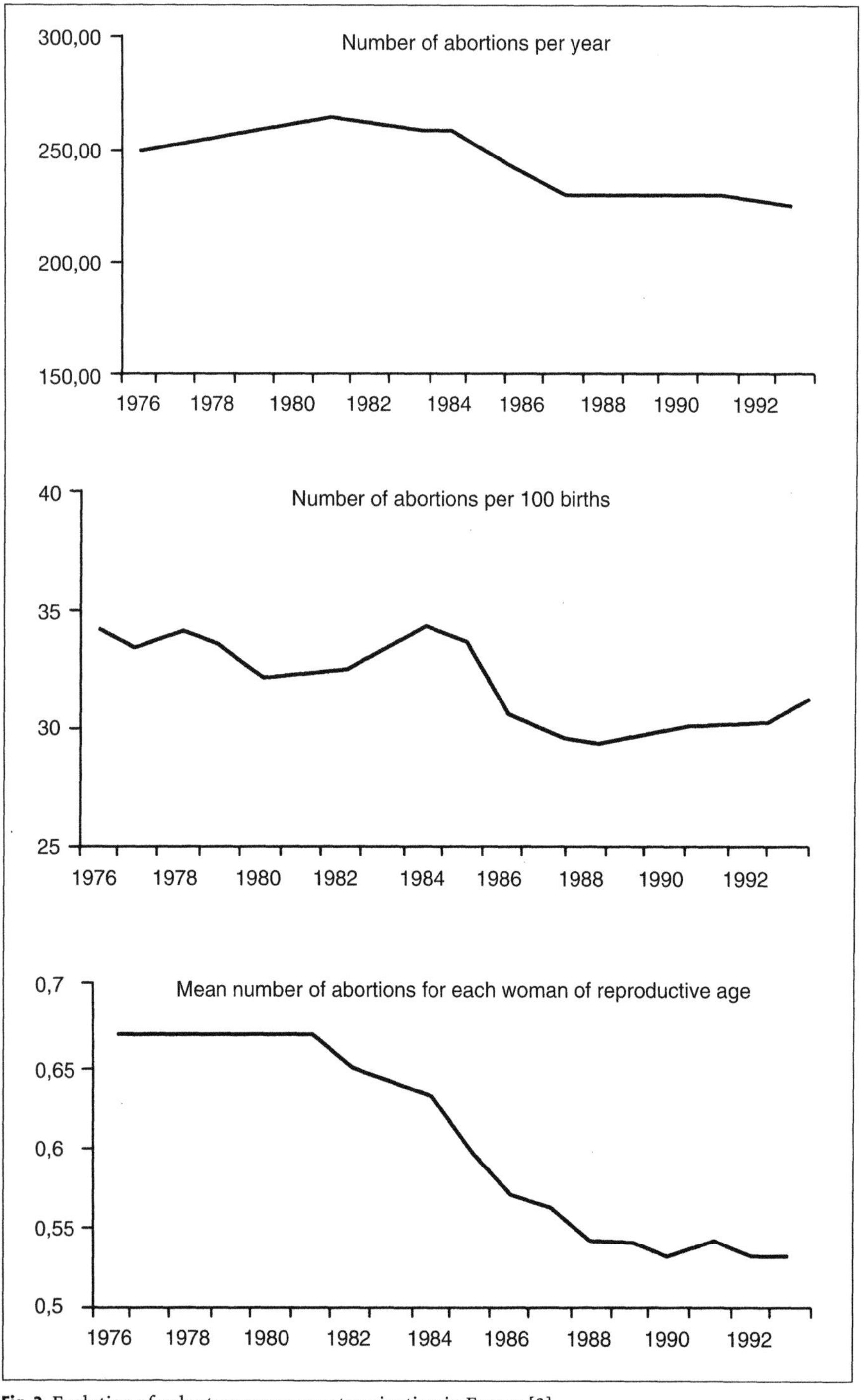

Fig. 2. Evolution of voluntary pregnancy termination in France [3]

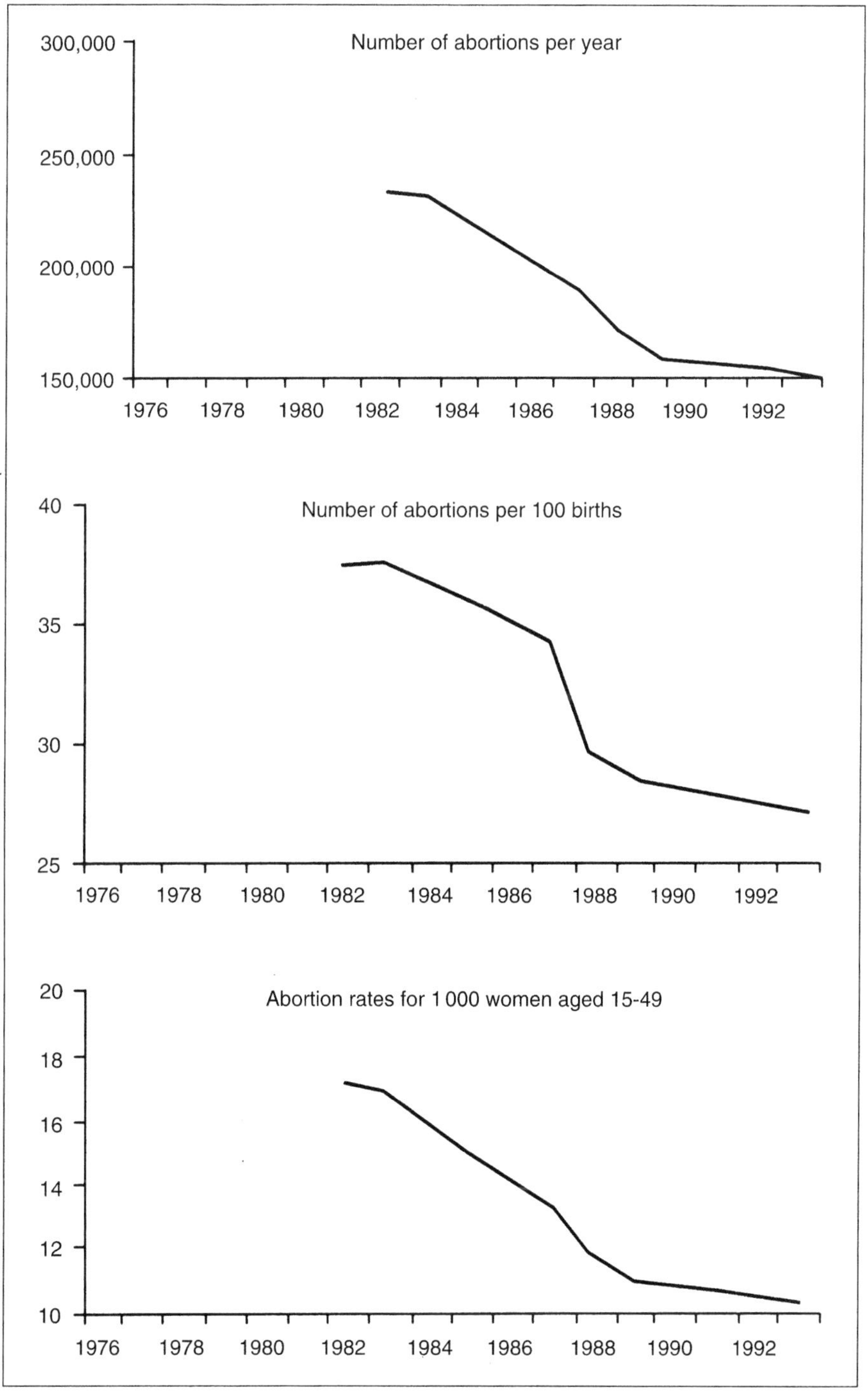

Fig. 3. Evolution of voluntary pregnancy termination in Italy [5]

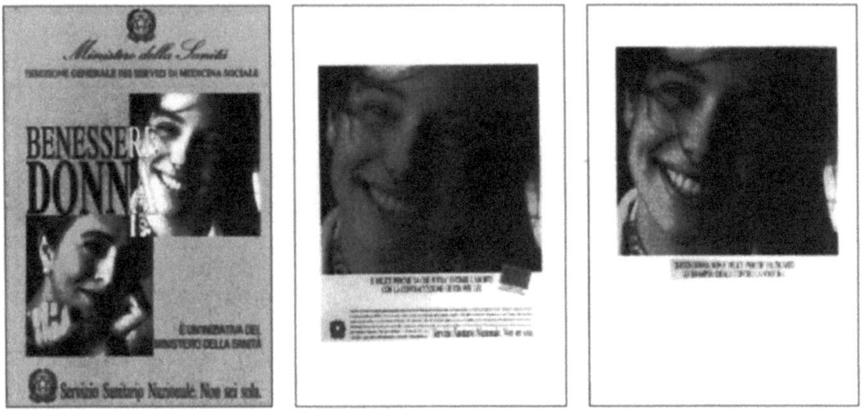

Fig. 4. The „Women Welfare“ initiative of the Italian Ministry of Health [6]

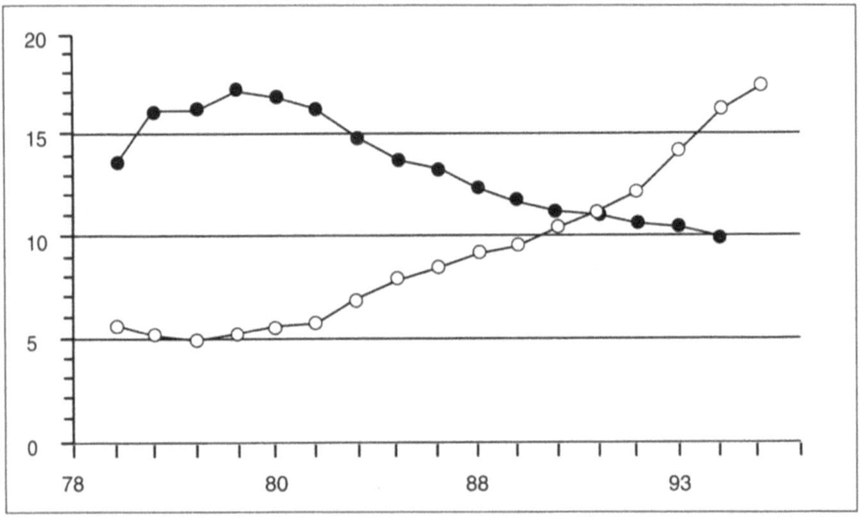

Fig. 5. Relationship between voluntary pregnancy termination (•) and oral contraceptive use (○) in Italy [7]

Figure 6 reports percentage utilization of the various contraceptive methods in Italy and the U.K. Although Italians seem to prefer more traditional methods (normally considered less effective), they nevertheless can manage their fertility very well – almost too well, one would say, since Italy has one of the lowest birth rates in the world [2].

Two examples will help in showing how restricting access to voluntary abortion does not, by itself, decrease the utilization of this procedure, or prompt women to prevent unwanted pregnancies; on the contrary, it may contribute to an increase in morbidity and mortality associated with pregnancy.

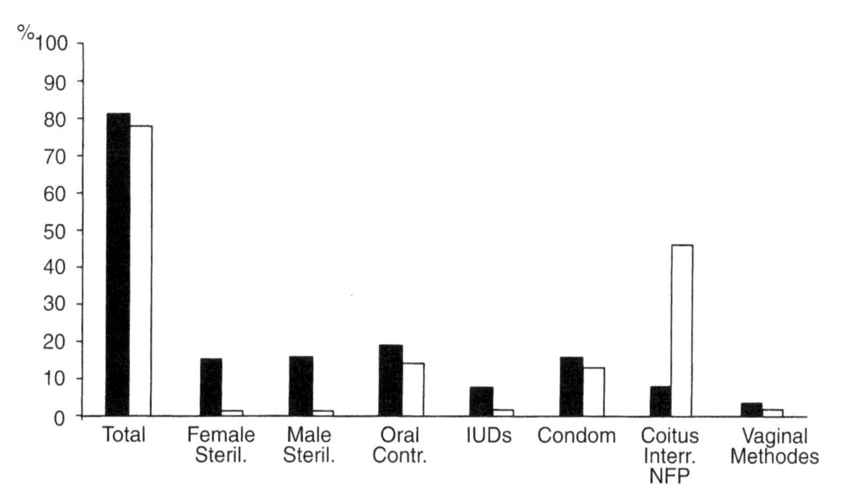

Fig. 6. Contraceptive prevalence by method in the United Kingdom (■) and in Italy (□)[2]

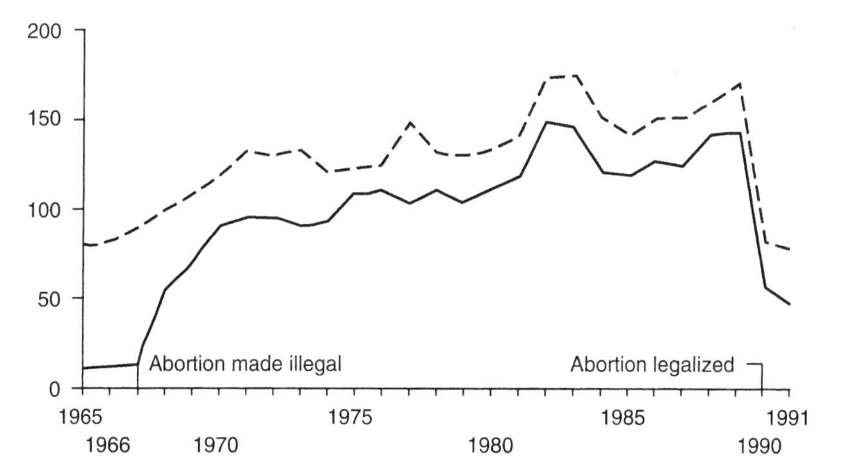

Fig. 7. Maternal mortality in Romania (years 1965-1991). All causes (– –) and abortion-related maternal deaths (——) are expressed per 100,000 live births [7]

The first example is that of Romania; it is a classic example, cited everywhere, because the situation (shown in Fig. 7) is dramatically clear [8]. Since 1966 and until 1989, the Romanian government has held strong pronatalist views; contraception was banned and abortion was all but illegal. Banning abortion resulted in the highest maternal mortality rates in Europe, with 85 per cent of deaths related to pregnancy attributable to unsafe abortions. In 1989, there were 159 maternal deaths per 100,000 live births; the next year, after abortion was legalized again and the procedure started becoming available in hospitals and being safer, mortality during pregnancy or delivery immediately fell to 83 per 100,000 live births.

The second good example is Poland, where parliament approved, in 1993, a law which permitted abortion only when the pregnancy threatened the life or health of the mother, when the foetus has a serious malformation or in cases of rape or incest. This led to a surge of illegal abortions on the one hand, and of women travelling to neighbouring countries for abortions on the other. Because of this reality, in 1996 the abortion law was relaxed again, although the situation is still under debate in the Supreme Court.

These facts underline an important concept: in most countries a law that forbids abortion does not – per se – decrease the number of women who recur to the procedure to stop an unwanted pregnancy. Such laws however have two important negative consequences. The first is an adverse effect on the reproductive health of women: illegal abortions are often unsafe and the consequences can be seen in increased rates of morbidity related to pregnancy and in higher secondary infertility and mortality among pregnant women [9]. The second negative consequence is the very clear tendency – evident everywhere – that, because abortion is illegal, nothing is done to actively reduce its incidence, or, rather, to reduce the reasons leading to the need for terminating a pregnancy [10]. Obviously the situation concerning decriminalization is complex and far from being clear-cut, as shown recently by the UN [11].

Going back to the Romanian example, an interesting feature is given by the evolution of birth rates in that country: following restrictive legislation, there was – as shown in Figure 8 – a steep increase in the fertility rate. This can probably be interpreted as evidence that the total number of abortions (both those performed illegally and those still performed for approved indications) must have sharply decreased. However, as the years went by, fertility started to progressively decrease, which seems to indicates that the "illegal sector" got – so to speak – organized and active, or that women travelled to other socialist countries to get an abortion. Therefore, in the long run, the impact of the Romanian law in decreasing the number of abortions is questionable, to say the least.

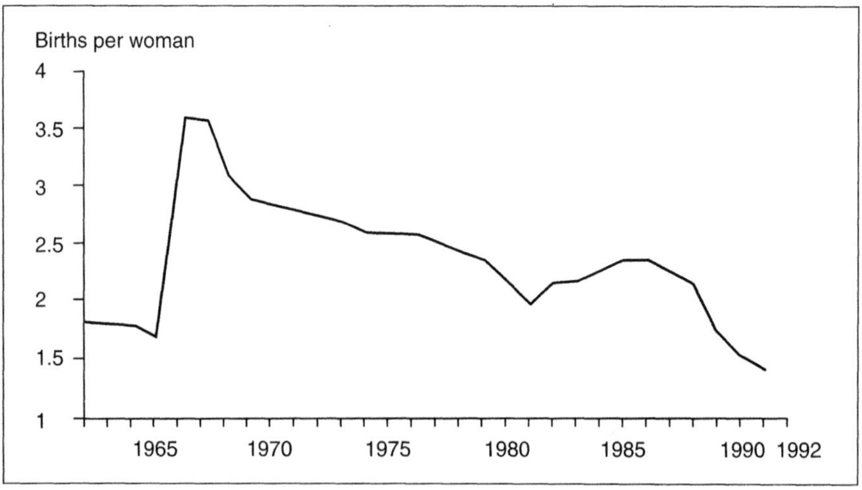

Fig. 8. Total fertility rates in Romania (1965-1992). Source: Demographic Yearbooks/UN and CHS/MOH Romania

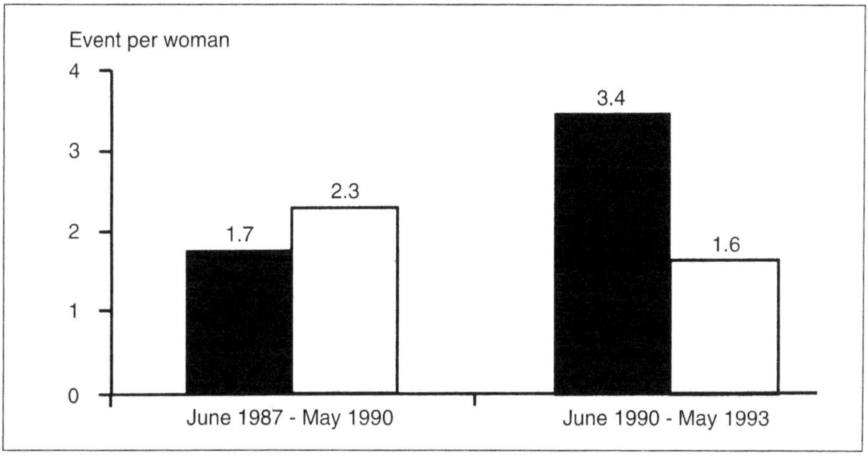

Fig. 9. Rate of induced abortions (■) and total fertility rates (□) in Romania, before and after change in the legislation [8]

The other peculiar feature is given by the comparison of abortions and fertility rates before and after the legislative changes, as shown in Figure 9. Consider that the abortions shown here are those officially performed. When you make a guess (from the maternal mortality figures) about the number of clandestine abortions and add those, then you have to conclude that – although fertility went down – this was the consequence of the new-found availability of contraceptives after 1990, rather than a decrease in abortions during the years of restrictive legislation.

One thing is certain: when, after the 1989 revolution, abortion was legalized again and safe abortion was made available, the reality of abortion used as a method of birth control surfaced again. Abortion rates in Romania are the highest in the world: in 1992, there have been 270 abortions per 100 births, most of them performed on married women who have reached the desired family size. Therefore, 25 years of criminalization of abortion did not change the pro-abortion mentality of Romanian women. It has to be said that, confronted with this grim reality, which for so long was ignored, the government is now actively working to change it.

To successfully move from abortion to contraception, people's attitudes and behaviour must be changed. This requires massive training and education programmes, as well as the will of governments to remove obstacles to a wide utilization of contraceptives. Decriminalization makes it possible to evaluate the true dimension of the problem and set in motion the process to reduce it.

Eastern Europe and the Asian Republics, once part of the Soviet Union, are among the countries where the move away from abortion is of primary importance. In this part of the world, there is still a very high prevalence of induced abortion [12]. The historical reason for this situation is a chronic non-availability of contraceptive methods; even where some could be obtained, there has been no real knowledge of them and abortion has been, for all practical purposes, the most important method of fertility regulation. As already stated, the highest abortion rate is found in Romania with 140/1000 women aged 15-44 per year; in the Russian Federation it is 82/1000, and in Hungary, 33/1000. For comparison, in Western Europe, France has a rate of 13/10001, Italy of 10.5/1000 and Finland 8/1000 [12].

Another way to look at abortion statistics is to compare them with birth rates: In 1993 in the Russian Federation, there have been as many as 214 abortions performed per 100 births. Also in this case however, there are regional differences and the ratio for the Baltic states is somewhat lower; for example, in Latvia in 1994, it was 129 per 100 births; the lowest ratio is found in the Central Asian Republics where, for example, it was 88 per 100 births in 1994 in Kazakstan [12]. In Eastern Europe and Central Asia we therefore have a major challenge to put into practice the solemn pact made during the Cairo Conference that "In no case should abortion be promoted", or used "as a method of family planning" [13].

There is no question that contraception is the corner-stone of our fight to reduce abortion, although – as already shown – the relationship between contraception and abortion is fairly complex. Data from several industrialized countries tell us that, where contraception is well established and utilized by the vast majority of people and where it is associated with a proper sex education, the need to resort to an abortion has substantially decreased. France, Finland (and the other Scandinavian countries) and the Netherlands are the best examples of this [4].

As already said, moving from abortion to contraception requires the positive intervention of governments. For example, in Estonia, where abortion is legal, the government has adopted a policy whereby women are charged for abortion services and this money is then used to subsidize contraceptives. Asking everyone to pay something to receive a legal abortion is definitely a possible strategy to discourage it, because even the poorest need to pay if they want an illegal abortion.

A very important way in which governments can be effective is in educating potential users and removing medical obstacles to a wide utilization. In addition, other obstacles, such as cost, should be removed, especially in countries with no local production, where the need to purchase them with hard currency makes contraceptives simply unaffordable. Here, education is the key, since a lack of knowledge about the real attributes of individual methods both within the population and the providers is at the basis of low prevalence. It is also necessary to fight misconceptions about the safety of modern contraceptives. For example, in Russia and Romania, many women believe that oral contraceptives are harmful to their health and should not be used. For this reason, more research concerning sexual behaviour and knowledge, attitudes and practice of contraception is needed in order to change the situation. Also, a proper training for providers and educational programmes for consumers are badly in demand.

The possibility for potential users to choose among methods is another very important issue. Italy is a good example of the fact that you can reduce both fertility and induced abortion with any method mix. This, however, implies the availability of a wide variety of methods, as well as education and advocacy. Contraceptive prevalence is directly linked to method availability: the greater the number of methods available, the higher the contraceptive prevalence, as shown in Figure 10 [14]. Indeed, the availability of a variety of methods encourages contraceptive continuation by allowing women and couples to switch to methods that better meet their changing needs. Finally, the availability of a variety of methods is the best way to reduce the so-called unmet need for contraception, which – in turn – will help decrease the need to terminate an unwanted pregnancy.

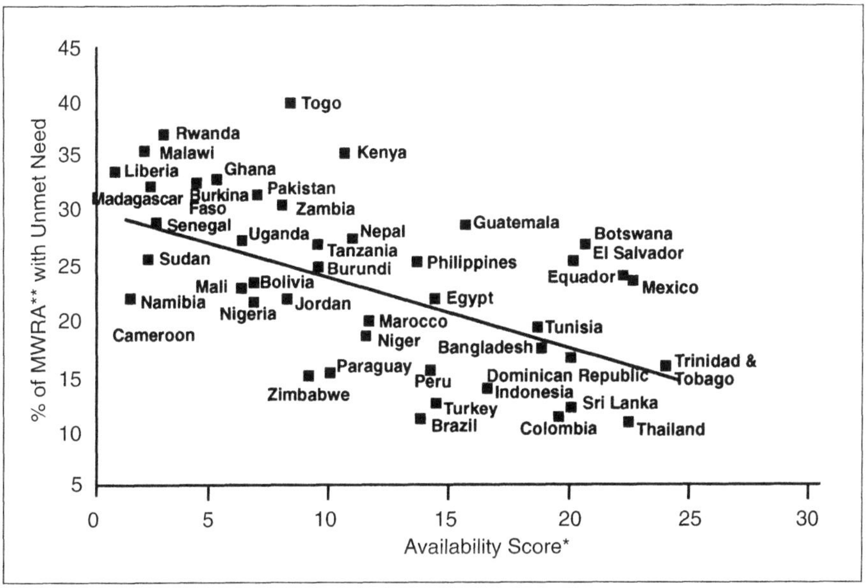

Fig. 10. Relationship between the number of contraceptive methods available and unmet needs. * Scores calculated on the basis of judgements about the availability of contraceptive methods by senior family personnel and observers in each country. ** MWRA, married women of reproductive age. Source: [14]

It must be stressed that ethical considerations influence the choice of strategies aimed at decreasing the need to terminate a pregnancy. A good example is the possibility to recur to emergency contraception. If we accept the definition of pregnancy laid out in the U. S. Code of Federal Regulations, under the title "Protection of Human Subjects", and endorsed by a World Health Organization (WHO) Scientific Group in 1992 [15], then emergency contraception – acting before nidation – does not interrupt a pregnancy and therefore is a means to prevent voluntary abortion. The problem with this definition is that it establishes biological criteria, not moral norms. Ethical judgment however should be based on biological facts, and the facts are sufficiently well established. As soon as fertilization occurs, a new human life begins. We know that this new life lacks individuality because, during the first days, a zygote or an early embryo, can give rise to more than one individual. We also know that typical fertilization rates are, in vitro, on the order of 70 to 90%, whereas the typical subsequent pregnancy rates are of the order of 20% [16]. Notwithstanding the fact that – in all likelihood – more than 50% of all fertilized ova do not end up as viable foetuses, we do not know which will do so. Therefore, we must presume – ethically – that they all have the potential to develop to become full human beings [17]. For this reason, we believe that emergency contraception can be ethically justified only as a lesser evil, when compared to abortion.

The situation is very different when discussing the so-called post-ovulatory methods, acting during the luteal phase of the cycle. There, one is intentionally allowing fertilization to occur, only to disrupt the process at an early stage. This may lead to what we would dare to call the unnecessary creation of new human life under circumstances when the intention is invariably to destroy it. Of course this is not – as some extremists claim – "voluntary manslaughter", but many – at least within the so-called western thinking – question the ethics of such a procedure.

One last group of methods that needs to be discussed is the so-called "menses inducers". I believe that, from an ethical point of view, methods aimed at "washing out the uterus at the time of the missed period", if acting after nidation, are to be included in the same category of the medical or surgical abortifacients. Therefore, the idea of using such a method on a regular monthly basis, should not be accepted.

Indeed, a survey published in 1992 in Human Reproduction [18], where women from several countries were asked what they felt about the idea of a pill which was to be taken only if menstruation was delayed by one or two days (that is, a pill which would cause an abortion), showed that only 24% of women in Scotland were attracted by this idea. In contrast to this, 58% of women in Slovenia and 80% in Romania thought that such a method of controlling fertility would be acceptable. Attitudes were not related to age, social class or marital status, but were influenced by religious beliefs and – in Scotland – by a history of prior abortion.

The last 25 years of the second millennium have been characterized by unprecedented advances in our ability to understand and manipulate fertilization and the early stages of life, up to recent furor over cloning. Our hope is that the beginning of the third millennium will be remembered as the time when all the necessary safeguards will be put in place by the international community to protect human life and ensure the continuation of its natural progression. An integral part of this strategy is a plan of action aimed at substantially decreasing the need to terminate a pregnancy. This is an achievable goal if we unite our forces rather than loose an opportunity by, instead, underlining what divides us. So let's work together, using as a common denominator our desire to reduce the need to recur to an abortion.

References

1. Clinton W, Discourses (1995)
2. Monnier A, de Guilbert-Lantoine G (1995) The demographic situation of Europe and developed countries overseas: an annual report. Population: an English selection 7:187-202
3. Bromham D, O'Brien T (1995) Information for health professionals further to the Committee on Safety of Medicine's advice on the safety of oral contraceptives. Faculty of Family Planning and Reproductive Health care and The Family Planning Association, London
4. Grunseit A, Kippax S (1993) Effects of sex education on young people's sexual behaviour. Unpublished review commissioned by the global programme on AIDS. The World Health Organization, Geneva.
5. Relazione del Ministero della Sanità sull'attuazione della Legge contenente norme per la tutela sociale della maternità e per l'interruzione volontaria della gravidanza (1995) Istituto poligrafico dello Stato, Rome
6. Servizio Sanitario Nazionale, Ministero della Sanità. Benessere Donna. Rome (1994) Istituto Poligrafico dello Stato
7. Spinelli A (1996) "Italia". In: Contraccezione e aborto alle soglie del 2000. A cura di G. Dalla Zuanna. Dipartimento di Scienze Demografiche, Università degli studi di Roma "La Sapienza", pp 189-208
8. Institute for Mother and Child Care, Bucarest, Romania & Centers for disease Control and Prevention, Atlanta, Georgia, USA (1995) Romania Reproductive Health Survey, 1993. Institute for Mother and Child Care (Bucarest, Romania)

9. The Prevention and Management of Unsafe Abortion. WHO/MSM/92.5,Annex I, World health organization, Geneva 1993
10. Studying Unsafe Abortion (1996) Under contract to: The World Health Organization, IPAS
11. Abortion Policies. A Global Review. vol III, United Nations, 1995
12. World Health Organization, Regional Office for Europe. & United Nations Population Fund: Family Planning and Reproductive Health in CCEE/NIS. Doc: EUR/ICP/FMLY 94 03/PB01.1995
13. United Nations. Population and Development. (Programme of action adopted at the International Conference on Population and Development, Cairo, 5-13 September 1994). New York: United Nations; Vol.1: 30-1, 1995
14. Division of Family Health of WHO. health Benefits of family Planning. Geneva: World health organization, 1995
15. The Code of Federal Regulations (CFR), Title 45, Public Welfare. DHHS/NIH;Office for the Protection from Research Risks. Title 46, Protection of Human Subjects, Revised as of March 8 1983
16. Edwards RG, Morcos S, Macnamee M, Balmaceda JP, Walters DE, Asch R (1991) High fecundity of amenorrhoeic women in embryo-transfer programmes. Lancet, 338: 292-294
17. Benagiano G, Pera A (1992) Il destino dell'uovo fecondato nei primi giorni del suo sviluppo. In: Quale statuto per l'embrione umano: problemi e prospettive, Mori M. (ed), Bibliotechne (Milano). 45-51
18. Rimmer C, Horga M, Cerar V, Alder EM, Baird DT, Glasier A (1992) Do women want a once-a-month pill? Hum. Reprod. 7: 608-611

3 Contraception: Historical Development, Current Status and Future Aspects

Thomas Rabe, Elena Vladescu, Benno Runnebaum

Since the birth of Christ, the world population has increased exponentially, although the real growth spurt only began in the early 19th century. The population increase in the so-called developing countries, e.g. Africa, India, China, accounts for 80% of the total population growth. Three children are born every second (98 million per year). By the year 2050, world population will have grown from a current 6 billion to 12.5 billion.

The number of children per family (fertility rate) has started to fall only recently due to international efforts. The number of children per family, which ranges between four and seven in developing countries, has already dropped below the stability level (2.1) in industrial countries and has fallen to 1.9 in Germany. History has proven that neither epidemics nor natural disasters or wars can make a decisive dent in population figures.

The following analysis is based on reviews by Djerassi 1980 [8], van Keep et al 1987 [42], Rao 1987 [30], Pannenborg 1987 [24], Fathalla 1993 [11], Benagiano and Shah 1997 [3], among others.

How Can the Population Explosion Be Stopped?

Only access to and adequate use of effective contraception can slow down population growth decisively. However, only about 40% of the 1.2 billion couples of reproductive age will have access to effective contraceptive methods by the end of the millenium, although only US $3 are required per couple per year (in China, oral hormonal contraceptives costs DM 0.10 per month). Diseases also have an impact on health and fertility. About one-third of the world population is chronically ill: malaria, enteritis, bilharzia, hepatitis, leprosy, AIDS. Malnutrition, lack of access to safe drinking water and, increasingly, pollution are also important for the reproductive health.

The acceptance of family planning methods depends largely on the implementation of women's rights as well as on the availability of a pension system; if a large number of children is the only way to provide security in old age, all efforts to spread contraceptives are in vain.

This chapter has been partially published in *Der Gynäkologe*, **31**, 5/1998, 461-476

Cultural Factors and Population Development

Politics, religion and education level (illiteracy) have a varying influence in the individual countries. In China, the one-child family is being enforced rigorously by the goverment, whereas in India and Africa, illiteracy and the total absence of a pension system (children provide for their parents) are an obstacle to the spread of new contraceptive methods.

Termination of Pregnancy as a Means of Fertility Control

Currently, about 60 million pregnancies per year are terminated, 40-50 million of them in China. In Europe, the highest number of terminations used to be performed in Romania and the former Soviet Union. Sometimes, no adequate contraceptives were available; in Romania, two terminations per year are cheaper (DM 15 x 2 = DM 30) than taking the pill for a year (12 x DM 5 = DM 60) (1997). In most cases, these interventions are illegal or carried out inadequately or without adequate anaesthesia, e.g. in the Phillippines, the abruptio placentae is manually induced by massage in the second trimester, and frequently the patients' lives are at risk. Each year, 200,000 women die as a result of an inadequate abortion procedure. During and after childbirth, 500,000 women die every year, 99% of them in developing countries. In countries with a low prevalence of oral contraceptive (OC) use, the incidence of pregnancy termination is high, e.g. Japan (1% OC, 84% abortions); US (9% OC, 28% abortions). In Japan, OCs were only introduced in 1997! (Table 1). In Germany, about 250,000 pregnancies are terminated each year.

Table 1. Pregnancy termination worldwide (1990)

	Percentage of women using oral contraceptives (15-44 years)	Terminations of pregnancy per 1 000 women (15-44 years)
Netherlands	36	5,1
Belgium	25	7,5
France	30	13,3
New Zealand	28	11,4
Australia	28	16,6
Great Britain	28	14,2
Sweden	23	19,8
Canada	19	12,1
Finland	18	11,7
USA	9	28,0
Japan	1	84,0

The acceptance and use of suitable methods of family planning depend on the availability of the method, the knowledge of the doctors consulted, family planning centres or health centres and the users themselves. The advantages and disadvantages of the various methods, the acceptance of possible side effects (also with respect to the religious or cultural background), the risk of unwanted pregnancy and the risk of infection by sexually transmitted pathogens also play an important role. Contraceptive advice, together with screening tests, can contribute greatly to disease prevention; they have come to be called reproductive health and are an important pillar of health policy [3]. Table 2 gives an overview of the current global distribution of various contraceptive methods.

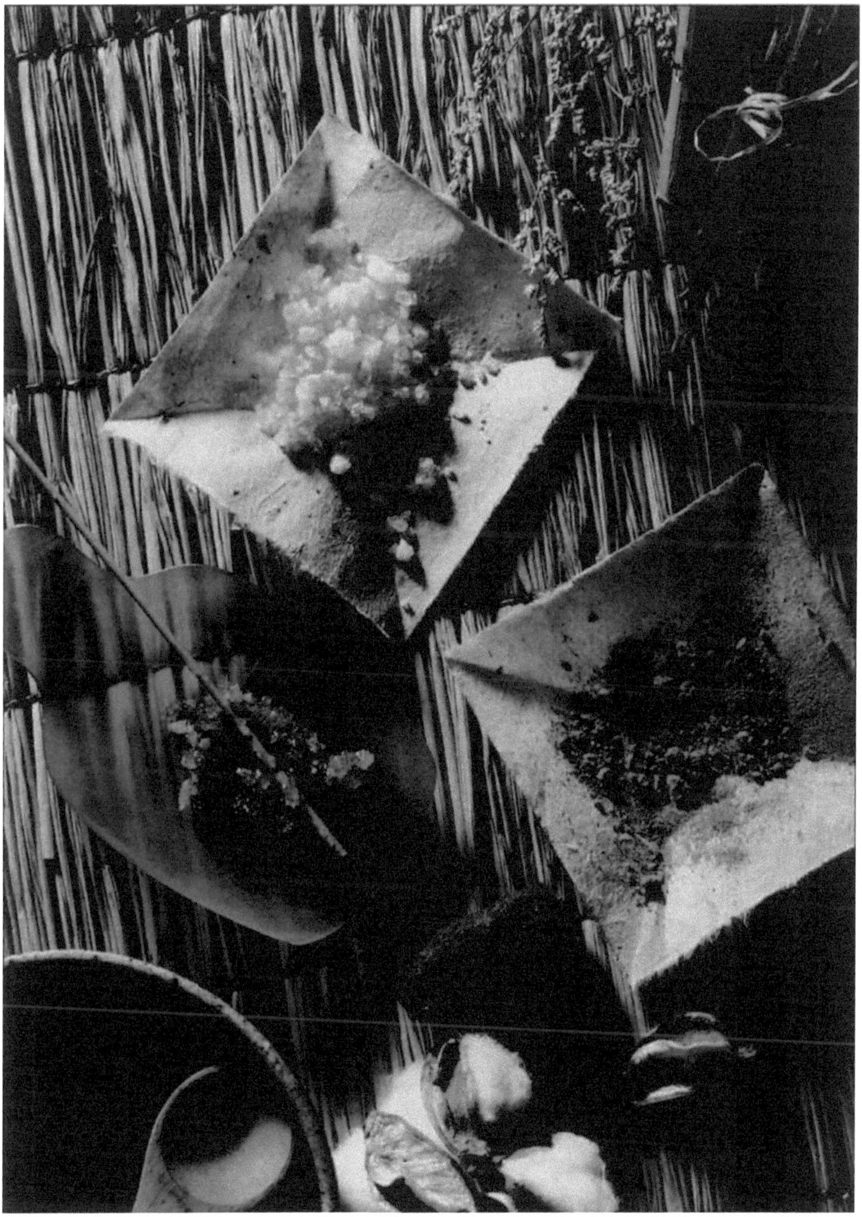

Fig. 1. Plants and plant extracts used for contraception (with kind permission from Percy Skuy: A Museum of Discovery: Tales of Contraception. Supported by Ortho-McNeil Inc.)

Table 2. Contraceptive methods (estimated numbers in millions) used worldwide

Method	1970	1980	1990	1997
Oral Contraceptives	30	55		60-80
Intrauterine device	12	15		
Other methods (diaphragma, spermicides, rhythm-method, coitus interruptus)	60	65		
sterilisation	20	80		
- Woman				108
- Man				60
Condom	25	35		
Termination of pregnancy	40	40	50-60	60

The Future of Contraception

New methods of contraception should be 100% reversible, inexpensive and easy to distribute, should not require any complex medical examination, should not disrupt the sex life and should be acceptable both religiously and culturally, e.g. in Ireland: no contraceptives for unmarried people; in Judaism: no coitus interruptus; in Islam: no method causing bleeding disorders [19]. They must not cause any adverse side effects and should, if possible, have positive side effects, such as protection from venereal diseases and inflammation in the small pelvis, protection from cancer, normalisation of the menstrual cycle, and positive effects e.g. on skin and hair. In many cases, the resistance of special interest groups must be overcome: for instance, Japanese gynaecologists managed to prevent the introduction of oral hormonal contraceptives for a long time because terminations of pregnancy are more lucrative.

Contraceptives prepared from plant extracts may gain more and more importance (Fig. 1).

Different Strategies of Contraception in Men and Women

There are different types of male and female contraception. In women, we distinguish between methods of ovulation suppression, prevention of fertilisation, prevention of the implantation of the fertilised egg in the uterus and the group of abortive drugs. In men, the distinction is made between methods influencing the formation of sperm and those interfering with fertilisation. Table 3 gives an overview of the most important contraceptive methods and preparatory and follow-up examinations (see also reviews [7, 10, 28, 32, 35 and 38]).

Contraceptive Methods

In the following sections, contraceptive methods in women (inhibition of ovulation, fertilisation and implantation) and men are listed by the function they target.

Table 3. Preparatory, control and follow-up examinations for various contraceptive procedures (main points; *diagnostic equipment allowing)

Method	Family history	Patient history	Gen. clinical examination	Examination finding	Laboratory test	Follow-up
Oral hormonal ontraceptives	Cardiovascular diseases, breast and ovarian cancer, diabetes mellitus	Cardiovascular diseases, diabetes mellitus, cancers, smoking	Heart defect, liver diseases, obesity, hypertension, diabetes mellitus	Gyn. cancers, bleeding disorders, exclusion of pregnancy	Depending on history: Blood glucose & oGTT, blood coagulation, lipids	Every 3-6 months
Intrauterine device	Not relevant	Risk for adnexitis, sexual behaviour, previous pregnancies, menstrual cycle	Signs of genital infection	genital infection, uterine anomalies, exclusion of cancer, exclusion of pregnancy	(BSR/leucocytes); (bacteriological smear, exclusion of chlamydia)	6 weeks after insertion, afterwards every 6 months, self-control
Progestin-only pill	Not relevant	Thromboembolism, vein thrombosis	No special diagnosis	Pregnancy exclusion	No special diagnosis	Every 6-12 months
Three-monthly injectable	Not relevant	Menstrual cycle	Not relevant	Pregnancy exclusion	Not relevant, (bone densiometry)	Every 2-3 months for the injection
Spermicides	Not relevant	Not relevant	Not relevant	Not relevant	Not relevant	Every 6-12 months
Natural family planning	Not relevant	Irregular menstrual cyle	Not relevant	Not relevant	Not relevant	Every 6-12 months
Sterilisation of the woman	Not relevant	No further children planned	Not relevant	Pregnancy exclusion	Fitness for general anasthesia	Only if unwanted pregnancy occurs
Morning-after pill	Not relevant	Menstrual cycle, time of intercourse, thrombosis risk	Not strictly necassary	Pregnancy exclusion	Not applicable	After next menstruation or if amenorrhea occurs
Condom	Not relevant	Not relevant	Not relevant	Not relevant	Not relevant	Every 6-12 months
Sterilisation of the man	Not relevant	No further children planned	Exclude systemic disease	varicocele, testicular tumors, infections	Sperm count	Monitoring of sperm count until negative

Contraception in Women

Inhibition of Ovulation

Prolonged Lactation

For developing countries, inhibition of ovulation due to an extended period of lactation is important. This method is used by 100 million women worldwide. According to this method, regular however exclusively breast-feeding during the first 6 months (max. 12 months) is a safe contraceptive in 98% of cases, if no menstruation occurs [45]. During lactation, the use of condoms is recommended for HIV-negative mothers who could be infected in order to prevent an infection of the child.

Oral Hormonal Contraception

Ovulation inhibition based on oral hormonal contraception (combination of synthetic ethinylestradiol and progestins) is currently the most common family-planning method. Around the world, 80 million women are using OCs.

The synthetic progestins contained in the pill are derived from two basic substances: the derivatives of 17α-hydroxyprogesterone and particularly cyproterone acetate has excellent antiandrogenic effect and is a suitable treatment for hirsutism; the derivatives of 19-nortestosterone (norethisterone) have a residual dose-dependent androgenic effect that is virtually undetectable in the more recent progestins (norgestimate, gestodene, desogestrel and dienogest).

Mechanism of action: Suppression of ovulation by synthetic progestins and oestrogens (i.e. ethinylestradiol) through inhibition of the hypothalamic secretion of gonadotropin releasing hormone (GnRH) and the pituitary secretion of gonadotropin; additional direct effects on the cervical mucus, the endometrium and tubal function.

When the pill was launched about 35 years ago, the issue of possible side effects was investigated across the world. As early as 1968, the link between the oestrogen and progestin doses and the occurrence of cardiovascular complications was identified and both dosages were lowered. The original preparations were introduced in the United States in 1958). In 1961, Anovular, containing 50 µg of ethinylestradiol (4 mg norethisterone acetate and 50 µg EE) was introduced in Germany. The first progestin-only pill (Microlut) was introduced in Germany in 1970, followed in 1973 by the first micro-pill at 30 µg ethinylestradiol and the ultra-low-dose pill containing 20 µg of ethinylestradiol in 1992. Even at such a low dose, oral hormonal contraceptives inhibit follicular development and oestrogen secretion, so that a protective effect against ovarian and endometrial cancer can be assumed. However, this remains to be confirmed by epidemiological studies. Depending on the duration of pill use, the risk of developing such cancers can be reduced by up to 50%. If the pill has been taken for 5 years, the protective effect will last for 10-15 years. Although breast cancer risk is slightly increased, particularly in young nulliparous women, the prognosis for patients with breast cancer is better in those who have taken the pill than in controls [26].

Today, combination, biphasic and triphasic contraceptive pills are available; using the same progestin, the triphasic pill contains the lowest steroid concentration per cycle. Individual examination is needed to find out which type of pill the patient tolerates best. Women with no risk factors, i.e. diabetes mellitus, fat-metabolism disorders, hypertension, cardiovascular diseases or smoking, may take the modern low-dose formulations up to the perimenopause.

Before the pill is first prescribed, the patient must be asked about any family risks of cardiovascular diseases, especially concerning the parents (before the age of 45 years).

Indications include:
- Reversible and safe contraception with good cycle control
- Medical indications such as dysmenorrhea, cycle disorders, acne, administration of drugs with a potential teratogenic effect

Contraceptive efficacy : Pearl index 0.05–0.9

Side-effects:
- Very rare (<0.01 %): thrombophlebitis, thrombosis (1 : 10,000); serious complications (thromboembolism, subarachnoidal bleeding, cardiac infarction) (1 : 100,000 women/year); death (1-3: 1 : 1,000,000 women/year)
- Rare (<1%): migraine and other headaches, depressive mood, urinary tract infection, candidial vaginitis, weight gain, hypertension, gall bladder diseases
- Frequent (1-10%): (during onset of therapy/after prolonged use of OC): intracyclic bleeding (5-20%/5%), nausea (5-10%/5%), breast tenderness (5-10%/5%)

Contraindications: for the most important contraindications, see current package leaflet and national pharmaceutical recommendations!

New products:
- See overview [29]
- Introduction or clinical trials of the triphasic pill containing third-generation progestins (desogestrel, gestodene, norgestimate and dienogest)
- Clinical trials with multi-phasic pills
- Oestrogen priming in the pill-free interval to suppress follicular growth, e.g. in combination with OCs containing 15-20 µg ethinylestradiol; same effect by a 24 day regimen
- Use of antiprogestins (their use as a mid-cycle pill has had little success since the time of ovulation changes in the next cycle) also in combination with traditional OC regimen
- Search for non-steroidal natural substances with oestrogenic or progestogenic effect (Fig. 1)

Apart from the synthetic oestrogens and progestins, the epiphyseal hormone melatonin has shown a contraceptive effect. In order to control the cycle, however, progestins are necessary. Dose-finding studies are underway, although it is clear that this combination is not suitable for contraception and that the rate of cyclic disorders is too high; it remains to be proven whether the contraceptive effect is not actually due to the progestin added.

In view of acceptance problems, it seems unrealistic to combine GnRH analogues for ovarian function suppression with natural oestrogens and progestins and also to add low-dose androgens for possible libido disorders (as suggested by Pike).

Inhibition of Fertilisation

Fertilisation can be inhibited using various mechanical, chemical, hormonal, intrauterine or behavioural methods. In future, specific immunological methods may also be an option.

Mechanical Methods (Overview)

Well-known mechanical methods are the vaginal diaphragm and the cervical cap. The costs of the female condom are much higher than the normal condom (five to tenfold), and its acceptance is controversial. Changes to the material, the shape, the size and the price may be able to improve acceptance [6]. Sterilisation methods have been improved by the introduction of minimally invasive surgical techniques, see reviews [4, 16]

Diaphragm

Method: elastic membrane with cavity rim is inserted into the vagina and prevents sperm contact with os (mechanical method). Additional use of spermicides required.

Mechanism of action:
- Mechanical barrier; and
- Inhibition of sperm ascension.

Indications:
- Pill intolerance;
- Presence of contraindication for the pill.

Contraindications:
- Anatomical changes (vaginal and uterine prolapse, vaginal operation, rectovaginal fistula);
- Puerperium;
- Vaginitis;
- Allergic reaction to rubber.

Side effects include (occasional) vaginal discharge.

Contraceptive efficacy: Pearl index 1-20 (depending on age and experience).

Advantages:
- Used only when needed
- No systemic side-effects

Disadvantages:
- High failure rate
- Reliability depends on accurate insertion
- Frequent manipulation required
- Discharge
- Pressure sores

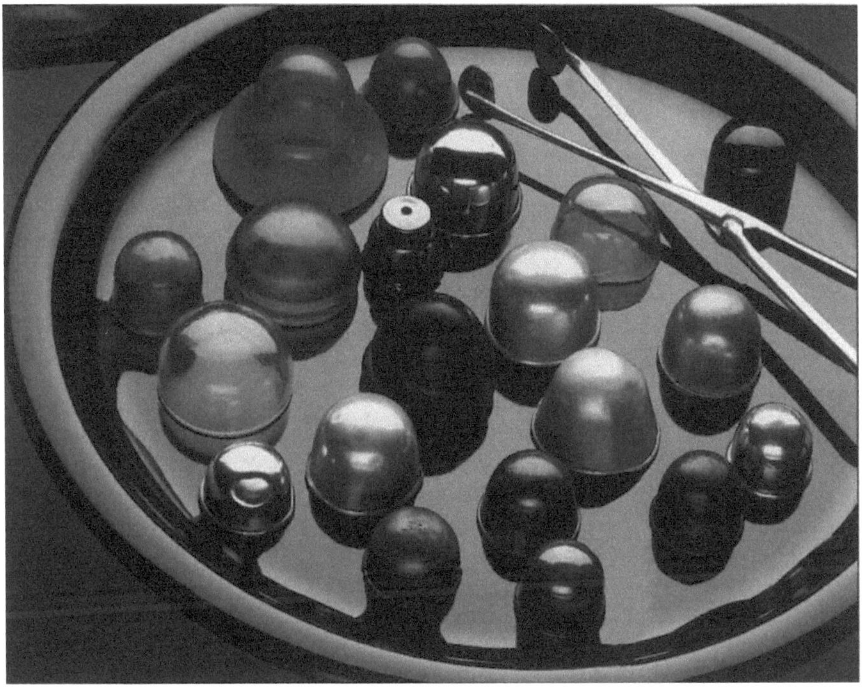

Fig. 2a. Cervical caps (historical development) (with kind permission from Percy Skuy: A Museum of Discovery: Tales of Contraception. Supported by Ortho-McNeil Inc.).

Conditions for use:
- Patient history: no genital infections, no urinary tract infections
- Clinical history (general): not relevant
- Clinical condition (gynaecological): no genital infections, no vaginal anomalies, no previous vaginal operations
- Lab: not relevant (only for special indication)
- Control examinations: every 3-6 months

Technique: horizontal insertion of the diaphragm by the woman between the posterior vaginal fornix and the symphysis before intercourse.

New developments: disposable diaphragms (pre-coated with spermicides) may become available in future [14].

Cervical Cap

Method: plastic or rubber cap placed over the os to prevent sperm contact (mechanically); spermicide must be added. An overview of the historical development of cervical caps is shown in Fig. 2a.

Indications: rejection or intolerance of other methods of contraception

Contraindications: cervicitis, vaginitis, vaginal endometriosis around the fornices and previous conisation.

Mechanism of action: mechanical barrier, inhibition of sperm ascension.

Contraceptive efficacy : Pearl index approximately 6 (higher when combined with spermicides).

Side effects include local intolerance and allergic reaction to rubber.

Advantages:
- No systemic side effects
- Infrequent insertion or manipulation
- May remain in place for up to 3 weeks

Disadvantages:
- Insertion frequently requires doctor
- Low contraceptive efficacy

Conditions for use:
- Patient history: exclusion of genital infection, pathological cytology of the cervical os, previous conisation
- Clinical history (general): not relevant
- Clinical history (gynaecological): no genital infections, vaginal anomalies, anomalies of the cervical os, cervical rupture, pathological cytology of the os
- Lab: not relevant (only for special indication)
- Control examinations: every 3-6 months

Technique: rubber hemisphere is placed over the os vaginalis uteri.

New developments:
- Customised cervical cap moulded from the individual os have been tested but have not become common.
- The Lea contraceptive (cervical cap with hole for the discharge of secretion) has not been successful either due to its size and moderate contraceptive efficacy (spermicides required) [33] (Fig. 2b).
- Disposable cervical cap (Fig. 2b).
- Fem Cap is a new cervical cap with a promising design (Fig. 2c).

Tubal Sterilisation

Mechanism of action involves mechanical (surgical) interruption of tubal continuity [44].

Indications: no further children desired; maternal risk from carrying a pregnancy to term.

Contraindications: excessive risk of the operation or anaesthesia; no irreversible contraceptive method indicated.

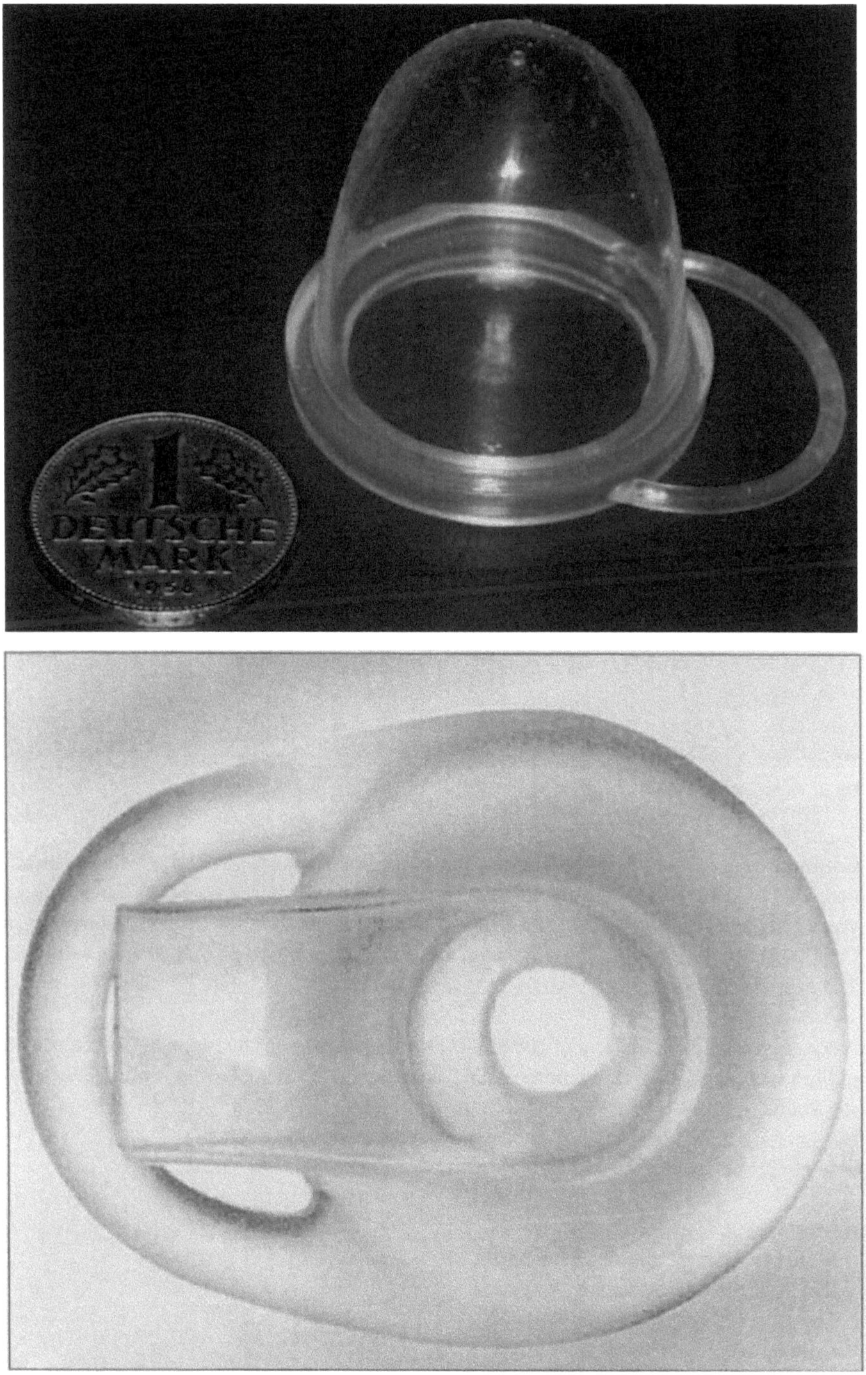

Fig. 2b. *Top* disposable cervical cap; *bottom* Lea contraceptivum: a cervical cap with secret drainage system. Both devices must be combined with spermicides. Moderate contraceptive efficacy

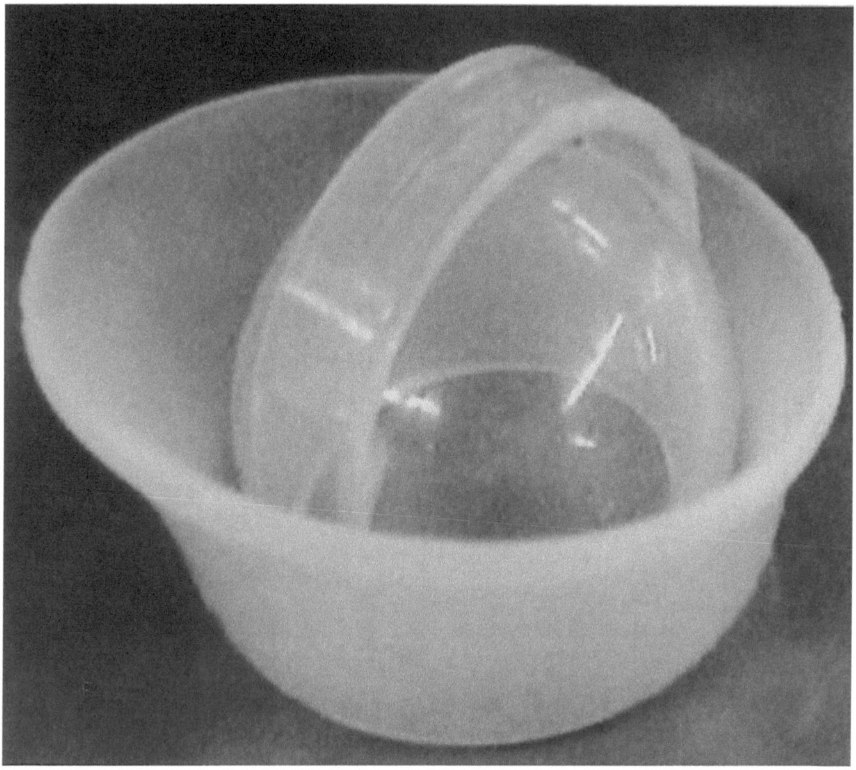

Fig. 2c. FemCap: new cervical cap

Contraceptive efficacy: high. In German literature, failure rate is given at 1/1000 sterilisations; US (1996 [25]): 143 failures in 10685 women, i.e. approximately 5% failures over 10 years with different methods of sterilisation; failure rate was highest after clip sterilisation (36.5/1000 sterilisations) compared with unipolar coagulation (7.5/1000 interventions) and partial salpingectomy (7.5/1000 interventions) [25].

Frequency: worldwide, a total of 108 million women have been sterilised; in Germany, 1.45 million women (8% of all women of child-bearing age) and 0.45 million men have been sterilised.

Side effects are caused by surgical intervention (see Disadvantages)

Advantages:
- Reliable, but not absolutely fail-safe
- No systemic effects on other organs.

Disadvantages:
- Reversible only by microsurgical or endoscopic refertilisation or assisted reproduction

- Surgical intervention required
- Risks of operation and anaesthesia
- Ovarian insufficiency and early onset of menopause in some patients due to the reduction in ovarian blood supply (ramus ovaricus a. uterina) in cases of extensive coagulation
- Contraceptive efficacy currently under debate (see above)
- Psychological problems after sterilisation

Conditions for use:
- Patient history: no genital infections
- Clinical history (general): previous operations, anaesthetic risk
- Clinical history (gynaecological): exclusion of pregnancy, evaluation of previous operations, adhesions in the small pelvis (evaluate operative risk and success prospects)
- Lab: fitness for general anaesthesia, pregnancy test if necessary
- Control examinations: usual cancerscreening

Techniques:
- Open surgery (now only in the form of a mini-laparotomy after childbirth or during Caesarean section) (techniques by e.g. Pomeroy, Madlener, Irving, Aldrige, Kröner, Uchida)
- Laparoscopic (currently the method of choice): techniques of bipolar tubal coagulation ± tubual dissection
- Alternative: clip methods (refertilisation may be easier) (e.g. Filshie clip)

New developments:
- Chemical sterilisation, e.g. with instillation of e.g. quinacrine (tubal adhesions caused by inflammation; already in use in some countries
- Improvement of clip-based methods
- Improvement and further development of intratubal silicon plugs (reversible)

Chemical Methods

Spermicides

Spermicides are used for contraception as gels, suppository or foams alone or in combination with a diaphragm, a cervical cap or a condom.

Substances: Nonoxynol-9, octoxynol-9, menfegol

Indications: intolerance to pill or IUP.

Contraindications: severe vaginal discharge.

Mechanism of action: chemical inactivation (destruction) of sperms.

Contraceptive efficacy: Pearl index 3-21 [41].

Side-effects:
- Foaming
- Increased vaginal discharge
- Local intolerance (allergic reaction (rare); hotness (frequent))

Advantages:
- No systemic side-effects
- For women with infrequent sexual relations
- Some bactericidal effect

Disadvantages:
- Suppository: Application required 10-30 min. before intercourse, duration of action 1 h
- Application must be repeated for repeated intercourse
- Hotness felt by some users
- Loss of spontaneity during intercourse

Conditions for use:
- Patient history: no genital infection
- Clinical history (general): not relevant
- Clinical history (gynaecological): no genital infection
- Lab: not relevant (only for special indications)
- Control examinations: not necessary

Technique: intravaginal application immediately before intercourse (gel, cream, foam) or 10-30 min before intercourse (vaginal suppository).

New developments:
- the spermicide nonoxynol offers some protection from venereal diseases;
- new spermicides should also afford good (100% !) protection from sexually transmitted diseases.

Progestin-Only Pill (POP)

Substances: Norethisterone (0.35 mg), levonorgestrel (0.03 mg), lynestrenol (0.5 mg), norgestrel (0.075 mg).

Technique: continuous daily use of a POP. The POP must be taken daily at the same time; the safety margin is 3 h (comment: effect on cervical factor subsides 22 h after last pill has been taken!)

Mechanism of action:
- Disruption of oocyte maturation and partial disruption of ovulation, luteal insufficiency
- Modification of the cervical mucus (main effect) (thickening)
- Endometrium: inhibition of implantation

Indications:
- Hormonal contraception while breast-feeding

- Intolerance to ethinylestradiol or contraindication to use it
- Contraception in the perimenopause

Contraindications:
- Lack of compliance (when patient cannot take the pill at the same time every day with an accuracy of 3 h)
- Progestin intolerance

Contraceptive efficacy: Pearl index 0.5-3 [40]; in younger women higher failure rate (3.1) than in older patients (0.3) [46]

Side effects:
- Poor cycle control; frequent breakthrough bleeding (30-40%), amenorrhoea (20%)
- Increased frequency of functional cysts [39]
- More frequent acne

Advantages:
- Low dosage
- No oestrogenic effect (apart from limited oestrogenic effect of the progestins)
- No significant central suppression
- Suitable during lactation
- Also suitable if oral hormonal contraceptives would cause cardiovascular risks
- In perimenopausal women, the ovarian status can be assessed by serum FSH even while the POP is taken

Disadvantages:
- Poor cycle control (intermediate bleeding, breakthrough bleeding, amenorrhoea)
- Accurate timing absolutely necessary (3 h interval: higher risk of application errors)

Conditions for use:
- Patient history: cardiovascular disease (only relevant for the decision OC versus progestin-only pill)
- Clinical history (general): not relevant
- Clinical history (gynaecological): exclusion of pregnancy
- Lab: possible pregnancy test
- No examinations required
- Control examinations: every 6 months

Comment: in the perimenopause, an increase in gonadotropin is possible with the pill. It can be detected by laboratory tests. If serum FSH is high, a control examination after 3 months is necessary since fluctuations are possible.

New developments: at low dosage, antiprogestins inhibit implantation (endometrial effect) and are suitable as a POP. However, their spread will probably be limited by their possible abuse as an abortive drug.

Injectables

Substances:
- 3-month injectable: depot medroxyprogesterone acetate (150 mg);
- 2-month injectable: norethisterone enanthate (200 mg);
- once-a-month injectable: norethisterone enanthate (50 mg) + oestradiol valerate (5 mg) (currently available in South America and Turkey only) [34].

Mechanism of action:
- Release of synthetic progestins from an injectable depot
- Changes in the cervical mucus (main effect)
- Reduction of sperm motility in the cervical mucus
- Inhibition of follicular development, no ovulation!
- Reduction of tubal motility

Indications:
- Hormonal contraception during lactation
- Intolerance to or contraindications for synthetic oestrogens

Contraindications:
- Intolerance to progestins (depressive mood, acne, disorders of hepatic metabolism, epileptic fits, voice changes)

Contraceptive efficacy: (Pearl index):

- Depot medroxyprogesterone acetate DMPA (150 mg)	0.3
- Norethisterone enanthate (200 mg, 60 days)	0.4
- Cyclofem (25 mg DMPA/5 mg oestradiol cypionate)	0.0
- Mesigyna (norethisterone enanthate 50 mg/5 mg oestradiol valerate)	0.2

Side effects:
- Cycle disorders (spotting) at beginning of therapy
- Amenorrhoea after ten injections in 50% of cases

Advantages:
- No oestrogenic effect (exception: monthly injectables)
- No significant central suppression
- Suitable during lactation
- Suitable for patients at cardiovascular risk from oral hormonal contraceptives
- Long-term concentration, e.g. in women with uterine myomata, endometriosis

Disadvantages:
- 2 to 3-month injectables: menstrual disorders at beginning of treatment or amenorrhoea after multiple use
- Possible negative effect on bone with depot medroxyprogesterone acetate
- Contraceptive effect may persist for several months after discontinuation

Conditions for use:
- Patient history: cardiovascular disease (if so, the patient must be informed about risks; this is no contraindication, but the individual risk may be increased)

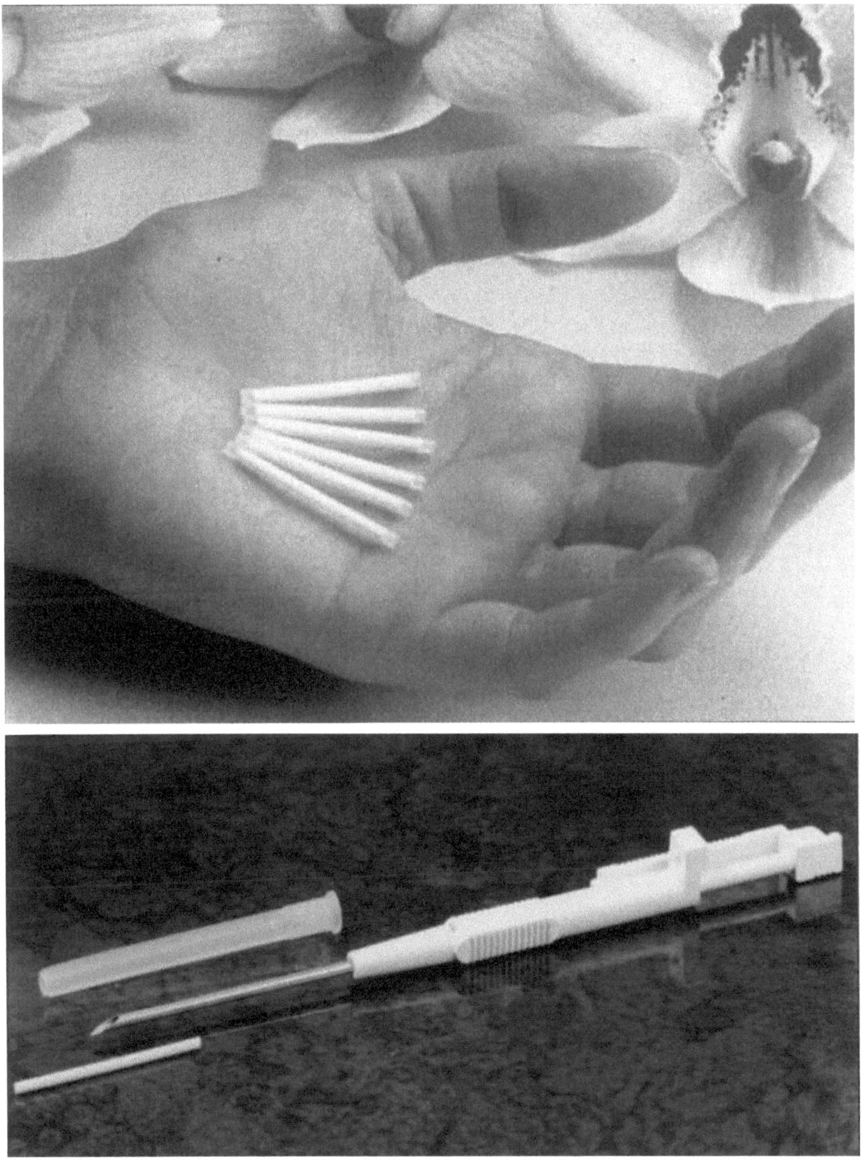

Fig. 3. Implantables. *Top:* Norplant: Six rods releasing levonorgestrel. Long-term contraception up to 5 years. During the first 6 months there is a high rate of intermenstrual bleeding. Contraceptive efficacy depends on body weight (contraindicated in women over 70 kg);
Bottom: Implanon: One rod releasing 3-ketodesogestrel. Implant and inserter.

- Clinical history (general): not relevant
- Clinical history (gynaecological): exclusion of pregnancy
- Lab: possibly pregnancy test; otherwise no examinations necessary
- Control examinations: every 6 months

Technique: depot injection at monthly, bimonthly or quarterly intervals.

New developments:
- One-month injectables. In various countries, studies are underway, e.g. involving women who have already given birth.
- Investigation of new formulations to optimise menstrual cycle control
- Evaluation of cardiovascular side-effects in the framework of epidemiological studies; comparison with oral hormonal contraceptives
- New injection systems: investigation into the stability of steroid hormones in aqueous solution (single-chamber system) or improvement of two-chamber systems (dry substance/solvents)

Hormonal Implants

Method: subdermal implantation of carrier systems containing progestins (levonorgestrel, desogestrel) and continuous release (depending on the system used, they are active for between 2 years (Implanon) and 5 years (Norplant) [20, 37] (Fig. 3).

Substances: levonorgestrel (Norplant) and 3-ketodesogestrel (Implanon; currently under clinical trial)

Mechanism of Action:
- Inhibition of sperm penetration by increasing viscosity of cervical mucus
- Inhibition of implantation by endometrial suppression
- Suppression of mid-cycle LH peak

Distribution: Norplant has been registered in Scandinavia as well as in Thailand, Indonesia and the US; 1-2 million users worldwide

Indications: long-term contraception, particularly if daily administration of the pill is undesirable or impossible.

Contraindications: progestin intolerance; obesity (>70 kg).

Contraceptive efficacy: cumulative pregnancy rate over 5 years: 0.2 [40], depending on body weight (<70 kg)

Side-effects: cycle disorders (especially spotting) and local haematoma caused by insertion (5%)

Advantages:
- Long-term effect of single procedure (up to 5 years)
- High contraceptive efficacy
- Reversible (non-biodegradable carriers may be removed any time)
- Constant hormone serum level (lower than with the progestin-only pill)
- Good acceptance
- No daily administration
- Independent of coitus

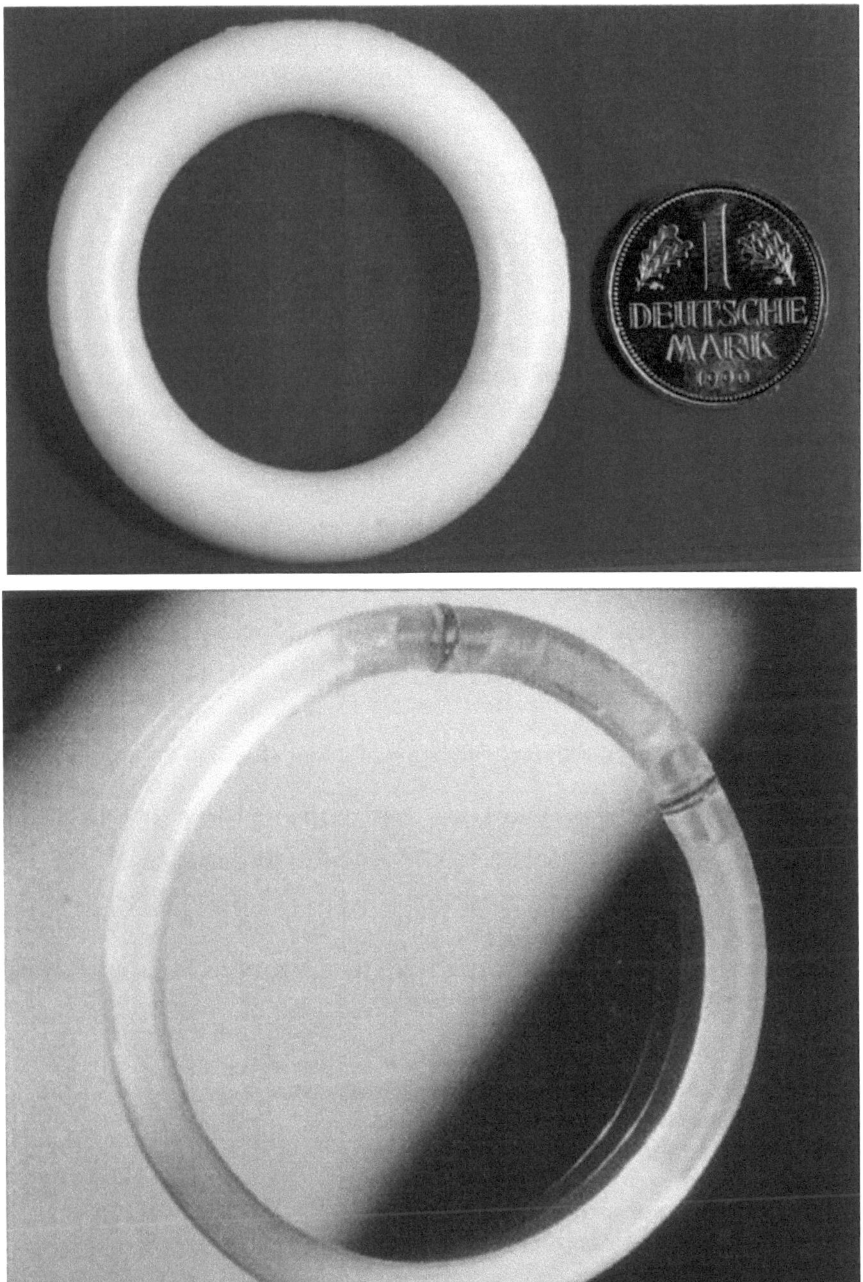

Fig. 4. Vaginal rings. *Top:* WHO ring releasing levonorgestrel. Local action like progestin-only pill. High rate of intermenstrual bleedings. *Bottom:* Organon ring. One compartment with ethinylestradiol and one with 3-ketodesogestrel. Acts by inhibiting ovulation. Good cycle control.

Disadvantages:
- Contraceptive effect can only be interrupted by doctor (removal of implant)
- Removal, e.g. of Norplant, is difficult and requires experience

Conditions for use:
- Patient history: menstrual history
- General clinical history: body weight (<70 kg)
- Gynaecological history: exclusion of gynaecological cancers, exclusion of pregnancy
- Lab: not relevant (only for special indication)
- Control examinations: initially every 3 months, later every 6 months

Technique: insertion under the skin of the inside of the upper arm under local anaesthesia by trocar (takes about 10-15 min.). Non-biodegradable implants: removal after palpation through a small skin incision; extraction after opening the fibrous capsule using a small curved clamp; compression dressing. If manual localisation is difficult, use ultrasound.

Vaginal Ring

Method: contraception through continuous local release of hormones (levonorgestrel: WHO ring; ethinylestradiol/3-ketodesogestrel: Organon ring) from an elastic vaginal ring over 3 weeks [20, 34] (Fig. 4).

Indications: women who want to avoid systemic hormonal effects.

Contraindications: acute or recurrent vaginal infections.

Mechanism of action:
- Levonorgestrel ring (WHO ring): inhibition of sperm ascension through localised progestogenic effect;
- Ethinylestradiol/3-ketodesogestrel ring (Organon ring): inhibition of ovulation.

Contraceptive efficacy: Pearl index: 3.5 (WHO ring); 0.05 (Organon ring)

Side effects:
- WHO ring: bleeding disorders in 25%
- Organon ring (in rare cases): vomiting, indigestion, vaginal discharge, mastodynia, foreign body sensation, candida infections

Advantages:
- Limited metabolic effect due to localised steroid action
- Hepatic metabolism is bypassed
- OTC product
- Not affected by intercourse
- No additional use of spermicides required
- Inexpensive, long-term treatment
- Self-insertion

Disadvantages:
- Monthly insertion
- WHO ring: fivefold EUG rate in cases of contraceptive failure
- Risk of ring expulsion; more frequent in older or multiparous women

Conditions for use:
- History: genital infections, pathological cytology of the cervical os, previous conisation
- General clinical history: not relevant
- Gynaecological history: genital infections, vaginal anomalies, shape of cervical os, previous cervical rupture, cervical cytology, exclusion of pregnancy, exclusion of carcinoma
- Lab: not relevant (only for special indication)
- Control examinations: every 3-6 months

Technique: self-insertion.

New developments:
- The vaginal ring in the WHO (levonorgestrel) or Organon (ethinylestradiol and 3-ketodesogestrel) form will join the range of contraceptives; within this group, the Organon ring is particularly promising as the WHO ring is associated with an increase in bleeding problems (25-50%).
- The levonorgestrel ring influences cervical mucus viscosity locally at the cervix, whereas the Organon ring (ethinylestradiol and 3-ketodesogestrel) inhibits ovulation; the Organon ring therefore has the same mode of action as oral hormonal contraceptives, but fluctuations in blood steroid level are generally avoided. This could mean improved tolerance and acceptance.
- For both systems, the local steroid effect in terms of vaginal infections or ascending genital infections must be studied (levonorgestrel ring: highly probable protective effect due to the progestinic effect on the cervix; currently, no published data are available for the Organon ring)
- Cell changes in the cervix have to be monitored closely, particularly in patients at risk for cervical neoplasia (e.g. heavy smokers, HPV infected patients etc.)
- The vaginal ring is a system for localised steroid release with an exclusively local effect (WHO ring: cervical factor) or a combined local and systemic effect (Organon ring: ovulation inhibition); it is an alternative to other release systems (e.g. implants, depot injections).
- New rings containing progesterone are under clinical trial and may be suitable for contraception in the puerperium

Intrauterine Devices (IUD) or Systems (IUS) (Inert IUD, Copper IUD, levonorgestrel-containing IUS)

Method: inert intrauterine plastic device with or without drug loading (i.e. copper, progestins) prevents sperm ascension, fertilisation or implantation.

Historical development: in the past, various intracervical pessaries (Fig. 5) as well as IUDs have been developed and tested clinically (Fig. 6a-b).

Mechanism of action:
- Inert IUDs: local effect on the endometrium (e.g. macrophage activation)
- Copper IUDs are plastic carriers wrapped in a copper wire. By acting on spermatozoic enzymes and the endometrium, they have a spermicidal effect and disrupt sperm-oocyte interaction, thus preventing fertilisation [17, 31]

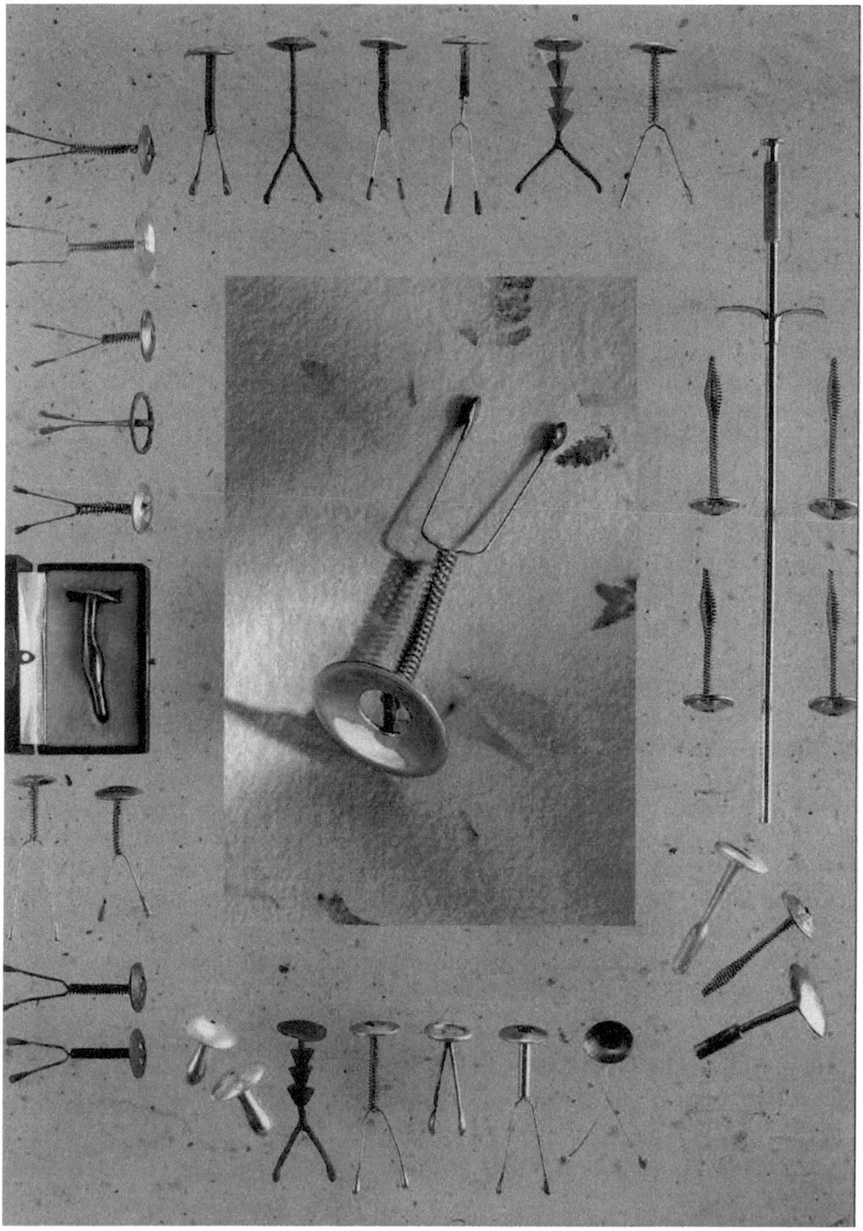

Fig. 5. Intracervical pessaries (with kind permission from Percy Skuy: A Museum of Discovery: Tales of Contraception. Supported by Ortho-McNeil Inc.)

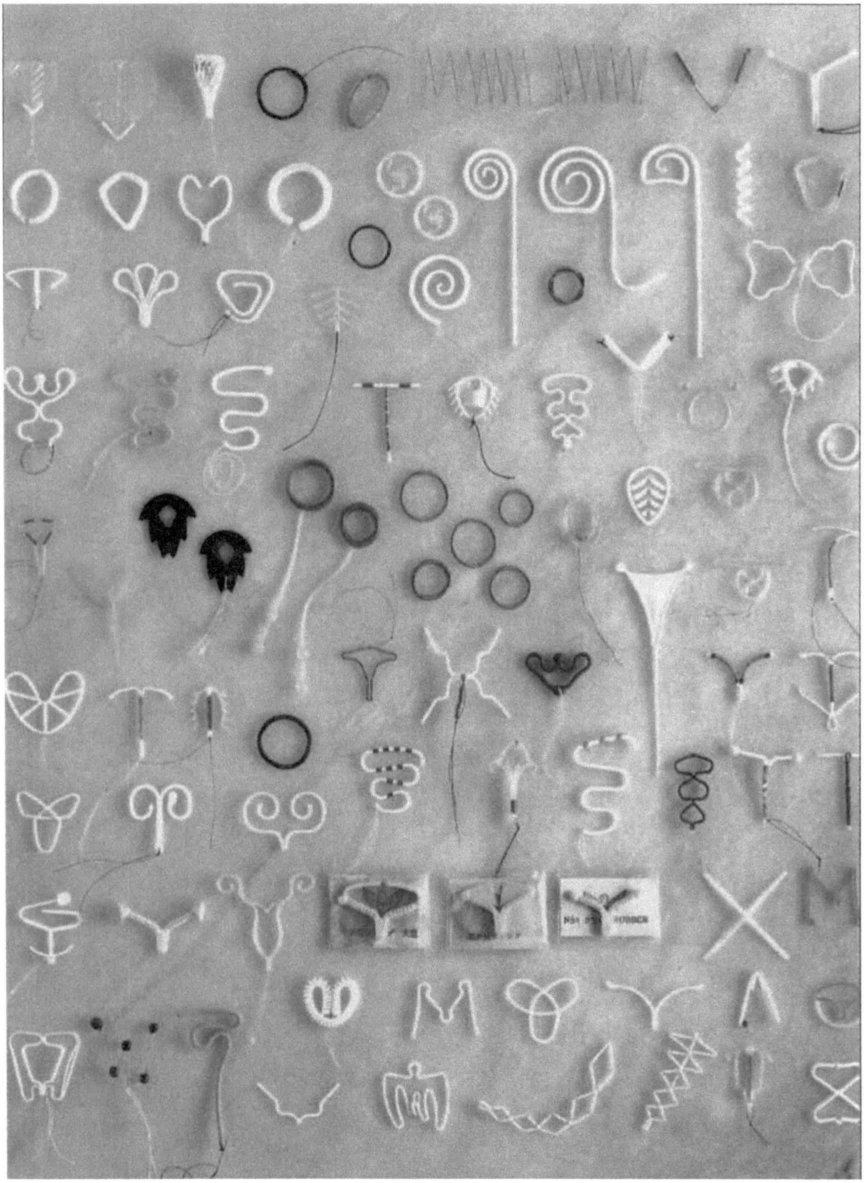

Fig. 6a. Intrauterine devices: historical development (with kind permission from Percy Skuy: A Museum of Discovery: Tales of Contraception. Supported by Ortho-McNeil Inc.)

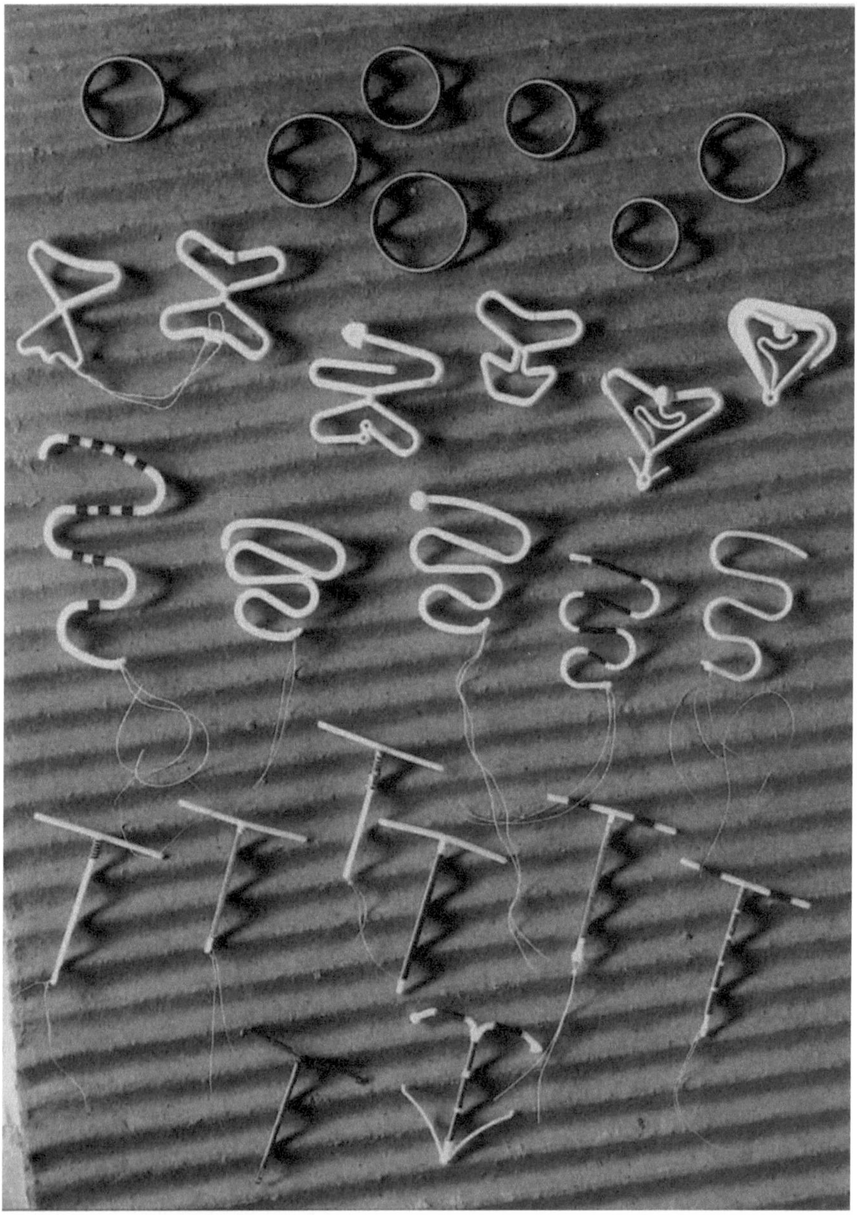

Fig. 6b. Intrauterine devices (continued) (with kind permission from Percy Skuy: A Museum of Discovery: Tales of Contraception. Supported by Ortho-McNeil Inc.)

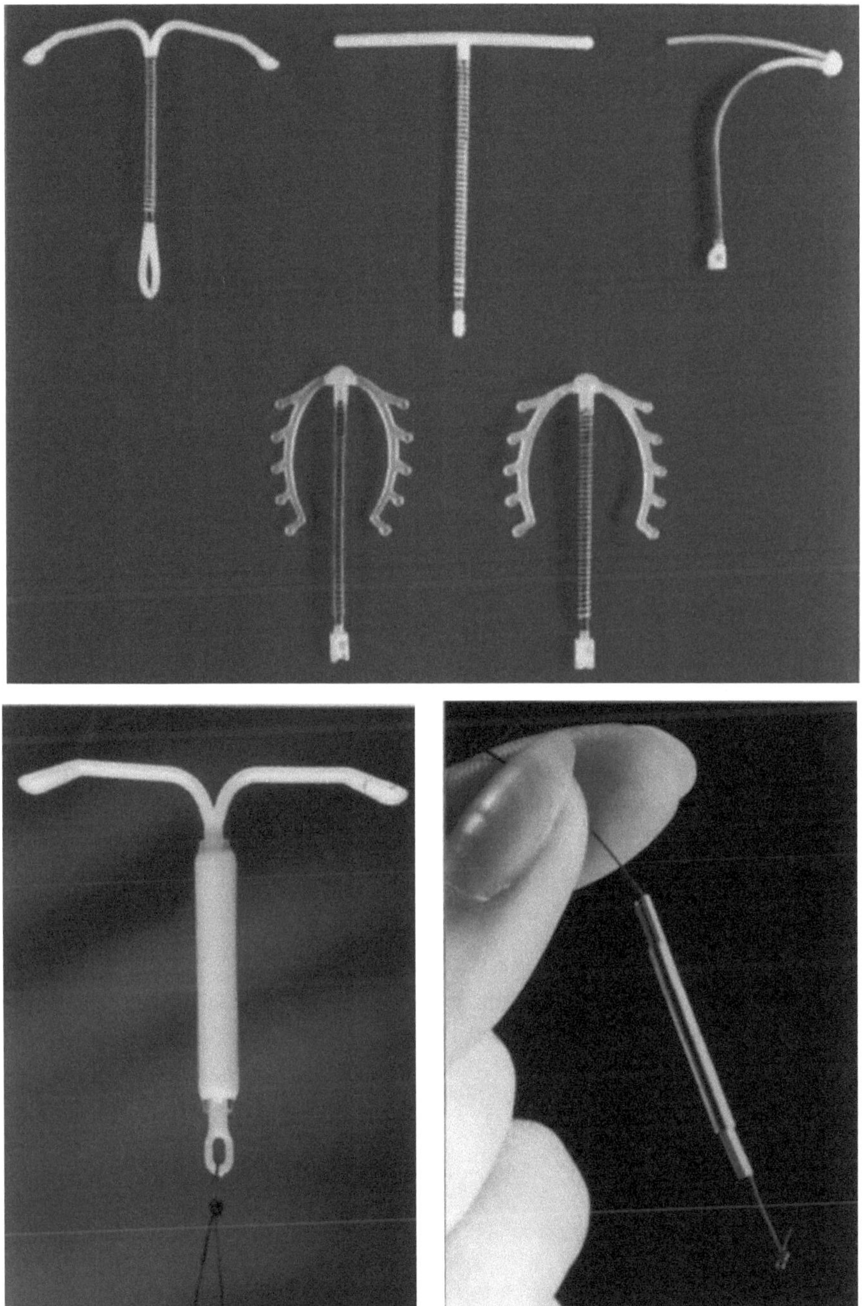

Fig. 6c. Modern intrauterine devices (*upper figure* from left to right). *First row:* Nova T, Kupfer T, Gravigard (German brand names). *Second row:* Multiload 250, Multiload 375. *Lower figure:* Left: Levonorgestrel IUS: Mirena. Right: GyneFix intrauterine device (IUD): six copper cylinders on a plastic string are anchored by a knote in the myometrium of the fundus uteri.

- Levonorgestrel-containing intrauterine systems (LNG-IUS) consist of a T-shaped polyethylene substrate and a cylinder containing levonorgestrel (52 mg). By continuously releasing the hormone locally, they affect the endometrium, leading to irregular secretion by the mucosa. Cervical mucus changes (reduction in viscosity) and capacitation inhibition have been described as additional effects [23].

Indications:
- IUDs or IUS are an alternative to hormonal preparations (intolerance or contraindications for the pill, possible drug interference)
- Women who are unable to time pill-taking precisely (due to their occupation, e.g. stewardess; or due to inadequate compliance)

Contraindications:
- Pregnancy
- Genital inflammation
- Uterine deformity and anomalies of the uterine cavity (bicornuate uterus, hypoplastic uterus, uterus subseptus, uterine myomata)
- Probe length <5 cm
- Undiagnosed bleeding disorders

Contraceptive efficacy: Pearl index: 0.9-3.0 (copper-containing IUD)
0.05-0.1 (levonorgestrel-containing IUS).

Side effects:
- Dysmenorrhoea (for LNG-IUS: reduction)
- Salpingitis (for LNG-IUS: reduction)
- Pelveoperitonitis (for LNG-IUS: reduction)
- Bleeding disturbances (break through bleeding, hypermenorrhoea) within the first 3 to 6 months of use
- Higher risk for ectopic (copper IUDs); lower risk for the Levonorgestrel-IUS
- Lost IUD
- Risk of uterus perforation

Advantages:
- Reversibility, no interference with the endocrine system, one intervention every 5 years only, no patient error possible, no disruption of libido, lowest mortality rate
- Protection from endometrial cancer afforded by copper IUD; not yet confirmed for LNG-IUS
- LNG-IUS: reduction in bleeding intensity, dysmenorrhoea and protection from pelvic inflammatory disease (PID)

Disadvantages:
Inert IUDs:
- Bleeding disorders (intermediate bleeding, spotting); no protection against PID

Copper IUDs:
- Frequent vaginal discharge (cervicitis), adnexitits, endometritis
- More frequent hypermenorrhea

Levonorgestrel IUS:
- Rare progestin-related side-effects (e.g., mild acne)
- Frequent bleeding disorders in the first six months of use

  - Amenorrhoea (20%), acceptance depends on patient information! (No health risk, no risk of osteoporosis since baseline oestrogens are high enough)
  - Diameter of inserter (4.8 mm) slightly higher than in copper IUD, therefore, insertion occasionally requires dilation of the cervix (possibly local anaesthesia)

Conditions for use:
- Patient history: stable relationship, sexual behaviour, risk of adnexitis, previous pregnancies
- General clinical history: signs of genital inflammation
- Gynaecological history: genital infection, uterine anomalies, recent cancer screening results, exclusion of pregnancy
- Lab: leukocytes, CRP, BSR, possible smears for chlamydia, mycoplasma
- Control examinations: 6 weeks after insertion followed by 6-monthly intervals; if available: ultrasound examination

Technique: insertion into the uterus during menstruation (2nd to 5th day of cycle) or at mid-cycle.

Remarks:
- Inert IUD: Lippes loop no longer available
- Copper IUD: ideal copper surface 380 mm^2; some with silver or gold core or copper cylinder on arms
- Levonorgestrel IUS: not worldwide available yet; relatively expensive

New developments: when intrauterine contraceptives with copper-containing spirals were developed, it was found that the ideal copper surface for maximum contraceptive effect is 380 mm^2. The silver core of the copper wire prevents wire breakage and changes of the spiral shape. It also reduces IUD-related side effects (pain, expulsion, perforation). Recently, gold cores have been introduced. Currently, the search is focused on suitable fixation systems for insertion after birth or pregnancy termination. An important step forwards in reducing expulsions, bleeding and unwanted pregnancies is the development of a new frameless intrauterine implant: the GyneFix. Through the advanced anchoring system together with the small insertion tube it is suitable both for nulliparous and parous women as well for imediate post abortum and post partum insertion [17].

Intrauterine contraception with a levonorgestrel-containing IUS (international brand name: Levonova; German brand name: Mirena) is promising. The local release of levonorgestrel (local antioestrogenic and antimitotic action) in the uterus has an excellent contraceptive effect (Pearl index 0.05-0.1) and alleviates both dysmenorrhoea and hypermenorrhoea, so that there is also a medical indication for this spiral. Shorter duration of menstruation; less menstrual blood loss and amenorrhoea is found in 20% of all users (after six cycles). Increase in haèmoglobin and serum iron. Low risk of ectopic pregnancy compared with copper- and progesterone-loaded IUDs and also compared with women not using contraceptives. Low risk of inflammation in the small pelvis (PID). Conception is not delayed: in 96%, conception occurs 12 months after removal. The role of this device in the postmenopause in terms of protection from endometrial cancer during oestrogen substitution therapy cannot yet be evaluated.

Future developments: further indications for protecting the endometrium. Peri- and postmenopausal women in phases II-III; breast cancer patients (phase II) taking tamoxifen.

Further improvements: new inserters, smaller Mirena (US) phase III.

Further intrauterine systems with other progestins are currently under development.

Natural Methods of Family Planning

Method: prevention of fertilisation or oocyte maturation based on the following methods [5, 13]:

Behaviour	Ejaculation outside the vagina (e.g. coitus interruptus)
Timing	Calculation or estimation of the fertile days and abstinence or use of mechanical methods (condom, diaphragm) during the fertile phase; periodic abstinence (Knaus and Ogino timing method), measurement of wake-up temperature, evaluation of cervical mucus (Billings method), combination of wake-up temperature measurement and evaluation of cervical mucus (Rötzer method).
Hormonal	- Prolonged breast feeding - Hormonal computer Persona: determination of fertile and infertile period of the menstrual cycle by urinary estradiol glucuronid and LH analysis

Mechanism of action: see Method.

Note: sperm survives in cervical mucus for up to 6 days [48]

Indications:
- Wish for natural family planning
- Hormone intolerance
- Patient at risk from oral hormonal contraceptives

Contraindications:
- High safety margin required
- Non-compliance
- Advantages of hormone treatment are desired, e.g. with respect to endometriosis
- Irregular cycle

Contraceptive efficacy: Pearl index by method:
- Coitus interruptus: 4-18 [41]
- Periodic abstinence:

  - Calendar-based method: 9 [41]
  - Wake-up temperature method (strict form): 0.8
  - Temperature method (loose form): 3
  - Symptothermal method according to Billings: 2 [41]
- Cycle computer: Persona cycle computer (measurement of LH and estradiol glucuronide in urine): pregnancy rate 6%!

Side effects:
- No systemic side effects
- Possible psychological side effects of coitus interruptus

Advantages:
- Natural contraception
- No systemic side effects.

Disadvantages: many sources of error, therefore, limited contraceptive efficacy.

Conditions for use:
- Patient history: menstrual history (regular cycle required)
- General clinical history: not relevant
- Gynaecological history: exclusion of pregnancy
- Lab: possibly, exclusion of pregnancy, no examinations
- Control examinations: if required, consultation every 3-6 months

Technique: requires patient cooperation and comprehensive information.

Future developments: some methods of natural family planning have been improved. Electronic thermometers (i.e. Evatherm, Roland, Babycomp/Ladycomp, Bioself, Cyclotest) have extended the scope of temperature measurement, e.g. single measurements. The role of integrated mucus resistance measurement as part of a computer analysis for fertility control cannot yet be evaluated; initial animal tests (cows, pigs) are promising (Fa. Rheintechnik,56170 Bensheim/Rhein, Germany).

Immunological Contraception

Suitable target organs for immunological contraception are oocyte and spermatozoal antigens. Scientists have now begun to characterise them, but no breakthrough has been achieved so far [1].

Inhibition of Implantation

The methods of implantation inhibition can be broken down into hormonal, intrauterine and immunological procedures.

Hormonal Methods

- As a morning-after pill, oestrogen/progestin combinations are suitable as an emergency measure [15, 47].
- Antiprogestins prevent implantation; they offset the progesterone effect in early pregnancy, thus inducing early abortion (possibly in combination with vaginal or oral prostaglandins). These substances should also be allowed for termination of pregnancy in Germany, especially since oral prostaglandins with similar effect (Misoprostol; indication: protection against stomach ulcer) are available on prescription.
- Low-dose antiprogestins may be able to change the surface structure of the endometrium in such a way that implantation is impossible without affecting the cycle. Implantation can also be prevented by antagonists.
- Antibodies against specific endometrial proteins also influence the implantation process.

Post Coital Contraception

Method: prevention of fertilisation or implantation by taking synthetic oestrogen/progestin combinations up to 36 hours after unprotected intercourse [15, 43, 47].

Mechanism of action: prevention of fertilisation or implantation by changing tubal motility, tubal secretions and the endometrium.

Contraceptive efficacy: Pearl index: 0.1.

Side effects: frequent nausea, vomiting, leg pain, oedema

Advantages:
- Readily available, relatively inexpensive
- Only taken in emergencies

Disadvantages:
- Nausea, vomiting
- Cycle disorders

Indications:
- Especially suitable for infrequent intercourse
- Emergency measure after unprotected intercourse at mid-cycle

Contraindications:
- History of thromboembolism
- No contraindications (exception: rare allergic reactions)
- Less suitable for frequent intercourse

Conditions for use:
- Patient history: not relevant
- Clinical history (general): not relevant
- Clinical history (gynaecological): not relevant apart from usual cancer screening
- Lab: not relevant

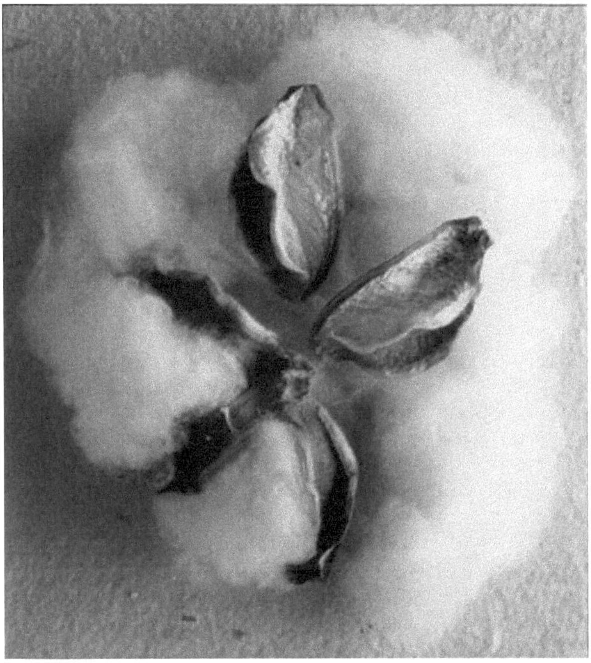

Fig. 7. Male contraception with an extract from the cotton wool seed (Gossypol) has been widely tested in China (courtesy of Percy Skuy, A Museum of Discovery: Tales of Tontraception. Supported by Ortho-McNeil Inc.)

Control examinations: not necessary; only when side effects or pregnancy occur

Note that, according to WHO recommendations, the regularity or timing of the cycle and a family or personal history of thrombosis or thromboembolism are not relevant.

Technique: Yuszpe method. Within 36 h after unprotected intercourse, 500 µg levonorgestrel/100 µg ethinylestradiol (two tablets of combined OC with 250 µg LNG/ 50 µg EE) are taken. Two further tablets should be taken after 12 h.

Comment: according to WHO recommendations, a gynaecological examination is not absolutely necessary.

New developments: postcoital contraception is also possible using antiprogestin [9], but the use is severely restricted because of its potential as an abortive drug.

Intrauterine Devices

Postcoital insertion of an intrauterine spiral is an emergency method that may be used up to the sixth postcoital day.

Immunological Methods

The hCG produced by the trophoblast can be deactivated by specific antibodies which do not cross-react with other gonadotropins; luteal progesterone production will

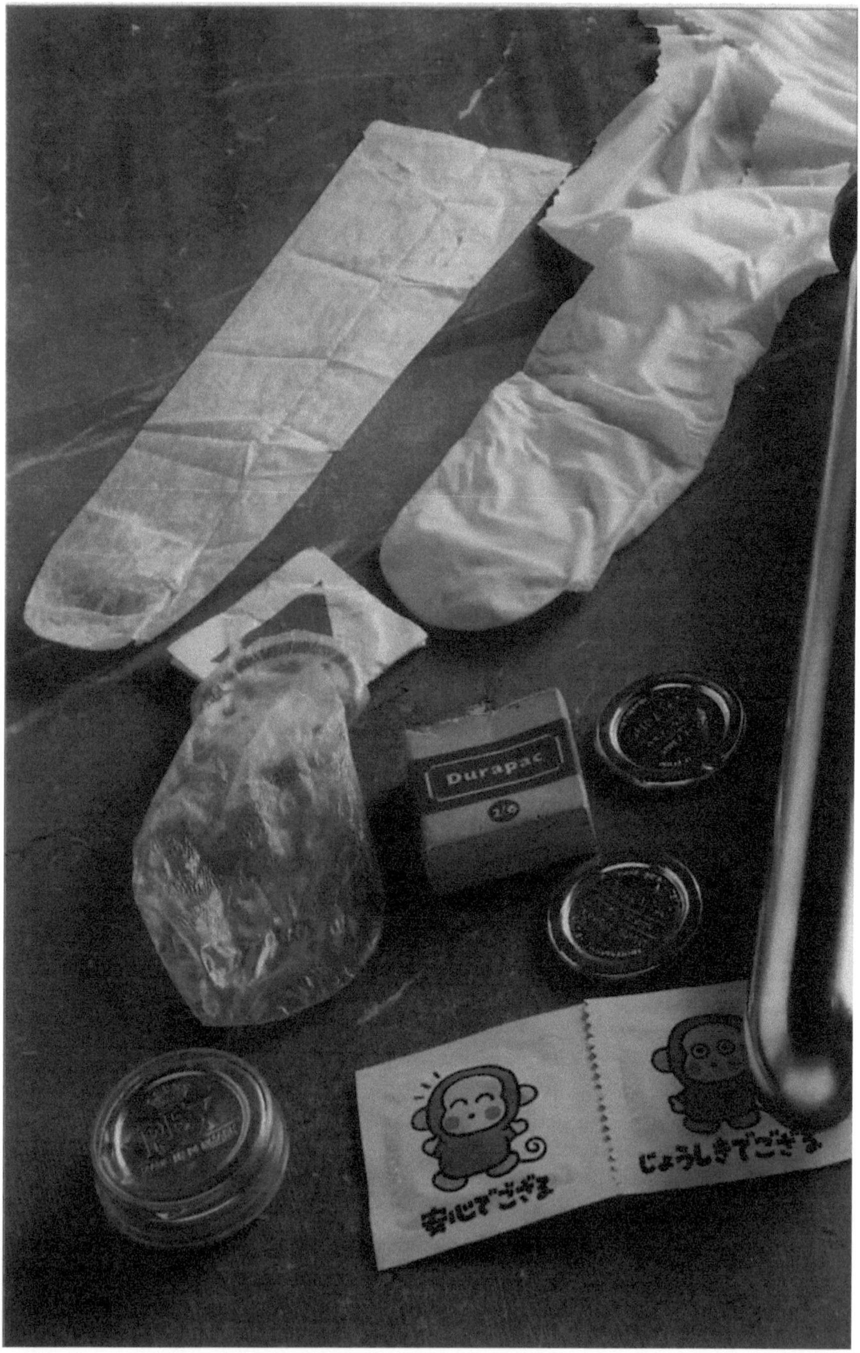

Fig. 8a. Historical condoms (with kind permission from Percy Skuy: A Museum of Discovery: Tales of Tontraception. Supported by Ortho-McNeil Inc.)

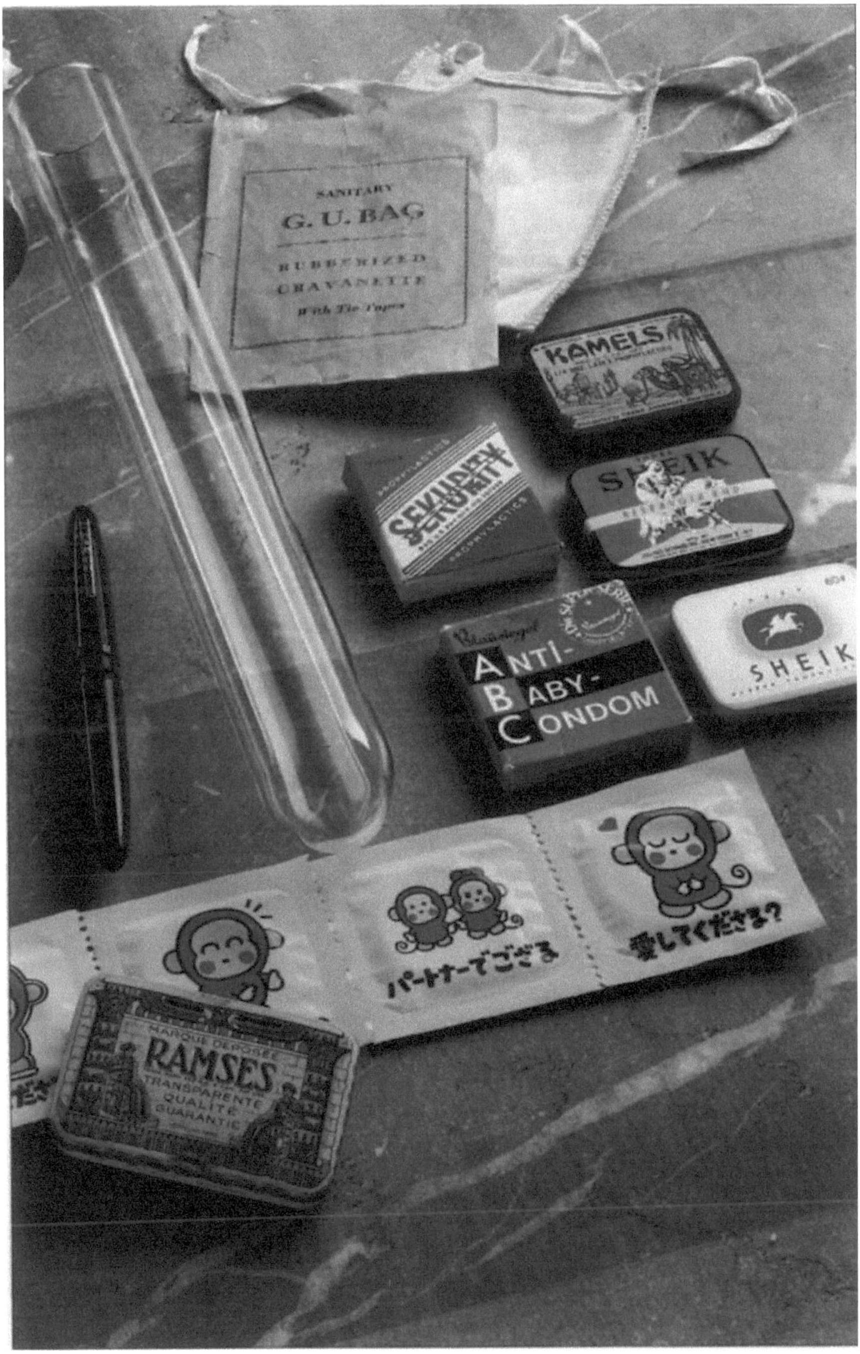

Fig. 8b. Historical condoms (with kind permission from Percy Skuy: A Museum of Discovery: Tales of Tontraception. Supported by Ortho-McNeil Inc.)

drop and early abortion will occur. It remains to be seen if triple vaccination against pregnancy, diphtheria and tetanus will be introduced, since the formation of HCG antibodies cannot be predicted precisely (antibody levels and duration of their increase). Antibodies against zona pellucida glycoproteins (ZP2 and ZP3) can prevent hatching of the embryo from the zona pellucida. Specific binding proteins or glycoproteins that are involved in implantation have been blocked by antibodies in animal experiments.

- Interaction with the interleukin 1 receptor (immunologically or through an antagonist) can also prevent implantation.
- Antibodies against specific endometrial proteins also influence implantation [1].

Male Contraception

- Vasectomy and the condom are the main means of male contraception. Various surgical techniques (silicon graft instillation, valve techniques) are currently under review.
- Behavioural methods (coitus interruptus) have varying degrees of acceptance and are not very effective. Drug-based inhibition of spermatogenesis (e.g., testosterone esters, Gossypol) must produce complete azoospermia for sufficient effect (Fig. 7).
- Hormonal methods (e.g. inhibition of spermatogenesis using GnRH analogues while replacing the testosterone deficit) are still in the stage of animal trials or under early clinical trials. The hepatotoxicity of the long-acting testosterone esters seems to be a problem. It remains to be seen whether testosterone patches are suitable for this purpose [21, 22].

The pill for men is not availible yet. For the time being, the condom will remain the method of choice in male contraception, especially since it also provides effective protection from venereal diseases.

The Condom

Method:
Latex-containing or latex-free condom (Fig. 8c). Condoms are tubes closed spherically on one side normally made of latex membrane with a wall thickness of 0.06-0.07 mm. Their manufacture is fully automatic. Each condom is tested for leaks electronically (quality label). For special purposes, condoms with twice the standard wall thickness have been introduced (cf. anal intercourse). Products with a thickened wall at the tip are also available. The tip of the condom is designed as a reservoir to receive the ejaculate.

"Waisted condoms" (with a tighter shaft portion) are harder to dislodge, but more difficult to test. Fluted condoms (with burls) cannot be accurately tested either. Condoms not carrying a quality label should not be used.

About 90% of all condoms are sold in a rolled-up state and are coated with water-soluble lubricants. Some lubricants contain spermicides. Some products contain still

Fig. 8 c. Modern condoms (selection). Upper left, quality control of condoms (with reservoir) by loading with water; upper right, in the design of the "united colors of Beneton"; bottom, female condom

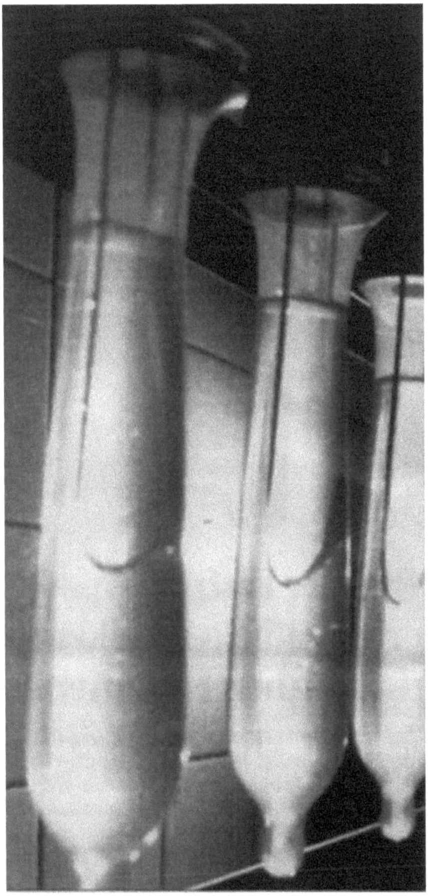

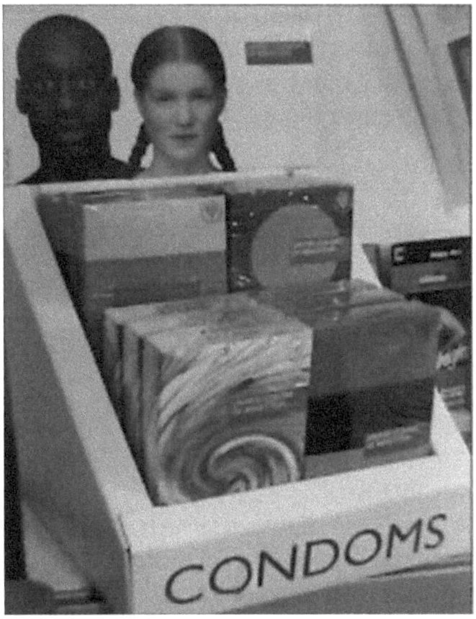
CONDOMS

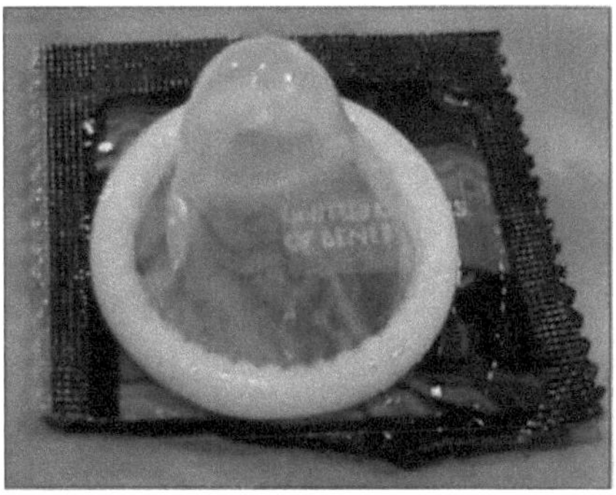

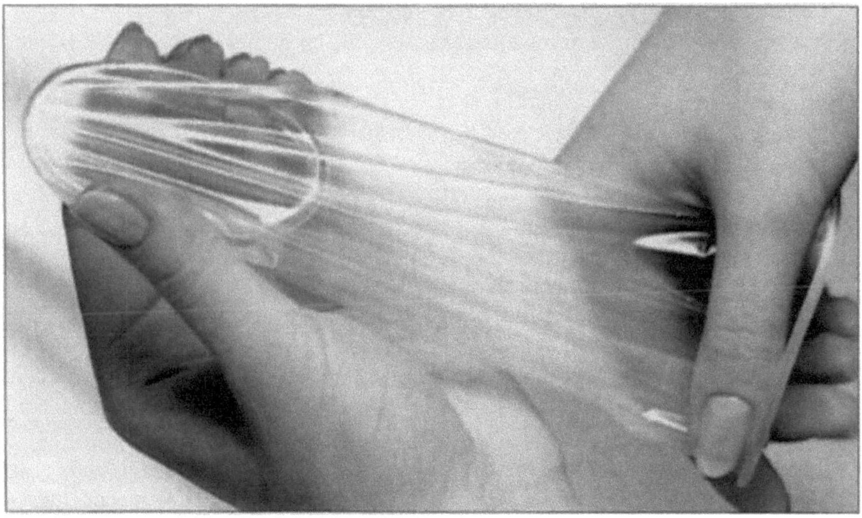

other additives in the lubricants: substances stimulating blood flow (claimed to be aphrodisiac), local anaesthetics (claimed to prolong stimulus to ejaculation) and flavours. As long as these products carry the quality label, there is no medical argument against them.

Historical development: an overview of some historical condoms is given in Figure 8a,b.

Mechanism of action: mechanical method of male contraception. Rubber sheath covers the penis, retaining the ejaculate and preventing contact with the vagina.

Contraceptive efficacy: Pearl index 2-12 [41].

Side-effects: contact dermitis in rare cases (latex condoms only).

Advantages:
- Readily available, relatively cheap (except for latex-free condoms)
- No medical risks
- Effective if used correctly
- No medical control needed
- Protection from venereal diseases
- No systemic contraception

Disadvantages:
- Moderate contraceptive efficacy
- Psychosexual interference with intercourse
- Rarely, contact dermatitis (vagina, penis) caused by condom or lubricant

Indications:
- Particularly suitable for infrequent intercourse
- Some protection from genital infections (e.g. venereal diseases, trichomonads, fungi, HIV) for people with casual sexual relationships
- For women who cannot or must not take the pill and do not tolerate the IUD

Contraindications:
- None (except for rare allergic reactions)
- Less suitable for frequent intercourse

Conditions for use:
- Patient history: not relevant
- Clinical history (general): not relevant
- Clinical history (gynaecological): not applicable; the usual cancer screening
- Lab: not relevant
- Control examinations: not necessary; there are no restrictions for the sale of condoms

Technique: condom is rolled on the penis by the man or the woman before intercourse. Contraceptive efficacy can be increased by the simultaneous use of spermicides or by using condoms with a spermicidal lubricant. Lubricating the condom increases sensitivity and reduces irritation or injury. Penis must be withdrawn from the vagina while holding the condom to the base of the penis as soon as the erection starts to subside. Shelf-life of 5 years (caution: reduced shelf-life at higher temperatures and humidity – protection from sunlight slows down ageing process). Caution: fingernails and rings may damage the condom [45].

New developments: latex-free condoms are already on the market; combination with new spermicides (maximum protection from sexually transmitted diseases would be desirable); female condoms (Fig. 8c).

Male Sterilisation

Method: sterilisation of the man.

Mechanism of action: interruption of the seminal duct by partial resection, ligation, silicon plug or post-inflammatory adhesion.

Distribution: globally, a total of 60 million men have received a vasectomy, 30 million of them in China. Strong variation: New Zealand 23%, US and Netherlands 10%, Germany 2%.

Vasectomy technique: palpate the ductus deferens under the scrotal skin, inject local anaesthetic, make skin incision, incise the sheath to expose the underlying ductus, lift up ductus loop, inject local anaesthetic into loop, dissect ductus after ligation, suture the skin.

Contraceptive efficacy: around 1 in 400 operated men remain fertile – Pearl index: 0.1-0.15 [41]. Azoospermia will take 3 months to occur. Control sperm count necessary. Recanalisation through surgical error; seminal duct diplogenesis

Side-effects:
- Psychological problems
- Complications of surgery (haematoma, infection)

Advantages:
- No systemic side effects
- Good access to seminal duct, low risk of operation

Disadvantages:
- Intervention is frequently irreversible (50-70%)
  Indications: man wants no further children and requests definitive sterilisation.

Contraindications:
- Young men whose family situation could change (e.g. divorce)
- Local infection
- Systemic diseases
- Varicocele, hernia

Conditions for use:
- Patient history: exclusion of genital infection
- Clinical history (general): not relevant
- Clinical history (andro): exclusion of genital infection, systemic disease, varicocele, hernia
- Lab: sperm count (see below)
- Control examinations: repeat sperm count until negative!

New developments: so-called "non-scalpel techniques" could gain in importance [12]

Recommendations for Contraception

Young Women (<18 years) [2]

Situation. Safe form of contraception is needed; frequent acne and seborrhoea; frequently changing partners; little experience with local methods of family planning; frequently unstable cycle (sometimes anovulatory), meaning that natural contraceptive methods are unsuitable. Considerable regional and ethnic differences.

OC. Most adequate method of contraception: safe contraceptive effect, good cycle control and low risk of inflammatory disease in the small pelvis (STD). Initial prescription of 20 (30) µg EE formulations. Acne is common in this age group (30-40% of all women below 20) and can be efficiently treated by antiandrogen-containing pills. OCs also afford good protection from certain diseases (e.g. polycystic ovary syndrome, ovarian cysts, ovarian cancer, endometrial cancer) and carry little risk.

It is unclear whether the long-term use of the pill before the first term pregnancy can produce a slight increase in the relative risk of women developing breast cancer (RR 1.27).

Spermicides and Condoms. In this age group, alternatives such as spermicides and condoms (ideally in combination) should also be considered. The recommendation is frequently given to combine oral hormonal contraceptives with the condom, since the condom alone is not safe enough at this age. Using only spermicides is not recommended in view of the waiting period of 10 min and the loss of contraceptive effect during repeated intercourse, which reduce the acceptance for and safety of this method. Protection from sexually transmitted disease through the use of condoms is an important aspect when the woman is not familiar with the partner or the partner is unreliable. In Germany, 9% of all couples (US 28%) use condoms in addition to OCs. In the US, the success of this approach is obvious: in 1987, AIDS ceased to be the main cause of death amongst 18-40 year-olds.

IUD. IUDs with copper release are only suitable in certain cases, since people with unstable relationships have an increased STD risk with the possibility of ascending bacteria and subsequent infertility due to infection of the fallopian tubes (e.g. adhesions, occlusion). If both partners are monogamous and have no STD risk, the IUD is an option for young women with no history of gynaecological infection if they do not prefer the other methods.

POP. Less suitable for young women because of bleeding and cycle disorders and the need for exact timing (time window of 3 h) and because of lower contraceptive efficacy.

Women Aged 18-35 Years [36]

Most couples in this age group use OCs with or without condoms, depending on the stability of the relationship and the risk of STD infections (see above). If intercourse is rare, they use condoms and spermicides. If no further children are wanted, see later.

Women Over 35 Years of Age [36]

Low dose OCs may be used by this age group if there are no risk factors. Risk factors include smoking (women over 30 years smoking more than ten cigarettes daily should be informed about their risk) and – independent of age – cardiovascular diseases, diabetes mellitus, hypertension and hyperlipidaemia. OCs are also used on a long-term basis for additional indications (e.g. bleeding disorders, dysmenorrhoea, endometriosis).

IUDs containing copper are appropriate for this age group, but the levonorgestrel-releasing IUS are even more suitable (cost consideration) because they reduce the intensity and duration of bleeding and improve dysmenorrhoea.

Depot injections are an alternative (so-called 3-monthly injectables), but amenorrhoea occurs in more than 50% of the cases after ten injections. It is still unclear whether long-term application gives rise to osteopenia or osteoporosis.

Post-Partum Contraception

The couple requests safe contraception without risk for the (breast-fed) baby or for the mother herself (e.g. increased risk of thrombosis in the puerperal period); intrauterine contraception is possible after uterine involution, but breast-feeding mothers, in particular, are liable to expel their device immediately after childbirth.

Prolonged Breast-feeding

- High contraceptive efficacy (98%) in exclusively breast-feeding mothers within the first 6 or 12 months [45]
- Ovulation occurs before the first period
- Risk of the child being infected by HIV if a previously HIV-negative mother is infected during the breast-feeding period (in Central Africa the use of condoms is urgently recommended)

POP

- May be taken immediately after childbirth or 6 weeks postpartum if the child is breast-fed
- Advantage: can be taken even when there are relative contraindications against OCs

OCs

- Low-dose OCs have no influence on the child (exception: prematurity), milk volume, milk composition or the breast-feeding period. Therefore, they may also be used immediately after childbirth (caution: increased risk of thrombosis in the puerperal period; OCs should only be taken if the mother is sufficiently mobilised).
- US recommendation: mothers should start taking OCs, at the earliest, 6 weeks after childbirth if the child is not breast-fed exclusively and if menstruation has started (before menstruation begins, the risk of pregnancy is low) [18].

IUD

- In principle, IUDs can be used immediately postpartum (caution: increased risk of expulsion).
- Alternatively, it can be inserted after uterine involution (about 6 weeks postpartum).

Depot Progestins

Depot progestins may also be given immediately postpartum and are reported to have no influence on breast-feeding.

STD protection

In countries with an increased risk of STD (e.g. Africa) and a prolonged breast-feeding period, the condom is recommended.

Women with no Desire for Future Childbearing

Women with no desire for future childbearing should only use OCs if there are no risk factors. These are smoking (risk information from age 30 years if more than ten cigarettes are smoked daily) and cardiovascular diseases, diabetes mellitus, hypertension, hyperlipidaemia (independent of age). In this age group, complementary indications often result in the prescription of OCs (e.g. bleeding disorders, dysmenorrhoea).

IUDs with copper are appropriate for this age group, but the levonorgestrel-releasing IUS are even more suitable (cost consideration) since they reduce the intensity and duration of bleeding and alleviate the dysmenorrhoea.

Hormonal depot injections are an alternative (3-monthly injectables), but amenorrhoea occurs after ten injections in more than 50% of the cases. It is still unclear whether long-term application causes osteopenia or osteoporosis.

Sterilisation is recommended if no (further) children are desired. However, the patient must be informed about the irreversibility (exception: microsurgery, endoscopic operations or in vitro fertilisation) and about the cumulative failure rate of around 5% in 10 years [25].

Postcoital Contraception

The following methods may be used in emergencies [43]

- The morning-after pill: Yuszpe method – 500 µg levonorgestrel/100 µg ethinyl estradiol immediately and after 12 h; treatment must start within 36 h of unprotected intercourse. According to WHO recommendations, it is not strictly necessary to perform a gynaecological examination.
- Postcoital IUD: may be inserted within 6 days of unprotected intercourse.
- Antiprogestins: may become available for this indication in the near future.

Summary

By the year 2030, of a total of 1.2 billion couples of reproductive age, 800 million will require adequate methods of family planning. Currently, 45 million abortions are performed in China and z60 million. Every year, 200,000 women die as a consequence of inadequate abortion procedures. The number of pregnancy terminations is inversely proportional to the use of contraceptives in the different countries. The antiprogestin RU 486 should be legalized in all countries. 500,000 women die every year during and after childbirth, 99% of them in developing countries.

Only 40% of all couples currently have access to adequate methods of fertility control although only 3 US dollars would be needed per couple per year. The main key to the acceptance of the different family planning methods is the implementation of women's rights combined with a pension system in each country; as long as a large number of offspring is the only guarantee for old age, all efforts to make contraceptives more popular will be in vain.

Contraceptives can be categorised by mechanism of action and user (man or woman). Female contraception may be based on prevention of ovulation, fertilisation, implantation of the fertilised egg in the uterus or on abortion. Male contraception can be broken down into methods influencing sperm production or fertilisation.

Oral hormonal contraceptives are currently used by around 60-80 million women – this method is one of the safest forms of female contraception and is especially suitable for young women who have no risk factors and may want children later. The copper-containing IUD is gaining in importance, as are levonorgestrel-containing intrauterine systems (IUS). The levonorgestrel-IUS is certainly the second most important contraceptive innovation after the pill, which was launched 30 years ago. Women with no desire for future childbearing are the best candidates for this kind of long-term contraception [29].

In the next 5-10 years, oral hormonal contraceptives will be the method of choice in fertility control. New methods, such as the monthly injectable, hormone implants and new sterilisation techniques for women and men, will become important for certain patient groups.

For male contraception, some interesting hormonal strategies (e.g. GnRH analogues and testosterone depot preparations) have been proposed to complement the condom and sterilisation. However, the promising initial clinical results have not been implemented on a larger scale yet.

In order to contain the risk of infection with sexually transmitted diseases in a new sexual relationship, „safer-sex" techniques should be used, including (latex-free) condoms.

References

1. Aitken RJ, Paterson M, Koothan PT (1993) Contraceptive vaccines. In: Drife JO, Baird DT (eds) Contraception. British Medical Bulletin, Churchill Livingstone, pp 88-99
2. Bailey P, Sanfilippo JS (1993) Contraception in the adolescent. In: Shoupe D, Haseltine FP (eds) Contraception. Springer-Verlag, Berlin Heidelberg New York, pp 93-111
3. Benagiano G, Shah I (1997) Contraception and health in Europe. In: Capdevila CC, Cortit LI, Creatsas G (eds) Contraception today. The proceedings of the 4th Congress of the European Society of Contraception. Parthenon, New York, pp 1-11
4. Bernstein GS (1993) Diaphragm, condoms, and sponge. In: Shoupe D, Haseltine FP (eds) Contraception. Springer-Verlag, Berlin Heidelberg New York, pp 158-168
5. Bonnar J (1994) Natural contraception through personal hormone monitoring. Proceedings of a symposium held at the XIV FIGO World Congress of Gynecology and Obstetrics, Montreal, Canada, September 1994. Parthenon, New York
6. Bounds W (1997) Female condoms. In: Capdevila CC, Cortit LI, Creatsas G (eds) Contraception today. The proceedings of the 4th Congress of the European Society of Contraception. Parthenon, New York, pp 161-165
7. Capdevila CC, Cortit LI, Creatsas G (1997) Contraception today. The proceedings of the 4th Congress of the European Society of Contraception. Parthenon, New York
8. Djerassi C (1980) The politics in contraception. Norton, New York
9. Donaldson MS, Dorflinger L, Brown SS, Benet LZ (1993) Clinical applications of mifepristone (RU 486) and other anti- progestins. Institute of Medicine. National Academy Press, Washington, D.C.
10. Drife JO, Baird DT (1993) Contraception. Churchill Livingstone, ppz.
11. Fathalla MF (1993) Contraception and women's health. In: Drife JO, Baird DT (eds) Contraception. British Medical Bulletin, Churchill Livingstone, pp 245-251
12. Filshie M (1997) No-scalpel technique for vasectomy. In: Capdevila CC, Cortit LI, Creatsas G (eds) Contraception today. The proceedings of the 4th Congress of the European Society of Contraception. Parthenon, New York, pp 222-230
13. Freundl G (1997) Rhythm methods and devices. In: Capdevila CC, Cortit LI, Creatsas G (eds) Contraception today. The proceedings of the 4th Congress of the European Society of Contraception. Parthenon, New York, pp 53-64
14. Hassan EA, Creatsas G (1997) Contraceptive barrier methods: new developments. In: Capdevila CC, Cortit LI, Creatsas G (eds) Contraception today. The proceedings of the 4th Congress of the European Society of Contraception. Parthenon, New York, pp 154-160
15. Kubba AA (1997) Hormonal postcoital contraception. In: Capdevila CC, Cortit LI, Creatsas G (eds) Contraception today. The proceedings of the 4th Congress of the European Society of Contraception. Parthenon, New York, pp 44-48
16. Laufe LE (1987) Mechanical contraception in the year 2001. In: van Keep PA, Davis KE, de Wied D (eds) Contraception in the year 2001. Proceedings of an Excerpta Medica Foundation symposium held at the Royal Netherlands. Academy of Sciences and Letters, Amsterdam 2-3 October 1986, International Congress Series 759 Excerpta Medica, Amsterdam, pp 127-139
17. Martinez F, Barri P (1997) The new generation of copper intrauterine devices. In: Capdevila CC, Cortit LI, Creatsas G (eds) Contraception today. The proceedings of the 4th Congress of the European Society of Contraception. Parthenon, New York, pp 131-136
18. Mitchell Jr. (1997) Combination OC formulations: Worldwide Conference Report. Symposium: contraception, FIGO, Copenhagen
19. Newton J (1987) The requirements for the ideal contraceptive. In: van Keep PA, Davis KE, de Wied D (eds) Contraception in the year 2001. Proceedings of an Excerpta Medica Foundation symposium held at the Royal Netherlands. Academy of Sciences and Letters, Amsterdam 2-3 October 1986, International Congress Series 759 Excerpta Medica, Amsterdam, pp 45-59
20. Newton J (1993) Long acting methods of contraception. In: Drife JO, Baird DT (eds) Contraception. British Medical Bulletin, Churchill Livingstone, pp 40-61
21. Nieschlag E (z) Kontrazeption beim Mann: Aktueller Stand und neue Entwicklungen. Gynäkologe, aus dem gleichen Heft
22. Nieschlag E, Knuth UA, Weinbauer GF (1987) Male contraception: possible endocrine approaches. In: van Keep PA, Davis KE, de Wied D (eds) Contraception in the year 2001. Proceedings of an Excerpta Medica Foundation symposium held at the Royal Netherlands. Academy of Sciences and

Letters, Amsterdam 2-3 October 1986, International Congress Series 759 Excerpta Medica, Amsterdam, pp 83-95
23. Odlind V (1997) Long-term experience of a levonorgestrel-releasing intrauterine system. In: Capdevila CC, Cortit LI, Creatsas G (eds): Contraception today. The proceedings of the 4th Congress of the European Society of Contraception. Parthenon, New York, pp 37-43
24. Pannenborg CO (1987) Contraceptive needs in the Third World: the present paradox of a future family planning - technology nexus. In: van Keep PA, Davis KE, de Wied D (eds) Contraception in the year 2001. Proceedings of an Excerpta Medica Foundation symposium held at the Royal Netherlands. Academy of Sciences and Letters, Amsterdam 2-3 October 1986, International Congress Series 759 Excerpta Medica, Amsterdam, pp 21-44
25. Peterson HB, Xia Hughes JM, Wilcox LS, Tylor LR, Trussell J (1996) The risk of pregnancy after tubal sterilization: findings from the U. Collaborative Review of Sterilization. Am J Obstet Gynecol 174:1161-1170
26. Pike MC, Spicer DV (1993) Oral Contraceptives and Cancer. In: Shoupe D, Haseltine FP (eds) Contraception. Springer-Verlag Berlin Heidelberg New York, pp 67-84
27. Population Reports (1978) Special topic monographs. Voluntary sterilization: world's leading contraceptive method. No. 2, M-37. Department of Medical and Public Affairs. George Washington University Medical Center, Washington
28. Rabe T, Runnebaum B (1994) Kontrazeption. In: Runnebaum B, Rabe T (eds) Gynäkologische Endokrinologie und Fortpflanzungsmedizin, Band 1, Springer, pp 411-512
29. Rabe T, Vladescu E, Runnebaum B (1998) Die Zukunft der oralen hormonalen Kontrazeption. Der Gynäkologe (im gleichen Heft)
30. Rao SLN (1987) Contraceptive needs in the 21st century: a demographic analysis. In: van Keep PA, Davis KE, de Wied D (eds) Contraception in the year 2001. Proceedings of an Excerpta Medica Foundation symposium held at the Royal Netherlands. Academy of Sciences and Letters, Amsterdam 2-3 October 1986, International Congress Series 759 Excerpta Medica, Amsterdam, pp 1-20
31. Rojnik B (1997) Mechanism of action of intrauterine devices. In: Capdevila CC, Cortit LI, Creatsas G (eds) Contraception today. The proceedings of the 4th Congress of the European Society of Contraception. Parthenon, New York, pp 117-121
32. Runnebaum B, Rabe T, Kiesel L (1988) Trends in hormonal contraception. In: Runnebaum B, Rabe T, Kiesel L (eds) Female contraception, update and trends. Springer-Verlag, Berlin Heidelberg New York, pp 109-121
33. Salzer H, Jinniate S, Tatschl S (1997) LeaR Contraceptivum: a new concept in female barrier contraception. In: Capdevila CC, Cortit LI, Creatsas G (eds) Contraception today. The proceedings of the 4th Congress of the European Society of Contraception. Parthenon, New York, pp 166-172
34. Shoupe D (1993) Injectable contraceptives and contraceptive vaginal rings. In: Shoupe D, Haseltine FP (eds) Contraception. Springer-Verlag Berlin Heidelberg New York, pp 144-157
35. Shoupe D, Haseltine FP (1993) Contraception. Springer-Verlag, Berlin Heidelberg New York
36. Shoupe D, Mishell DR Jr. (1993) Oral contraceptives for women over the age of 35. In: Shoupe D, Haseltine FP (eds) Contraception. Springer-Verlag, Berlin Heidelberg New York, pp 85-92
37. Sivin I (1993) NORPLANTR contraceptive implants. In: Shoupe D, Haseltine FP (eds) Contraception. Springer-Verlag Berlin Heidelberg New York, pp 131-143
38. Speroff L, Darney Ph. (1992) A clinical guide for contraception. Williams & Wilkins,
39. Tayob Y, Adams J, Jacobs HS, Guillebaud J (1985) Ultrasound demonstration of increased frequency of functional ovarian cysts in women using progestogen-only oral contraception. J Obstet Gynaecol 92:1003
40. Trussell J & Kost K (1987) Contraceptive failure in the United States: a critical review of the literature. Stud Fam Plann 10:117
41. Trussell J, Hatcher RA, Cates W Jr, Stewart FH, Kost K (1990) Contraceptive failure in the United States: an update. Stud Fam Plann 21:51
42. van Keep PA, Davis KE, de Wied D (1987) Contraception in the year 2001. In: van Keep PA, Davis KE, de Wied D (eds) Contraception in the year 2001. Proceedings of an Excerpta Medica Foundation symposium held at the Royal Netherlands. Academy of Sciences and Letters, Amsterdam 2-3 October 1986, International Congress Series 759 Excerpta Medica, Amsterdam
43. van Look PFA, von Hertzen H (1993) Emergency contraception. In: Drife JO, Baird DT (eds) Contraception. British Medical Bulletin, Churchill Livingstone, pp 158-170

44. Vancaillie TG (1993) Female Sterilization. In: Shoupe D, Haseltine FP (eds) Contraception. Springer-Verlag, Berlin Heidelberg New York, pp 169-180
45. Vekemans M (1997) Postpartum contraception: the lactational amenorrhea method. In: Capdevila CC, Cortit LI, Creatsas G (eds) Contraception today. The proceedings of the 4th Congress of the European Society of Contraception. Parthenon, New York, pp 65-74
46. Vessey MP, Lawless M, Yeates D, McPherson K (1985) Progestogen-only contraception: findings in a large prospective study with special reference to effectiveness. Br J Fam Plann 10:117
47. Webb AMC (1997) Gestagens, danazol and antiprogestogen in emergency contraception. In: Capdevila CC, Cortit LI, Creatsas G (eds) Contraception today. The proceedings of the 4th Congress of the European Society of Contraception. Parthenon, New York, pp 49-52
48. Wilcox AJ, Weinberg CR, Baird DD (1995) Timing of intercourse in relation to ovulation. Effects on the probability of conception, survival of pregnancy, and sex of the baby. N Engl J Med 333:1517-1521

4 The Future of Oral Hormonal Contraception

Thomas Rabe, Benno Runnebaum

Each second, the world population increases by three newborn babies (98 million per year); nine out of ten are born in developing countries. In 2050, the total population will be 12.5 billion instead of the 6 billion of today. No war, no disease, but only access to and the acceptance of effective methods of fertility control can stop the growth of the world population. Additionally, religious aspects, the realisation of female rights, equal access to education and jobs for women and men, availability of pensions (no further need for support by a big family) will be the pillars of a successful family policy. Furthermore, a better health care system for women (500,000 deaths annually during pregnancy and childbirth) and safe techniques of pregnancy termination (200,000 deaths annually per 50 million abortions) are necessary. Oral hormonal contraceptives (OCs) are one of the methods of fertility control which is highly effective, safe, well accepted and available in most countries worldwide.

Oral hormonal contraceptives have been available since 1959 in the US (brand name: Enovid) and since 1961 in Germany (brand name: Anovlar). Until now, more than 150 million women have taken OCs and, today, 60–80 million women are using OCs daily for contraception.

The future of oral hormonal contraceptives (OC) is determined by their safety, non-contraceptive benefits, costs, and the users' attitude towards OCs when compared with other contraceptive methods. These individual items will be discussed in this review (reviews see: Rabe & Runnebaum 1982; 1996; Runnebaum et al. 1988a, b; 1991; Speroff & Darney, 1992).

Safety

Contraceptive Efficacy

The contraceptive efficacy of different contraceptive methods is specified by means of the Pearl index (number of unwanted pregnancies per 100 woman-years) or a life table analysis, e.g. analysis of the contraceptive efficacy and the side effects, depending on the duration of use.

The contraceptive efficacy of tubal sterilisation – taken as a gold standard – has been assumed to be 1-2 pregnancies per 1000 sterilisations. This number must be recon-

This chapter originally appeared in congress proceedings: Research on Human Reproduction, 25 years of achievement with the WHO Special Programme of Research, Development and Research Training in Human Reproduction. Edited by L. Kovacs and B.A. Resch, 1997, Albert Szent-Györgyi Medical University Press, Szeged, Hungary and in *Der Gynäkologe*, **31**, 5/98, 451-460.

sidered. In a recently published US study, a higher cumulative pregnancy rate (n=143), ranging from 2% to 5%, was observed in 10,685 women undergoing a tubal sterilisation by various methods: highest failure rates followed clip sterilisation (36.5/1.000 cases) compared with unipolar coagulation (7.5/1.000 cases) and partial salpingectomy (7.5/1.000 cases) (Peterson et al. 1996).

The highest contraceptive efficacy can be achieved by use of the levonorgestrel containing Intrauterine System (IUS) (Pearl index: 0.1); the Pearl index for OCs ranges between 0.05 and 0.1 for methodological failure and between 0.1 and 0.9 due to user's failure. Higher contraceptive failure rates have been found in non-European countries: up to 3% in US studies (Trussel et al. 1990). For young clients who desire high contraceptive efficacy, this is provided by regular use of OCs. Interactions with drugs, vomiting and diarrhoea must be considered individually, as should the potential for unwanted pregnancies. For natural family planning methods, a Pearl index between 0.8-3 (strict method) and up to 20 (Knaus-Ogino method) has been determined, but all behavioural methods are rather unsafe due to the long survival time of spermatozoa in the cervical mucus (up to 6 days) (Wilcox et al. 1995).

No Negative Metabolic Impact

During the last 20 years significant attention has been drawn to OC effects on metabolism (lipids, carbohydrates and blood coagulation). Changes of various metabolic parameters caused by low doses of oral hormonal contraceptives may be statistically significant when compared with untreated controls or to pretreatment values of patients in a study, but, in most cases, these changes are clinically irrelevant.

Lipids

Changes of some lipids in OC users have been reported: cholesterol (-10% to +15%); triglycerides: (-10% to +50%); HDL-cholesterol (-10% to +10%); LDL-cholesterol (-20% to +15%) (Rabe et al. 1988), but no increased atherogenesis has been found in these women; in cynomolgous monkeys, OCs even have a protective effect against coronary atherosclerosis (Kaplan et al. 1995).

Carbohydrates

A slight hyperglycaemia and mild hyperinsulinaemia (without and after oral glucose loading) can be found in OC users; effects are so minimal, that they are believed to be without clinical relevance (Gaspard & Lefebvre 1990; Bowes et al. 1989; van der Vange et al. 1987; Skouby 1988).

Blood Coagulation

OCs affect factors of blood coagulation and fibrinolysis in the same way, so that the blood clotting process remains balanced (Bonnar 1988; Notelovitz 1993). OC effects in patients with antithrombin III-, protein C-, protein S-deficiency and/or APC resistance will be discussed in Sect. 1.4.

No Co-Carcinogenesis

Epidemiological studies with OCs containing 50 μg or more EE showed a marked reduction of endometrial and ovarian cancer, with a persisting protective effect even after withdrawal of OCs. A slight increase in cervical neoplasia needs further clarification. OC steroids promote but do not induce breast cancer.

Breast Cancer

- No increase in incidence after introduction of OCs into market
- Total incidence in women below age 59 years is not increased
- Slight increase in young women (<20 years of age) RR 1,22 (± 0.044); current users (all age groups): RR 1,24 (± 0.038)(Collaborative Group on Hormonal Factors in Breast Cancer 1996)
- No significant excess of having breast cancer diagnosed 10 or more years after stopping use (RR 1.01; 0.96-1.05)(Collaborative Group on Hormonal Factors in Breast Cancer 1996)
- No higher breast cancer risk in OC users with and without family history of breast cancer (Collaborative Group on Hormonal Factors in Breast Cancer 1996)
- The cancers diagnosed in women who had used combined OC were less advanced clinically than those in never users (Collaborative Group on Hormonal Factors in Breast Cancer 1996)
- OCs are not initiators; may be promoters of breast cancer
- Bias through more intensive clinical breast screening in OC users; OC selection for contraception is influenced by lifestyle; until now tumour histology and spread has not been considered; long time interval (15-30 years) between steroid exposure and tumour diagnosis.

Endometrial Carcinoma

- Decreased risk depending on duration of use: after 1, 2, 4, 8 and 12 years, the risk is decreased by 23%, 38%, 51%, 64% and 70%, respectively (Centers of Disease Control 1983b, 1987b)
- Beginning of protective effect (studies incoherent): 0-10 years after first OC use (Centers of Disease Control 1983b, 1987b)
- Duration of protective effect 15 years and more, if OC have been used for at least 5 years: RR 0.3 (0.2-0.6) (Centers of Disease Control 1983b, 1987b; review by Vessey 1991b; Rabe & Runnebaum 1996).

Ovarian Carcinoma

- OCs protect against malignant and borderline tumours of the ovaries
- Higher doses of combined OCs decrease risk: 13/15 case-control studies showed a

decrease in risk; e.g. RR 0.3 (0.1-0.7) and 0.6 (0.3-1.4) in two UK studies in relation to duration of use; RR 0.2 (0.1-0.4) (Cash Study) in users of more than 10 years. Protective effects start with delay of several years after first OC-use. No differences between various formulations (Centers of Disease Control 1983a, 1987a; review by Vessey 1991b; Rabe & Runnebaum 1996)
- For low dose OCs, no epidemiological data are available; inhibition of follicular maturation (oestrogen synthesis) and ovulation could be shown for formulations containing 20 μg EE in combination with desogestrel (Rabe et al. 1997), gestodene (Fitzgerald et al. 1994) or levonorgestrel (Spona et al. 1996)
- Protective effect depends on inhibition of ovulation due to progestin dominance (Fathalla 1971; Casagrande et al. 1979)
- OCs are the only pharmaceutical drug with a protective effect in view to ovarian cancer.

Cervical Cancer

- Slight increase in intraepithelial neoplasia and invasive cervical carcinoma in OC users (studies are biased because sperm exposure in controls is inhibited by use of diaphragm); Cu ions may influence cell growth at the cervical os (note: Cu IUDs are protective against endometrial cancer)
- In 51 studies (21 case control-studies, 18 comparative- and 12 cohort studies): RR 1.5 (1.3-1.8) for cervical dysplasia and carcinoma in situ, RR 1.2 (1.1-1.4) for invasive cervical cancer (review by Rabe & Runnebaum 1991).

No Health Risks

Cardiovascular Risks

Epidemiology

Cardiovascular disease, such as myocardial infarction, stroke, deep venous thrombosis (DVT) and pulmonary embolism, have been related to OC use since the first studies in the UK published by Jordan (1961) and Inman & Vessey (1968), who showed a correlation between OC use and pulmonary embolism. Originally, cardiovascular morbidity and mortality has been attributed to the venous part of the vascular system (thrombosis) and related to the dosage of ethinylestradiol – leading to a decrease of EE in OCs from 150 μg to 50 μg per tablet in the 1970s. Later on, the study of the Royal College of General Practitioners (1974) showed a relationship between progestin dosage and hypertension, and it has been assumed that progestins mainly influence the arterial part of the cardiovascular system. Recently, cardiovascular risk has been related to changes in the lipid metabolism, the carbohydrate metabolism and blood coagulation.

Most recently seven national and international studies have looked at the cardiovascular risk of modern OCs. Initial studies (12/95-1/96): WHO Collaborative Study (WHO 1995; WHO 1996a, b), (Boston Collaborative Drug Surveillance Program (Jick et al. 1995; Jick et al. 1996); Leiden Thrombophilia Study (Bloemenkamp et al. 1995), Transnational study (Spitzer et al. 1996, Lewis et al. 1996a, b). Later studies (6/96-6/97): Danish case control study (Lidegaard et al. 1997a; Lidegaard & Kreiner 1997b), Pharma database (Herings et al. 1996), Mediplus UK (Farmer et al. 1997), MediPlus Germany (Farmer et al. unpublished observations); re-analysis Transnational study (Sulssa et al. 1997).

The potential cardiovascular risk in OC users based on results of these studies led to extensive confusion, both on the part of doctors and patients. The relevance of these epidemiological studies has been discussed intensively with respect to bias (systematic failure) and confounding factors (interfering factors, risk factors):

- Evaluation of epidemiological studies should be performed according to the criteria of Bradford-Hill (1965)
- The progestin classification into three groups is not based on pharmacological criteria (except 1. generation), but on availability of the products on the market – therefore, epidemiological data must be linked to individual progestins and not to a heterogenous group of third generation of progestins
- All information on OC and VTE (venous thromboembolism) is based on case-control studies, in which controls must be selected according to known risk factors for the disease analysed. Data from case-control studies are valid until new risk factors are found which have not been considered for selecting appropriate controls. This is the reason why the case-control studies of OCs and VTE are biased. In cases with VTE, a genetic predisposition of up to 60% for thrombosis has been found, whereas in controls VTE risk of the average population can be assumed (e.g. APC resistance 5%)
- Another bias is the "healthy user"-effect; pre-selection bias and as confounding factors (Lewis et al. 1996; Spitzer 1997)

In the last statement of the CPMP (London) (22.1.1997), it has been mentioned that in seven published studies concerning the risk of venous thromboembolism, the differences between progestin of the so-called second (levonorgestrel) and the so-called third generation (e.g. gestoden, desogestrel) could not be finally evaluated due to bias and confounding factors. VTE seems a rare event (1 per 10,000 women per year). Until now, no clear therapeutic guideline has been issued by the CPMP; this should be done by the individual countries themselves. The suggestion was made that additional information on beneficial effects and thromboembolic risks should be provided.

The relevance of the seven epidemiological studies was called into doubt recently by a court in Berlin/Germany, which led to the cancellation of prescribing restrictions for desogestrel and gestodene containing oral contraceptives (Pressemeldung des Verwaltungsgerichts, Berlin).

Risk Factors

Reversible risk factors are hypertension, hypercholesterinaemia, hyperglyceridaemia, smoking, hyperglycaemia, hyperhomocystemia, obesity; increased cardiovascular risk by chlamydia pneumoniae infection may be important as an additional risk factor. Irreversible risk factors are: sex, age, genetic risk factors, thrombocyto- and coagulopathy.

Risk factors act in a synergistic manner; the risk increases exponentially. APC resistance: missing inhibition of the conversion of factor Va to Xa leads to increased thrombogenesis. In 97% of cases with a genetic defect (substitution of the aminoacid arginine in position 506 by glutamine), factor Va (=factor Va-Leiden) is the underlying condition (see Witt & Kraus, 1996). The incidence in Europe is about 4.4% with regional differences (Greece 7%, Germany 4%) and in Asia 0.6%. It is not found at all in USA, Australia and Africa (Rees et al. 1995). Thromboembolic risk: in patients with a heterozygous defect without OC use RR = 3-8 (Ridker et al. 1995; Rosendaal et al. 1995; Vandenbroucke et al. 1994), in OC users RR = 30; in patients with homozygous defect without OC use RR = 80-100 (Ridker et al. 1995; Rosendaal et al. 1995; Vandenbroucke et al. 1994); with OC use RR >200 (Bertina 1994).

It is possible that the relative risk has been overestimated; new studies from Germany will be published soon (note: life expectancy in patients with APC resistance is not influenced) (Hille et al. 1997). General screening has not been recommended in Germany; what is important is the family history (see below); only 1 of 1000 women with APC resistance develops a thrombosis (Kierkegaard 1980; Nylander & Olivecrona 1976).

In women with thrombosis the incidence of APC resistance ranges between 21% (deep venous thrombosis) and 50%-60% (familial venous thrombosis) (Griffin et al. 1993); the incidence of thrombosis in pregnancy is up to 60% and in the control population 5-7%. Note: therefore, all case control studies in which controls have been selected without considering the genetic risk are biased because the most important risk factor, a familial thrombophilia due to genetic predisposition, has not been considered.

Antithrombin-III deficiency: in patients with antithrombin-III deficiency thrombosis occurs during the first 2 years of OC use (Pabinger-Fasching & Schneider 1994); it is important to know whether the patient has an antithrombin-III deficiency in view to operations, because this factor can be substituted.

Protein C and S deficiency: clinical importance may be limited – additional information is necessary.

Cardiovascular Risk and OC Use

Cardiovascular Risks

Moderate	1/10 000	woman-years
Severe	1/100 000	woman-years (Vessey 1991a,b)
Fatal	1-3/1 000 000	woman-years (Lidegaard 1997, personal communication)

A reevaluation of data from the transnational study confirmed the interim analysis (Sulssa et al. 1997). The relative risk of severe cardiovascular complications (40% death) in OC users is independent of the progestin generation and about 2.0 compared with non users. It is such a rare event (0.5 cases per 10,000 women) that for young healthy women without cardiovascular risk factors (especially smoking) it has no clinical impact.

Risk factors for cardiovascular diseases include smoking (arterial myocardial infarction, stroke), obesity (all), hypertension (arterial myocardial infarction, stroke), LDL-cholesterol (arterial myocardial infarction.

OC dosage and cardiovascular risk:

- RCGP and Swedish reports indicate that women using 50 μg EE pills have a higher incidence of venous thrombosis than those using lower dose pills (Meade et al. 1980; Bottinger et al. 1980).

- Recently Medicaid data from the state of Michigan, USA, confirmed the fact that the risk of venous thrombosis is increased by the 50 µg EE dose (Gerstman et al. 1991).
- The cardiovascular risk of former users is not increased (Stampfer et al. 1990; Rosenberg et al. 1990; Croft & Hannaford 1989).

Venous thrombosis: diagnosis and therapy of a deep venous thrombosis are influenced by:
- Age (incidence increased; decrease of antiplasmin 2a)
- Wrong diagnosis in 70% of cases
- Wrong treatment in 50% of cases

  but if the disease and the sequelae can by detected and treated in time, only in 1 of 100 patients with thrombosis does pulmonary embolism occur with a mortality of 1 per 100 cases.

Pathogenesis and risk factors:
- Endogenous risk factors: genetic risk factors are APC resistance, antithrombin III-, protein C- and S-deficiency
- Exogenous risk factors: immobilisation, smoking, OC.

OC use and venous thrombosis:
- The total risk of VTE is about 1 per 10,000 women per year; in users of modern oral contraceptives, it is 3-4/10,000 and 6/10,000 in pregnancy
- OC use leads to a fourfold risk of deep venous thrombosis and a 2 times higher risk of superficial thrombosis
- The risk of venous thromboembolism (VTE) in relation to OC declined since the 1970s
- Dose-related to oestrogens
- Limited to current users only.

Myocardial infarction:
- Risk in OC-users: 0.5 per 10,000 women per year
- Risk is increased synergistically by OC use and other risk factors (hypertension, hypercholesterinemia, cigarette smoking, obesity and diabetes mellitus) in women over age 35 years
- OC use does not lead to atherogenesis (proven by coronar angiography in women with myocardial infarction).

Stroke:
- Risk in OC-users: 1 per 10.000 women per year
- Thrombotic stroke is increased threefold by OC use by and hemorrhagic stroke twofold (depending on older studies)
- Modern oral contraceptives lead to a slightly increased risk of stroke (compared with non users) and also of thromboembolic stroke (threefold increased risk), but this event is quite rare in women below age 45 years (less than 1 case per 10,000 women per year).

Summary

For healthy young women without cardiovascular risk factors especially with controlled or normal blood pressure, the cardiovascular risk induced by OCs can be neglected. Additional risk factors, such as cigarette smoking, obesity and immobilisation should be avoided; before an operation it is important to inform the treating physican about a potential risk of thrombosis, including a positive family history (thromboembolism, deep venous and pelvic thrombosis, myocardial infarction of the mother, cerebrovascular insults of the parents below age 45 years or of brothers and sisters). In patients with a positive family history, specific screening tests, e.g. APC resistance, antithrombin III-, protein C-, protein S-deficiency can be performed; informed consent and heparinisation are required in surgical cases. Cardiovascular complications in the patient are a contraindication for OC-use. In patients with a family history of diabetes mellitus, diabetes screening is recommended – with familial lipid disorders cholesterol and trigylcerides (HDL-cholesterol, LDL-cholesterol) should be measured in view of dietary restrictions and health recommendations, e.g. exercise, body weight, smoking)

Non-contraceptive Benefits (see review Vessey 1991a)

Good control of menstrual cycle: incidence of breakthrough bleeding and spotting during initial use (first 3 months) of OCs is increased with decreasing dosage of ethinylestradiol (EE) in combined OCs (50 μg EE: 5-10%; 30 μg EE: 10-15%; 20 μg EE: 20-30%). OCs with the same content of EE show comparable effects on menstrual cycle, e.g. amenorrhoea; breakthrough bleeding, spotting.

No weight gain: for low dose OCs, weight changes within ±1-2 kg are possible. No metabolic impact can explain weight changes; psychological factors and steroidal effects modulate appetite.

No skin reactions: OCs based on norethisterone and its metabolites may cause slight skin impurities, such as acne and seborrhoea, even though EE induces hepatic SHBG synthesis and decrease of free testosterone. OCs containing antiandrogens, e.g. cyproterone acetate, chlormadinone acetate and dienogest, show, depending on the antiandrogenic efficacy, a pronounced beneficial effect in patients with hyperandrogenism (acne, hirsutism, seborrhoea); in patients with mild and moderate acne vulgaris also norgestimate/ethinylestradiol (Redmond et al. 1997) and in cases with mild acne vulgaris all low dose oral hormonal contraceptives can be used: positive metabolic impact.

Protection against pelvic inflammatory disease (PID): PID risk decreases by 50%-60% in current OC users after at least 12 months of use (Eschenbach et al. 1977; Panser & Phipps 1991). But this protection is limited to goenococcal disease, whereas chlamydial infection may even be enhanced. Fifteen of 17 studies published since 1985 report a positive association of OCs with lower genital tract chlamydial cervicitis (Cates et al. 1985; Speroff & Darney 1992); nevertheless, the combined use of OCs and condoms or safer-sex techniques are recommended in relationships with unknown risk of transmission of sexually transmitted diseases (for example, 28% of OC-users in the US use condoms at the same time; only 8% in Germany).

Protection against cancer: see earlier section

Protection against cardiovascular diseases: older OCs with high-dose oestrogens have been associated with an increase in blood pressure in 1-2% or all OC users (Crane et al. 1971; Fisch & Frank 1977; Weir et al. 1970, 1971; Weir 1982). Newer low-dose OC formulations have no clinical relevant impact on blood pressure

The anti-mineralocorticoid action of progesterone is appreciated for hormonal replacement in the premenopausal age; new progestins with a pronounced anti-mineralocorticoid effect would be valuable in view to prevent hypertension and additionally offering a cardiovascular protection. New oestrogens with inhibitory effects on vascular nitrogen monoxide formation/action must be analysed (Brosnihan et al. 1994).

Costs

Standard formulations must be available at reasonable prices worldwide; cheap re-imports from countries with low prices to high priced industrialised countries are threatening research and innovation, which must be based on profit with new products.

If new products offer significantly higher health benefits than older products, it is unethical to inhibit availability to bar worldwide by a high price policy in poor countries! Due to fixed prices in specific trade unions (e.g. Europe) a price refound system for the contraceptive users might be one solution.

Users' Attitude

The users' attitude will be the key to successful continuation – because the client must be convinced about the method. Information can come from doctors, nurses, friends, books, newspapers and TV. The attitude should not be influenced by tabloid press, e.g. publication of unauthorised papers presented in internal discussions before official public release.

Acceptability of oral hormonal contraception by users will be based on possible effects of OCs on carcinogenesis, especially breast cancer: 1/7-1/10 of all women are affected during lifetime and not on cardiovascular risks:

Moderate	1/10,000 woman-years
Severe	1/100,000 woman-years
Fatal	1-3/1,000,000 woman-years

Scientific information should be filtered by adhoc commitees of public health authorities, e.g. in Germany, "Special Study Group of Gynecological Endocrinology and Reproductive Medicine" (AGGEF) of the German Society of Gynecology and Obstetrics

(DGGG), "Study Group for Hormone Toxicology" of the German Society of Endocrinology. Disagreements within the scientific community should be settled "behind closed doors" and not in the media (TV, newspapers etc.).

New Developments

Ideal Contraceptive

Contraceptives with clear advantages over OCs must fulfil the criteria for an ideal contraceptive:
100% reversible
100% effective
100% easy to practice
0% side effects
100% protection against sexually transmitted diseases
Great additional benefit: good availability and easy handling.
These methods are targeting ovulation, fertilisation and implantation in the female reproductive process.

Oral Hormonal Contraceptives

- New (non-steroidal) oestrogens will selectively block folliculogenesis and/or ovulation.
- New regimen (combination with e.g. antiprogestins) will provide a better control of menstrual cycle at lower steroid dosages of OCs.
- Use of antigestagens will improve contraceptive efficacy and control of withdrawal bleedings and new progestins offer a better choice for women with specific health problems:
  - Drospirenon: a progestin with anti-mineralocorticoidal and antiandrogenic characteristics. Only little impact on body weight and blood pressure; positive oestrogenic side effects due to partial anti-mineralocorticoidal action, which antagonizes the effect of water retention by oestrogens. Combination with ethinylestradiol in oral contraceptives intended. Possible indication: premenstrual syndrome. Phases I and II completed. Phase III will be finished in 1997, permission probably in 1999-2000.
  - Better characterisation of risk groups (e.g. thrombophilia; breast cancer)
  - Better follow-up procedures for at-risk patients using OCs
  - Better understanding of prophylactic effects of OCs (e.g. endometriosis, polycystic ovary syndrome, uterine myoma)
  - Better consumer information about risks and benefits

Other Contraceptive Methods

Targets for Uterine Contraception

New developments of methods blocking fertilisation depend on the two targets:

1. Cervical os:
   - Intracervical devices (large variety developed; progestin loaded devices may be suitable)
   - Intrauterine devices: progestins released by intrauterine devices also act at the level of cervical mucus (e.g. levonorgestrel (IUS)
   - Hormone-loaded vaginal ring: progestins (mode of action like progestin-only pill (POP); poor bleeding pattern), oestrogen/progestins (inhibition of ovulation, good bleeding control, but systemically active) – may be a choice in selected subgroups
2. Endometrium:
   - Intrauterine system (IUSs): inert OC, medicated IUSs: copper, progestins; most promising are progestin (e.g. levonorgestrel; not progesterone!) loaded IUSs

LNG-IUS (Levonorgestrel intrauterine system)

Contraceptive efficacy depends on the local progestin release in utero up to 5 years:
- Thickening of the cervical mucus
- Biochemical changes of the utero-tubal fluid
- Suppression of formation of the endometrium
- Weak foreign body reaction of the endometrium
- In 5-15% anovulatory cycles without inhibition of endogenous oestrogen production
- High contraceptive efficacy compared with copper IUDs (Pearl index = 0.1)

Beneficial effects:
- Local antioestrogenic and antimitotic effects of LNG:
- Shorter duration of menstruation; lower menstrual blood loss and amenorrhoea in 20% of all users (after six cycles)
- Decrease of dysmenorrhoea
- Increase of haemoglobulin and serum iron
- Lower risk of ectopic pregnancies compared with copper- and progesterone loaded IUDs and also with women without contraceptives
- Lower PID risk
- Full reversibility:
  - Conception without delay
  - 96% conception rate within 12 months after removal
  - Normal course of pregnancy.

LNG-IUDs: future developments. Further indications for endometrial protection:
- Peri- and postmenopausal phase II-III women
- Breast cancer patients phase II taking tamoxifen
- Further improvement of the device and inserter:
  - New inserter 1998
  - Small Mirena (german brand name) (IUS) phase III
  - Dosage finding studies phase I-II

Steroid Hormones (orally)

Progestins (POP available since 1993); high rate of intermenstrual bleedings (40%); daily administration within 3 h), antiprogestins (good efficacy but high potential for misuse in view of induction of abortion)

Steroid Hormones (parenterally)

Steroid hormones can be administered by injection of slow-release formulations (e.g. depot medroxyprogesterone acetate, norethisterone enanthate, estradiol valerate, estradiol cypionate) in 3-, 2- or 1-month intervals (once-a-month injectables) or in terms of biodegradable or non-biodegradable implantables releasing various progestins (e.g. levonorgestrel, 3-ketodesogestrel, norethisterone).

Once-A-Month Injectables

Method: Monthly injection of oestrogen/progestin-combinations.
Products:
- Mesigyna: 50 mg norethisterone enanthate + 5 mg estradiol valerate
- Cyclofem: 25 mg depot medroxyprogesterone acetate + 5 mg estradiol cypionates.

Advantage: better cycle control: relative low rates of intermenstrual bleedings. Disadvantage: injections every 4 weeks required.

Subdermal Progestin Implantables

Principle: release of progestins for several years exerts a progestational effect on the cervical mucus and endometrium, comparable to the POP. Products: Norplant system: six capsules (34x2.4 mm) containing 36 mg levonorgestrel (5 years efficacy); Implanon: one capsule containg 3-ketodesogestrel (1 year efficacy).

Advantage: long-term contraception (up to 5 years).
Disadvantages:
- not available in Germany
- irregular menstrual bleedings in up to 2/3 of Norplant users during initial phase; in 1/3 of users premature removal due to bleeding disturbances
- 1/3 will benefit from amenorrhoea; a minor surgical procedure is needed for removal
- local complaints possible, in the region where the implantable has been placed.

Trends:
- Usage of different progestins
- Biodegradable carrier substances
- Number of implantables will be decreased
- Easy to handle inserter

Gene Therapy

Experimental transient infection with genes regulating endometrial susceptibility to implantation.

Quality Control

Quality management in medicine (evidence-based medicine) is accepted worldwide. Prospective randomised double-blind cohort studies are necessary for "evidence-based medicine". Results of case-control studies are largely influenced by selection criteria used for controls and invalid if new risk factors for the specific disease investigated are determined. Evaluation of epidemiological studies according to the criteria of Bradford-Hill (1965).

In a meta-analysis, the mean or median relative risk given together with the standard deviation may be misleading because no information is provided by this type of analysis about the significance (95% confidential range) of the original study!

The correct use of statistical tests in scientific studies submitted for publication must be proved as part of the peer review procedure by experts in this field.

All clinical trials performed for drug licensing by health authorities must fullfil criteria of good clinical practice, including performance of the study, documentation and availability of the database for audits or reanalysis. In studies independent of drug licensing, each investigator can publish data in an uncontrolled way, or controlled by peer review committees, but access to the original database may not be allowed by the investigator. Therefore, quality control for non-pharmaceutical clinical trials is necessary.

Quality control should include epidemiology:

Epidemiological studies with impact on public health should be evaluated by two independent epidemiologists.

No scientific paper should be published without written consent of the author to open his database to health authorities and other scientists on request.

Final Conclusions

OCs are one of the safest, most reliable and globally accepted methods of female contraception. Additional benefits include protection against ovarian and endometrial cancer, pelvic inflammatory disease, dysmenorrhoea and regulation of the menstrual cycle. No overall increase in breast cancers has been demonstrated, although the incidence in young women before the first full-term pregnancy is slightly higher. This must be proven for all new OC formulations by large scale epidemiological trials. Cardiovascular risk is considerably low (1/100 000 events per woman-year) and linked to a large extent to genetic risk factors, such as antithrombin III-, protein-C-, protein S-deficiency, APC resistance, factor-V-leiden disease, and classical risk factors such as hypertension, diabetes mellitus, cigarette smoking, hyperlipidaemia and immobilisation. New screening programs should exclude women belonging to specific risk groups, e.g. women at risk of cardiovascular diseases and breast cancer. New progestins will provide additional health benefits (e.g. lowering blood pressure); research in contraceptive oestrogens must be intensified. Combining antiprogestins with conventional OCs might improve bleeding control at low steroidal levels.

The worldwide acceptance of these methods should not be undermined by unproven reports on health hazards published by tabloid papers. Quality control of epidemiology is necessary as a part of quality management in medicine in general (evidence-based medicine). All investigators publishing medical data with an impact on public health should agree to provide underlying data of their studies to health authorities upon request. This self-control is important to strengthen the confidence in the contraceptive methods available (used by healthy women) and to avoid uncontrolled fear of undesired but not clinically established side effects. Emotionally caused withdrawal of OCs due to fear of breast cancer or cardiovascular disease led to thousands of unintended pregnancies in the last year.

Within the next 5-10 years, oral hormonal contraceptives will be the number one option for fertility control in women. New methods such as progestin-releasing IUDs, once-a-month injectables, implantables and new techniques for female and male sterilisation will gain importance for specific subgroups of patients. To avoid infection by sexually transmitted diseases in uncertain relationships, safer-sex techniques should be used including the use of condoms (and spermicides).

Worldwide availability of safe contraceptive methods is necessary for the control of population growth. US $3 are needed for each couple per year and it is a challenge for all of us to motivate government agencies to provide this amount of money - in the interest of peace: "If we radiate godness, we will receive godness in return" Chinese proverb.

References

Bertina RM, Koeleman BPC, Koster T, Rosendaal FR, Dirven RJ, de Ronde H, van der Velden PA, Reitsma PH (1994) Mutation in blood coagulation factor V associated with resistance to activated Protein C. Nature 369:64-67

Bloemenkamp KWM, Rosendaal FR, Helmerhorst FM, Büller HR, Vandenbrouke JP (1995) Enhancement by factor V Leiden mutation of risk of deep vein thrombosis associated with oral contraceptives containing a third generation progestagen. Lancet 346:1593-96

Bonnar J, Daly L, Sabra A, Carroll A (1988) Effects of oral contraception on blood clotting. In: Runnebaum B, Rabe T, Kiesel L (eds) Female contraception, update and trends. Springer-Verlag, Berlin Heidelberg New York, pp 56-59

Bottinger LE, Boman G, Eklund G, Westerholm B (1980) Oral contraceptives and thromboembolic disease. Effects of lowering oestrogen content. Lancet i:1097

Bowes WA, Katta LR, Droegemueller W, Braight TG (1989) Triphasic randomized clinical trial. Comparison of effects on carbohydrate metabolism. Am J Obstet Gynecol 161:1402

Bradford-Hill (1965) Criteria of causality. Proceedings of the Royal Society of Medicine 58:295-300

Brosnihan KB, Moribuchi A, Nakamoto H, Dean RH, Ganten D, Ferrario CM (1994) Estrogen augments the contribution of nitric oxide to blood pressure regulation in transgenic hypertensive rats expressing the mouse Ren-2 gene. Am J Epidemiol 7:576-582

Casagrande JT, Pike MC, Ross RK, Louie EW, Roy S, Henderson BE (1979) Incessant ovulation and ovarian cancer. Lancet ii:170-173

Cates W Jr, Washington AE, Rubin GL, Peterson HB (1985) The pill, chlamydia and PID. Fam Plann Perspect 17:175

Centers for Disease Control (1983a) Oral contraceptive use and the risk of ovarian cancer. JAMA 249:1596-1599

Centers for Disease Control (1983a) The reduction in risk of ovarian cancer associated with oral contraceptive use. N Engl J Med 1987a 316:650-655
Centers for Disease Control (1987a) The reduction in risk of ovarian cancer associated with oral contraceptive use. N Engl J Med 1987a 316:650-655
Centers for Disease Control (1987b) Combination oral contraceptive use and the risk of endometrial cancer. Dominant social status and contraceptive hormone treatment inhibit atherogenesis in premenopausal monkeys. Arterioscler. Thromb. Vasc. Biol 15:2094-2100
Collaborative Group on Hormonal Factors in Breast Cancer (1996) Breast cancer and hormonal contraceptives: collaborative reanalysis of individual data on 53 297 women with breast cancer and 100 239 women without breast cancer from 54 epidemiological studies. Lancet 347:1713-27
Crane MG, Harris JJ, Winsor W (1971) Hypertension, oral contraceptive agents, and conjugated estrogens. Ann Intern Med 74:13
Croft P, Hannaford PC (1989) Risk factors for acute myocardial infarction in women: evidence from the Royal College of General Practitioners' oral contraception study. BMJ 298:165-168
Eschenbach DA, Harnisch JP, Holmes KK (1997) Pathogenesis of acute pelvic inflammatory disease: role of contraception and other risk factors. Am J Obstet Gynecol 128:838
Farmer RDT, Lawrenson RA, Kennedy JG, Hambleton IR (1997) Populations-based study of risk of venous thromboembolism associated with varis oral contraceptives. Lancet 349:83-86
Fathalla MF. Incessant ovulation– a factor in ovarian neoplasia? Lancet 1971; ii:163
Fisch I, Frank J (1977) Oral contracptives and hypertension. JAMA 237:2499-2503
Fitzgerald C, Feichtinger W, Spona J, Elstein M, Lüdicke F, Müller U, Williams C (1994) Comparison of the effects of two monophasic low dose oral contraceptives on the inhibition of ovulation. Adv Contracept 10:5-18
Gaspard UJ, Lefebvre PJ (1990) Clinical aspects of the relationship between oral contraceptives, abnormalities in carbohydrate metabolism, and the development of cardiovascular disease. Am J Obstet Gynecol 163:334
Gerstman BB, Piper JM, Tomita DK, Ferguson WJ, Stadel BV, Lundin FE (1991) Oral contraceptive estrogen dose and the risk of deep venous thromboembolic disease. Am J Epidemiol 133:32
Griffin JH, Evatt B, Widerman C, Fernandez JA (1993) Anticoagulant protein C pathway defective in majority of thrombophilic patients. Blood 82 1989-1993
Herings RCM, Boer A de, Urquhart J, Leufkens HGM (1996) Non-causal explanations for the increased risk of venous thromboembolism among users of third generation oral contraceptives. Pharmacoepidemiol Drug Safety 5:S 88
Hille ET, Westendrop RG, Vandenbroucke JP, Rosendaal FR (1997) Mortality and causes of death in families with the factor V Leiden mutation (resistance to activated protein C). Blood 89:1963-1967
Inman WHW, Vessey MP (1968) Investigation of deaths form pulmonary, coronary and cerebral thrombosis and embolism in women of child-bearing age. BMJ 2:193-199
Jick H, Jick SS, Gurevich V, Myers MW, Vasilakis C (1995) Risk of idiopathic cardiovascular death and nonfatal venous thromboembolism in women using oral contraceptives with differing progestagen compents. Lancet 348:1589-1593
Jick H, Jick SS, Myers MW, Vasilakis C (1996) Risk of acute myocardial infarction and low-dose combined oral contraceptives. Lancet 347:627-8
Jordan WM (1961) Pulmonary embolism. Lancet 2 II: 1146-1147
Kaplan JR, Adams MR, Anthony MS, Morgan TM, Manuck SB, Clarkson TB (1995) Dominant social status and contraceptive hormone treatment inhibit atherogenesis in premenopausal monkeys. Arterioscler Thromb Vasc Biol 15:2094-2100
Kierkegaard A (1980) Incidence of acute deep vein thrombosis in two districts. Acta Chir. Scand 146:276-9
Lewis MA, Heinemann, LAG, MacRae KD, Bruppacher R, Spitzer WO (1996a) Transnational Research Group on oral contraception and the health of young women. The increased risk of venous thromboembolism and the use of third generation progestagens; role of bias in observational research. Contraception 54:5
Lewis MA, Spitzer WO, Heinemann LA, MacRae KD, Bruppacher R, Thorogood M (1996b) Third generation oral contraceptives and risk of myocardial infarction: an international case-control study. BMJ 312:88-90
Lidegaard O, Edström B, Kreiner S (1997a) Oral contraceptives and venous thrombosis: a case-control study. Eur J Contracept Reprod Health Care 2:73 (abstracts of the XV FIGO World Congress of Gynaecology and Obstetrics. Copenhagen, 3-8 August)

Lidegaard O, Kreiner S (1997b) Cerebral thromboembolism and oral contraceptives: a case-control study. Abstract no 297 in 13th International Conference on Pharmacoepidemiology Orlando. Florida USA. August 1997 (submitted for publication)

Lidegaard, O (1997c) Danish study on cardiovascular mortality. personal communication, OC-Symposium Madrid

Meade TW, Greenburg G, Thompson SG (1980) Progestogens and cardiovascular reactions associated with oral contraceptives and a comparison of the safety of 50- and 30-μg estrogen preparations. BMJ 280:1157

Notelovitz M (1993) Oral contraceptives. Effect on hemostasis. In: Shoupe D, Haseltine FP (eds) Contraception. Springer-Verlag, Berlin Heidelberg New York, pp 42-59

Nylander G, Olivecrona H (1976) The phlebographic pattern of acute leg thrombosis within a defined urban population. Acta Chir Scand 142:505-511

Pabinger-Fasching I, Schneider B (1994) Thrombotic risk of women with hereditary antithrombin III-, protein C- and protein S-deficiency taking oral contraceptive medication. Thromb Haemost 71:548-552

Panser LA, Phipps WR: Rees DC, Cox M, Clegg JB (1995) World distribution of factor V Leiden. Lancet 346:1133-1134

Peterson HB, Xia Hughes JM, Wilcox LS, Tylor LR, Trussell J (1996) The risk of pregnancy after tubal sterilization: findings from the U. S. Collaborative Review of Sterilization. Am J Obstet Gynecol 174:1161-70

Rabe T, Grunwald K, Kiesel L, Runnebaum B (1988) Oral contraceptives and lipid metabolism. In: Runnebaum B, Rabe T, Kiesel L (eds) Female contraception, update and trends, Springer-Verlag, Berlin Heidelberg New York, pp 64-90

Rabe T, Nitsche D, Runnebaum B (1997) The effects of monophasic and triphasic oral contraceptives on ovarian function and endometrial thickness. Eur J Contracept Reproduct Health Care 2:39-51

Rabe T, Runnebaum B (1996) Kontrazeption. In: Runnebaum B., Rabe T (eds) Gynäkologische Endokrinologie und Fortpflanzungsmedizin. Springer, Berlin Heidelberg New York, pp 411-512

Rabe T, Runnebaum B (1982) Kontrazeption. Springer, Berlin Heidelberg New York

Redmond GP, Olson WH, Lippman JS, Kafrissen ME, Jones TM, Jorizzo JL (1997) Norgestimate and ethinyl estradiol in the treatment of acne vulgaris: a randomized, placebo-controlled trial. Obstet Gynecol 89:615-622

Rees DC, Cox M, Clegg JB (1995) World distribution of factor V Leiden. Lancet 346:11330-11340

Ridker PM, Hennekens CH, Lindpaintner K, Stampfer MJ, Eisenberg PR, Miletich JP (1995) Mutation in the gene coding for coagulation factor V and the risk of myocardial infarction, stroke, and venous thrombosis in apparently healthy men. N Engl J Med 332:912-917

Rosenberg L, JRP, Lesko SM, Shapiro S (1990) Oral contraceptive use and the risk of myocardial infarction. Am J Epidemiol 131:1009-1016

Rosendaal FR, Koster T, Vandenbroucke JP, Reitsma PH (1995) High risk of thrombosis in patients homozygous for factor V Leiden (Activated Protein C Resistance. Blood 85:1504-1508

Royal College of General Practitioners (1974) Oral contraception and health; an interim report from the oral contraception study of the Royal College of General Practitioners. Pitnam New York

Runnebaum B, Rabe T, Kiesel L (eds) (1988) Female contraception, update and trends, Springer-Verlag, Berlin Heidelberg New York

Runnebaum B, Rabe T, Kiesel L (eds) (1991) Female contraception and male fertility regulation, vol. 2. Parthenon, New York

Skouby SO (1988) Effects of oral contraceptives on carbohydrate metabolism in healthy women. In: Runnebaum B, Rabe T, Kiesel L (eds) Female contraception, update and trends, Springer-Verlag, Berlin Heidelberg New York, pp 60-63

Speroff L, Darney P (eds) (1992) A clinical guide for contraception, Williams & Wilkens, Baltimore

Spitzer WO, Lewis MA, Heinemann LAJ, Thorogood M, MacRae KD (1996) Third generation oral contraceptives and risk of venous thromboembolic disorder: an international case-control study. BMJ 213:83-8

Spitzer WOS (1997) The 1995 pill scare revisited: anatomy of a non-epidemic. Hum Reprod 12:2347-2357

Spona J, Feichtinger W, Kindermann Ch, Wünsch C, Brill K (1996) Inhibition of ovulation by an oral contraceptive containing 100 μg Levonorgestrel in combination with 20 μg ethinylestradiol. Contraception 54:299-304

Stampfer MJ, Willett WC, Colditz GA, Speizer FE, Hennekens CH (1990) Past use of oral contraceptives and cardiovascular disease: a meta-analysis in the context of the Nurses' Health Study. Am J Obstet Gynecol 163:285-291

Sulssa S, Blair L, Spitzer WO, Cosson J, Lewis M, Heinemann LAJ (1997) First-time use of newer oral contraceptives and the risk of venous thromboembolism. Contraception 56:141-6

The European Agency for the evaluation of medicinal products. Human Medicines Evaluation Unit (1997) Position statement of the CPMP on oral contraceptives containing desogestrel or gestodene. Press Release: Annex III to CPMP - Jan. 97◊

Trussell J, Hatcher RA, Cates W Jr, Stewart FH, Kost K (1990) Contraceptive failure in the United States: an update, Stud Fam Plann 21:51

van der Vange N, Kloosterboer HJ, Haspels AA (1987) Effects of seven low-dose combined oral contraceptive preparations on carbohydrate metabolism. Am J Obstet Gynecol 156:918

Vandenbroucke JP, Koster T, Briet E, Reitsma PH, Bertina RM, Rosendaal FR (1994) Increased risk of venous thrombosis in oral-contraceptive users who carriers of factor V Leiden mutation. Lancet 344:1453-1457

Verwaltungsgericht: Der Präsident des Verwaltungsgerichts Berlin: Pressemitteilung. Grünes Licht für die Pille der dritten Generation. Beschlüsse der 14. Kammer des Verwaltungsgerichts Berlin (VG 14 A 360.97, VG 14 A 361.97, VG 14 A 379.97), 19.12.1997

Vessey (1991a) An overview of the benefits and risks of combined oral contraceptives In: Runnebaum B., Rabe T, Kiesel L (eds) Female contraception and male fertility regulation, Parthenon, Lancester, England, pp 63-76

Vessey (1991b) Oral contraceptives and cancer. In: Runnebaum B, Rabe T, Kiesel L (eds.): Female contraception and male fertility regulation, Parthenon, Lancester, England, pp 77-79

Weir R, Briggs E, Mack A, et al. (1971) Blood pressure in women after one year of oral contraception. Lancet; 316:467-470

Weir RJ, Wilson ESB, Cruikshank J, Tree N, Fraser R (1970) Effects on blood pressure of low dose oestrogen and progestagen only oral contraceptives. J Hypertens; 1[Suppl 2]:100

WHO Collaborative Study of Cardiovascular Disease and Steroid Hormone Contraception (1995) Effect of different progestagens in low oestrogen oral contraceptives on venous thromboembolic disease. Lancet 346:1582-1588

WHO Collaborative Study of Cardiovascular Disease and Steroid Hormone Contraception (1996a) Ischaemic stroke and combined oral contraceptives: results of an international, multi-centre, case-control study. Lancet; 348(ii):498-405P

WHO Collaborative Study of Cardiovascular Disease and Steroid Hormone Contraception (1996b) Haemorrhagic stroke, overall stroke risk, and combined oral contraceptives: results of an international, multi-centre, case-control study. Lancet; 348(ii):505-510P

Wilcox AJ, Weinberg CR, Baird DD (1995) Timing of intercourse in relation to ovulation. Effects on the probability of conception, survival of pregnancy, and sex of the baby. N Engl J Med 333:1517-1521

Witt I, Kraus M (1996) APC-Resistenz: Klinik, Pathophysiologie und Diagnostik. Hämostaseologie 16:60-75

5 Cardiovascular Risks Associated with Oral Contraceptives

Lothar A.J. Heinemann, Edeltraut Garbe

Introduction

Methods of steroid hormone contraception have been available since the 1960s and are now thought to be used by more than 100 million women worldwide [1]. The overwhelming majority of women use steroid hormone contraceptives in their oral application. One can estimate that, currently, 93 million women are users of combined oral contraceptives (OCs).

Diszfalucy, a pioneer of "reproductive health", has coined the term "contraceptive revolution" in this context [2]. Indeed, steroid hormone contraceptives have improved family planning and by that reproductive health of women worldwide and considerably. One should remember the important public health impact of contraceptive use regarding common diseases and mortality particularly in developing countries. The World Health Organisation (WHO) estimates say that many of the following listed events could be prevented by use of steroid hormone contraceptives: maternal deaths (585,000 per year), cases of severe maternal morbidity (20 million per year), perinatal deaths (7.6 million per year), unsafe abortion (20 million per year), couples with unmet family planning needs (120 million per year) and so on [3].

The first indications that OCs might be associated with an increased risk of cardiovascular diseases were published in the early 1960s. In 1961, a case of pulmonary embolism in a woman being treated for endometriosis was published [4], followed by several other case reports. In 1962, a report appeared describing the occurrence of a brain lesion in a woman being treated for dysmenorrhea with OCs [5]. A possible relationship between OC use and these events was first interpreted with great caution, because the events occurred a rather long time after the start of OC treatment, and the number of pill users had increased dramatically during this period of time [6]. In the following years, numerous epidemiological case-control studies appeared and showed that such an association obviously really exists.

Since the introduction of OCs, there have been many changes in the composition of steroid hormone contraceptives, but also regarding the utilisation pattern for these preparations. For instance, the content of oestrogens in these preparations was very much reduced. Multiphasic preparations were developed, and several new progestagens introduced. OC users became younger and due to the results of epidemiological studies more carefully medically selected and monitored than in the past (for instance regarding the exclusion of women with important cardiovascular risk factors) [1]. These changes may also have impact on the OC-associated cardiovascular risks reported in earlier studies.

Information is now available from several large and only recently completed studies in which the cardiovascular risks have been evaluated for newer OC preparations.

A recently performed expert meeting by the WHO came to the conclusion that the relative risk estimates for cardiovascular diseases reported from the recent studies should not be used in isolation to guide counselling for family planning, but more in the balance of risks and benefits [1]. The choice of contraceptive method by the individual woman does, however, not only depend on the objectively measurable benefits and risks, but also on the subjectively perceived risks and benefits associated with different methods of contraception. Moreover, social, economic, psychological and socio-cultural considerations may also contribute to the choice of the contraceptive method [1].

Safety and Risk

Several types of measures for risk are used in epidemiology, each of which has a different meaning, thereby contributing to the confusion about the term risk [7, 8]:
- The *absolute risk* is the likelihood for an individual to develop an event in a defined period of time and is equivalent to the incidence of this event.
- The difference in incidence for the exposed and nonexposed group is called *excess risk*.
- The *relative risk* is the ratio of the incidence in the exposed group divided by the incidence in the nonexposed group; the relative risk is estimated by the odds ratio in case-control studies.

The relative risk (odds ratio) is important in considering questions of causation as, for example, the question whether a causal relationship exists between OC use and the risk of venous thromboembolism. If the relative risk is high, it will be more suggestive of causality than a low relative risk, although several other criteria need also to be considered to support the claim of causality [9]. The excess risk, i.e. the difference of the risk in the exposed and nonexposed group is used to answer questions concerning the public health importance of an exposure. It may for instance be used to answer the question what the public health impact of a fourfold increased relative risk might be. If the absolute risk in the nonexposed group is very low, even a fourfold increase in the relative risk for the exposed group will still be absolutely low.

For the individual person, risk is no clear-cut term, but rather a perceived value [7, 8, 10]. Although risk is primarily the probability of an outcome during a certain defined period of time, as mentioned earlier, it is secondarily and *subjectively* first of all the value of this outcome for the person who may experience this risk. For instance, an individual may perceive the drug-related risk of a very rare cancer stronger than the risk of a severe cardiomyopathy, even when the associated risk of severe cardiomyopathy is higher and the prognosis of both events equally poor. The perception of risk involves a personal and social judgement [10].

As a consequence of these considerations, we are faced with two problems: (1) the absolute risk must be measured (usually done with epidemiological methods) and (2) the acceptability of the respective risk must be judged on the individual and social level. Strom correctly pointed out that everything in life is associated with some risk and that certainly no drug is completely safe [10]. This, however, is neither easy to communicate to patients nor to their physicians. An unrealistic expectation persists in the public that drugs should be without any risks at all [10].

On the individual level, patients are confronted with the following questions before taking a drug: Can I accept the possible risks of the prescribed drug? Or do I rather live on with the problems, complaints and symptoms of the disease instead? In this respect, some disease risks create more fear and emotions than others as, for example, AIDS, cancer, and also cardiovascular outcomes [10]. The acceptability of certain risks will be higher in patients who suffer a lot from their disease than in healthy or asymptomatic patients. The latter is of particular importance for the evaluation of the acceptability of cardiovascular risks associated with OC use, since these drugs are mainly used by healthy young women.

Study Designs for the Evaluation of Risks

In practice, there are several types of studies available to describe and analyse a risk [8, 10, 11]: case series (several case reports), descriptive observational studies (monitoring, surveillance or follow-up investigations), analytic observational studies (correlation studies, case-control studies and cohort studies), randomised clinical trials and meta-analyses.

Case reports including reports from spontaneous adverse event reporting systems are useful to raise the suspicion that an adverse event might be associated with a certain drug. This information can only be used for hypothesis generation. Information of this kind is, nevertheless, important, because it generates a signal (warning) at relatively low cost. The evaluation of the suspicion of a drug-related adverse reaction, however, usually requires additional epidemiological studies.

Descriptive observational studies are similarly rather used for hypothesis generation than for hypothesis testing. In studies of this type, the course of a disease in a patient is usually observed in sentinel practices or clinics over a longer period of time (*monitoring or surveillance studies*). The patients are often highly selected which will result in restricted generalisability of the findings. A surveillance study may provide an estimate of the frequency of an event or an outcome; however, there is no control group to compare the frequency of the event with.

Analytical observational studies, such as *correlation studies* (so-called ecological studies), compare two variables at an aggregated level. In these studies, an association between exposure and outcome can be investigated relatively quickly. However, the association resulting from this type of study is quite uncertain, since there are no data available on the individual level which can be compared. Because of the insufficient information on the individual level, which makes adequate control of bias and confounding impossible, this type of study should also only be used for hypothesis generation.

In an *analytical cohort study*, two or more groups of patients (cohorts) that are different with respect to their exposure status are followed over time to look for differences in their outcomes. The incidence of the outcome in the exposed cohort is then compared with the incidence of the outcome in the nonexposed (or differently exposed) cohort. These studies are generally called "prospective" because of the time sequence of 'first exposure' and 'then outcome'; ideally these studies are also prospective in the sense that the data gathering occurs concurrently ("concurrent prospective cohort study"). However, under certain circumstances, a historic cohort study may also be very useful. In such a study, patients are prospectively followed from a historic point in time. This is only possible, if for each patient sufficient information on exposure and confounders has been documented in the past as well as adequate information on the incidence of the outcome of interest during the follow-up period ("historic prospective cohort study").

The cohort approach permits the calculation of incidence rates. Concurrent cohort studies provide the opportunity to measure exposure and confounders relatively accurately with negligible danger of recall bias, which is a problem whenever data are gathered retrospectively. Cohort studies, however, are extremely expensive (as to time and money). This study type can therefore only be applied to evaluate relatively common outcomes (diseases). As a consequence, the prospective cohort approach does not appear to be suitable for investigating rare cardiovascular risks in women of reproductive age unless the cohort data were collected for other reasons (administrative databases of insurance companies, sickness funds or sentinel networks of doctors).

Case-control studies provide a valuable alternative to cohort studies if one cannot afford the high expenses necessary to conduct a cohort study (huge number of persons/ patients needed; many years necessary to complete the study). In case-control studies, one compares a group of diseased persons (the so-called "cases") with another group of nondiseased persons (the so-called "controls") with regard to their antecedent ex posure to one or more risk factors. After ascertainment of cases and controls, all persons will be asked whether they have previously been exposed to the risk factor under study. Cases and controls are ascertained either population-based or in certain medical settings, e.g. in hospitals. The control group should be selected from the same population from which the cases originate. Since this is not always easy to accomplish, valid selection of controls constitutes a major challenge in case-control studies.

Case-control studies are suitable for investigating the association of a specific exposure (risk factor) with a rare outcome. It is possible to examine the association of multiple exposures with one outcome within one study, that is using the same cases and controls. In comparison with cohort studies, case-control studies may be conducted more quickly and are logistically easier to handle. Regarding the time sequence of cause and effect, the conclusions will be drawn in a "retrospective" way. Besides valid control selection, this study design has particular problems with potentially biased exposure and confounder data, since these data are collected retrospectively and "recall bias" may therefore play an important role.

Randomised clinical trials (RCTs) are not of observational but experimental nature in that treatment allocation is under the control of the investigator. Patients will be randomly assigned to the exposure under study (experimental regime) or to a control exposure (control regime, possibly placebo). Random assignment of exposure makes it likely that the study groups are comparable with respect to potentially confounding variables which are unknown or unmeasurable. Blinding of the investigator and the study participants regarding the type of treatment received helps to minimise information bias. Randomised clinical trials are, however, time-consuming and very expensive; they require a high logistical effort and are feasible only for frequent outcomes. As a consequence of the strict inclusion and exclusion criteria, the study design of the RCT is often artificial, leading to results that may not be applicable to medical practice in general. Due to the rarity of serious adverse drug reactions and the high costs associated with the RCT, this study approach is unfortunately hardly ever useful to study questions of drug safety. This is also the case, because unexpected adverse drug reactions may occur only years after the first exposure or may be caused by interaction with other concomitant diseases or treatments which are often excluded from those trials.

Meta-analyses are more and more used to obtain a precise estimate of the effect of a drug, a medical intervention or a risk factor. In a meta-analysis, the results of many, mainly smaller studies, which very often – due to their limited sample size – could not find statistically significant results, are summed up, resulting in one summary estimate for the effect. The calculation of one effect estimate has obvious advantages, but also many problems. One advantage is that the "statistical noise", which is dominating in smaller studies in such a way that it hides potential effects, can be very much reduced by pooling numbers. The obvious disadvantage is that by pooling small risks which may be insignificant for clinical practice or public health these risks will gain statistical significance and lead to an overestimation of their real public health impact. There are many well-known epidemiologists who rather prefer an in-depth discussion of the results of many individual studies from which they can then draw conclusions based on their clinical and epidemiological experience to the result of a mega-meta-analysis which may not always be comprehensible. One should also remember that the method of meta-analysis was primarily developed for pooling the results of smaller randomised clinical trials and not for aggregating the results of observational studies. However, presently the method is increasingly being used also for observational studies.

Absolute Risks of Cardiovascular Diseases in Women of Reproductive Age

Cardiovascular diseases in women of reproductive age are extremely rare. However, if they occur, they have severe and long-lasting consequences: Reduced quality of life, chronic impairment, disability as well as increased mortality may result.

The absolute risk of cardiovascular complications (myocardial infarction, stroke and venous thromboembolism) in women under the age of 45 years ranges between 22 and 50 per 100,000 women-years, whereas the related mortality is in the magnitude of only few cases per 100,000 women-years.

The incidence of venous thromboembolism (VTE) is about 10 cases per 100,000 women-years (ranging from 4-20 in noncurrent user of OCs). The majority of VTE occurs in the context of pregnancy, delivery and operations [7]. The case fatality rate is within about 1%, relatively low (that is about 1 death per 1 million women-years). VTE is less frequent in certain geographic regions (Africa, Eastern Mediterranean, South-East Asia) than in Europe and North America. Disability is an extremely rare sequelae; a few cases will develop a postthrombotic syndrome as chronic condition.

The absolute risk of *thromboembolic stroke* for women of reproductive age is in the same order of magnitude as the risk of VTE: 10-16 cases per 100,000 women-years [12]. However, the case fatality rate is between 10% and 20% and chronic conditions and disability are major problems for survivors.

The absolute risk of *haemorrhagic stroke* (subarachnoidal bleeding and intracerebral bleeding) is less frequent in women under the age of 45 years and ranges approximately between 6-8 cases per 100,000 women-years. The case fatality rate is, however, higher.

Acute myocardial infarction is relatively rare in women of reproductive age: 4-6 cases per 100,000 women-years. However, a case fatality rate of approximately 50% has been reported from Germany (including those women who die before hospital admission) [13, 14]. Survivors may suffer from chronic disability and impairment of their quality of life.

Based on the figures of the absolute risk of the various cardiovascular diseases and their possible health outcomes as, for example, the possibility of chronic conditions, disability or mortality, arterial thromboembolism appears to have a higher public health importance than venous thromboembolism, although the absolute risk of arterial thromboembolism is still fairly low [7, 8].

In order to set these figures in relation to other risks, one can compare them with commonly accepted risks of daily life. One can for example compare one VTE case per 10,000 women-years and one fatal case per 1 million women-years with one fatal accident per 12 200 middle-aged women per year; or with one car accident per 21,000 women per year [15]; or with one fatal accident in the household per 33,000 women per year [16]; or with fatal events in the context of pregnancy and delivery of about one case per 1 million women and year and with maternal mortality of 1 per 10,000 births [15].

OC Use and Cardiovascular Risks

Acute Myocardial Infarction

The relative risk estimates for the occurrence of acute myocardial infarction (AMI) associated with OC use ranged between 0.3 and 15 with a median between 2 and 4 in earlier studies [17]. In about 40% of the case-control studies, the relative risk of AMI was two- to fourfold increased in OC users, and in about 10% of the studies a four- to eightfold increased relative risk was reported. In about 7% of the studies, the relative risk was increased more than eightfold. The respective risk estimates for cohort studies were a relative risk under 2 in 40% of the studies, a relative risk between 2 and 4 in one-third of the studies and a relative risk of more than 4 in about 25% of the studies. Some of the studies also examined the risk of coronary heart disease (CHD). In about two-thirds of the studies, the relative risk of CHD was less than twofold increased in OC users [17].

Table 1 gives an overview about case-control studies and cohort studies that investigated the risk of AMI associated with OC use. In one of the largest studies, the relative risk of AMI was increased 3.5-fold (2.2-5.5) in OC users compared with nonusers [18]. This study also showed a 1.5-fold (0.4-6.0) increase in relative risk for 25- to 39-year-old women with past use of OCs for more than 10 years, whereas the increase in risk in women aged 40-49 years was slightly higher (OR=2.5; 1.5-4.1). Another relatively large study in North Italy showed a relative risk of 1.8 (0.3-11.5) for current OC users, and a relative risk of 1.9 (0.8-4.7) for past users of OCs [19]. The broader confidence intervals for current users of OCs in the Italian study reflect the lower incidence of myocardial infarction in Italy in comparison with most of the other European and North American countries, and also the relatively low prevalence of OC use in Italy. A risk of similar magnitude as in the Italian study was found in a case-control study in

Table 1. Relative Risk (Odds Ratio) of myocardial infarction in current users of oral contraceptives compared with nonusers (Table modified and supplemented after M. Thorogood [6]). CC Case-Control-Study; CO Cohort Study

Author, Year	Study Type	No. of Cases with AMI	Relative Risk (Odds Ratio)
Inman, 1968 [84]	CC	69	2
Vessey, 1969 [85]	CC	17	1
Mann, 1975/76 [86, 87]	CC	72	4.2
Mann, 1975 [88]	CC	47	2.8
Jick, 1978 [89]	CC	26	14
Shapiro, 1979 [90]	CC	234	4
Rosenberg, 1980 [91]	CC	156	1.8
Krueger, 1980 [92]	CC	163	1.2
Slone, 1981 [18]	CC	556	3.5
Ramcharan, 1981 [93]	CO	24	1.1
Adam, 1981 [94]	CC	139	1.4
La Vecchia, 1987 [19]	CC	168	2
Mant, 1987 [95]	CO	25	0.9
Croft, 1989 [96]	CO/CC	158	1.8
Talbott, 1989 [97]	CC	16	3
Rosenberg, 1990 [21]	CC	910	1.1
Thorogood, 1991 [22]	CC [a]	161	1.9
D'Avanzo, 1994 [98]	CC	251	2
Sidney, 1996 [20]	CC	130	1.7
WHO, 1997 [25]	CC [b]	198	5
Lewis, 1997 [13]	CC	182	2.4#
Lidegaard, 1997 [26]	CC	94	1.3*

[a] Study included only fatal cases of myocardial infarction
[b] Only European cases and controls
Risk for second generation OCs only
* All OCs: Own calculations from details of the publication

North-America in the early 1990s [20]. In this study, the relative risk of AMI was 1.65 (0.45-6.06) for current users of low-dose oral contraceptives. There was no increase in risk observed with past use of OCs.

In the 1990s, a number of new studies of OC use and myocardial infarction were published [13, 21-26]: in two of these studies, which were carried out in the United States and the United Kingdom, a crude relative risk estimate of 1.1 was published [21, 22]. After adjustment for cardiovascular risk factors, these risk estimates increased to about 2. These studies also showed that OCs with an oestrogen content of 50 µg or more have a higher risk of AMI than OCs with a lower content of oestrogen. The relative risk of AMI for high-dose oestrogen OCs was increased 4.2-fold (0.5-39.2) in one of the two studies [22]. Both studies found a nonsignificantly increased risk for past users of oral contraceptives. The relative risk of myocardial infarction in OC users compared with nonusers was in most of the newer studies around 2-fold increased, but was higher in the WHO study with a 5-fold increased relative risk. OCs with a higher oestrogen dose (>50 µg) showed in one of the recently published studies [26] a higher relative risk than low-dose preparations (<50 µg), but this was not the case in another study [25].

A number of the most recently published studies also assessed the effect of the type of progestagen on the AMI risk, following the "pill scare" in 1995. In these studies,

Table 2. Relation of the relative risk of myocardial infarction (odds ratio) for users of OCs with newer progestagens (Gestodene, Desogestrel) compared with users of OCs with older progestagens (mostly Levonorgestrel)

	Desogestrel or Gestodene vs. Older (LNG)	No. of Cases/Controls with Desogestrel/Gestodene	Significance
WHO, 1997 [25]	0.97 (0.1;6.9)*	3/5	No
Lewis, 1997 [13]	0.28 (0.1;0.9)	7/49	Yes
Jick, 1996 [24]	0.7 (0.1-8)	2/11	No
Lidegaard, 1997 [26]	0.63 (0.2-2)*	7/18	No

* Own calculations from details of the publication
LNG Levonorgestrel

either a statistically significantly [13]or a nonsignificantly [24-26] decreased risk of preparations with newer progestagens (desogestrel and gestoden) compared with traditional progestagens (particularly levonorgestrel, see Table 2) was found. Therefore, it cannot be ruled out that the use of OCs with newer progestagens is less often complicated by AMI than use of the older preparations, although this needs to be confirmed in further studies. Cautious interpretation of the results of these studies is currently recommended: there were only a few studies with small numbers of cases which investigated OCs with newer progestagens. Only one study published so far showed statistically significant results [13]. Some studies have not yet been published completely and, therefore, the design and results of these studies have not been discussed extensively in the scientific community. Although the possibility of bias and confounding was primarily raised for the studies investigating the VTE risk associated with OC use, bias and confounding may also have played a role in the myocardial infarction studies.

The pathophysiological mechanisms by which the AMI risk could be reduced in users of newer progestagens are currently not clear. There is some evidence that desogestrel (and very likely gestoden as well) have a low affinity to androgen receptors [27] and do not inhibit the oestrogen-related increase in sex-hormone-binding globulin (SHBG) [28]. A lower level of SHBG was reported to be associated with a higher frequency of hypertension and cardiovascular mortality [29]. It is not yet clear if these observations can be used to explain the effect on the AMI risk. Besides, it is known that the modern progestagens positively influence the lipid metabolism due to an increase of HDL cholesterol [30, 31]. This effect may, however, not be relevant for AMI in young women, since hypercholesterolemia and low HDL levels are risk factors for arteriosclerosis, whereas AMI in OC users are in the majority caused by thrombosis in nonarteriosclerotic vessels rather than by arteriosclerotic lesions [32]. In summary, the statement that newer progestagens are associated with a lower AMI risk than traditional progestagens requires further confirmation from epidemiological studies as well as from basic research to search for potential physiological mechanisms.

Table 3 displays estimates of the relative risk of AMI for various classical cardiovascular risk factors using data from the Transnational Study [13]. Women of reproductive age with cardiovascular risk factors such as hypertension, lipid metabolism disturbances, a family history of myocardial infarction, diabetes mellitus and smoking women had a much higher relative risk of myocardial infarction than women without

Table 3. Relative risk (odds ratio) of myocardial infarction in young women in relation to (reported) cardiovascular risk factors. Table from the Transnational Study [13]

Risk characteristics	Exposed Cases	OR (95% CI)
Smoking	146	9.7 (5.6-16.9)
Hypertension	42	3.3 (1.7-6.3)
Disturbance in lipid metabolism	20	4.2 (1.7-10.7)
Body mass index (BMI>30)	42	4.8 (2.1-11.1)
Diabetes	14	2.5 (0.8-8.0)
Family history of AMI	39	3.7 (1.9-7.1)

these risk factors. For some of these classical risk factors, the relative risk of AMI was markedly higher than the risk for OC use. This finding is particularly interesting since an angiographic study has demonstrated that AMI in OC users is only in one third of the cases associated with coronary arteriosclerosis whereas in two thirds of the cases it appears to be due to a thrombosis in a nonarteriosclerotic coronary vessel [32]. The same angiographic study reported that women not currently using OCs who suffered a myocardial infarction had a coronary arteriosclerosis in 75% of the cases.

Two recent studies demonstrated that women who smoke and use the pill have a markedly increased risk of AMI [13, 25]: in pill users who smoked ten or more cigarettes a day, the relative risk of myocardial infarction was 20-80-fold increased compared with women who did neither smoke nor use the pill (Table 4). Compared with women who smoked but did not use the pill, the relative risk of AMI was about 2.5-fold [13] to 8-fold [25] increased in smoking pill users. For systemic hypertension, an interaction with OC use was not as clear: in the WHO study [25], pill users with a history of high blood pressure showed a more than 60-fold increased risk of AMI compared with nonusers without selfreported history of high blood pressure, but this was not found in the Transnational Study [13].

The importance of an interaction of OC use with other cardiovascular risk factors for the risk of AMI was underlined by another observation: one could regard the measurement of blood pressure prior to the first prescription of OCs as a marker for general attention to cardiovascular risk factors before prescribing OCs. In women who did not smoke and underwent blood pressure measurement before the prescription of an OC, OC use did not carry a significantly increased risk of AMI (Table 5) [13, 25].

Table 4. Relative risk (odds ratio) of myocardial infarction in relation to the use of oral contraceptives. Interaction with cardiovascular risk factors. (Reference [=1.0]: Without hypertension or without smoking)

	WHO [25]**	Transnational Study [13]*
Hypertension		
OC Use: No	5.4 (2.4-12.4)	4.4 (1.8-10.8)
OC Use: Yes	68.1 (6.2-751)	0.9 (0.04-24.3)
Smoking >10 Cigarettes		
OC Use: No	11.1 (5.7-21.8)	9.3 (4.6-18.9)
OC Use: Yes	87.0 (29.8-254)	23.6 (7.2-77.7)

* Calculations by LAJ Heinemann based on the method used by WHO [25]
** Data from Europe

Table 5. Relative risk (odds ratio) of myocardial infarction in relation to OC use: influence of the marker "Blood Pressure Check" (reference [=1.0]: nonsmokers without current OC use

	No Blood Pressure Check	Blood Pressure Check
WHO [25]**		
Nonsmokers	16.4 (3.1-87.7) [a]	1.1 (0.1-9.7) [a]
Smokers	71.4 (16.5-309) [a]	26.6 (7.0-101) [a]
Transnational Study [13]*		
Nonsmokers	4.3 (0.4-42.6) [b]	2.4 (0.4-15.6) [b]
Smokers	84.8 (21.7-332) [b]	20.2 (6.1-66.3) [b]

[a] Conditional Analysis
[b] Unconditional Analysis
* Calculations by LAJ Heinemann based on the method used by WHO [25]
** Data from Europe

However, women who smoked and had no blood pressure check prior to pill use had a 20- to 80-fold increased relative risk compared with nonusers. Some of the reported higher relative risk estimates for myocardial infarction in OC users may therefore be due to an interaction of OCs with smoking or with other cardiovascular risk factors.

For healthy nonsmoking young women under the age of 35 years, the absolute risk of AMI is around 0.8 per 1 million women-years, for OC users it is approximately 3.6 per 1 million women-years [25]. The excess risk of 2.7 AMI per 1 million women-years could be further reduced, if cardiovascular risk factors would get more attention prior to the prescription of OCs. The message for women who desire oral contraceptives and for their physicians seems to be clear: there is no appreciably increased risk of myocardial infarction associated with modern OCs in healthy young women. However, cardiovascular risk factors need to be checked prior to prescribing the pill, and monitored thereafter [1, 7].

Stroke

An association between OC use and the occurrence of stroke was first reported in the 1960s and early 1970s in Europe and the USA (Table 6). In cohort- and case-control studies prior to 1985, the median of the relative risk estimates for stroke associated with OC use versus no use ranged between two and four [17]. Approximately one-fourth of the cohort studies showed a risk estimate under 2, about one third between 2 and 4, one fourth between 4 and 8 and the rest of the studies above 8. In case-control studies, 40% of the risk estimates were under 2 and one fifth each between two and four and four and eight [17].

The relative risk estimates for haemorrhagic stroke associated with OC use versus no use were in around 50% of the earlier studies under 2, in almost one third of the studies between two and four and in the rest above four. For ischaemic stroke, the respective figures were in one third of the studies under two and in 25% each between two and four and four and six [17]. However, since this early period the composition of OCs has changed, the oestrogen dose was reduced and some new progestagens were introduced. It became also clear that an important interaction exists between OC use and smoking with respect to stroke.

Table 6. Results of epidemiological studies of the relationship between oral contraceptive use and the risk of thromboembolic and haemorrhagic stroke (table modified and supplemented after M. Thorogood [6]).

Author, Year	Study Type	No of Cases	Relative Risk for OC Users
A. Thromboembolic			
Inman, 1968 [84]	CC	10	5
Collaborative Group, 1975 [43]	CC	140	9
Jick, 1978 [99]	CC	14	26
Vessey, 1984 [33]	CO	31	3-4#
Chang, 1986 [100]	CC	323	4
Oleckno, 1986 [101]	CC	40	4.6
Alvarez, 1989 [102]	CC	137	2.3
Lidegaard, 1993 [38]	CC	320	3.0
Hannaford, 1994 [35]	CO	14	3.5
Carolei, 1996 [103]	CC	146	1.7
WHO (Europe), 1996 [40]	CC	141	3.0
Petitti, 1996 [39]	CC	144	1.2
Haapaniemi, 1997 [104]	CC	140	4.2
Heinemann, 1997 [12]	CC	220	2.9
B. Haemorrhagic			
Collaborative Group, 1975 [37]	CC[c]	196	2
Petitti, 1978 [36]	CC[a]	11	7
Vessey, 1984 [33]	CO[a]	13	1.2
Thorogood, 1992 [34]	CC[a]	296	1.1
	CC[2)]	105	1.2
Hannaford, 1994 [35]	CO/CC[a]	12	1.5
	CO[b]	2	1.1
WHO (Europe), 1996 [41]	CC[c]	247	1.4
Petitti, 1996 [39]	CC[c]	151	1.1

CC Case-Control-Study; *CO* Cohort Study
[a] Subarachnoidal hemorrhage
[b] Other than subarachnoidal hemorrhage
[c] Cerebral hemorrhage
secondarily estimated odds ratio

Haemorrhagic Stroke

Table 6 gives an overview of studies investigating the risk of haemorrhagic stroke associated with OC use. In these studies, the risk of subarachnoidal bleeding and OC use showed a rather changing picture. Three studies in the UK found no significantly increased risk of fatal subarachnoidal bleeding for ever-users of oral contraceptives [33-35]; however, a smaller study showed a 7-fold increased relative risk [36]. A large study of nonfatal haemorrhagic strokes (all types of bleeding) in the USA found a 2-fold increased relative risk [37].

Several large studies were conducted in the late 1980s and early 1990s in order to evaluate the risk of haemorrhagic stroke under modern combined oral contraceptives [12, 34, 38-42]. Use of low-dose OCs was not associated with a significantly increased risk of haemorrhagic stroke in a North-American case-control study including 151 women (RR=1.1; 0.6-2.2) [39]. In a large case-control study carried out by WHO in industrialised and developing countries, the association of OC use with stroke was investigated in 1068 cases and 2910 controls (worldwide) in the age range of 20-44 years. OC use was associated with a small increase in risk of haemorrhagic stroke: in developing countries, the risk was 1.8-fold (1.3-2.3) increased, whereas the increase in risk was not significant in Europe (OR=1.4; 0.8-2.3). The modern low-dose OCs (<50 μg oestrogen) showed a smaller increase in risk (OR=1.4; 0.9-2.2) in Europe than OCs with a higher oestrogen dose (OR=2.7; 1.7-4.3) [41]. Women under 35 years of age who smoked and used the pill had a 2.7-fold (1.04-6.8) increased risk of haemorrhagic stroke, whereas women who did not smoke, but used the pill had no significantly increased risk (0.7; 0.3-12.1) [41]. For OC users over 35 years of age, an increased risk of hemorrhagic stroke was demonstrated. In nonsmoking OC-users over 35 years of age, the risk was 2.4-fold (0.9-6.4) increased. The respective risk estimate for smoking OC users over 35 years was 3.9 (1.5-9.9) [41]. Other cardiovascular risk factors were also related to the magnitude of the risk: women with a history of hypertension who had used OCs had a substantially higher risk than normotensive women: 10.3 (3.3-32.3) for hypertensive women versus 1.05 (0.6-1.8) for normotensive women [41].

In other words, the cardiovascular background risk is likely to be more important for the risk of haemorrhagic stroke than exposure to OCs which was similarly shown for the risk of AMI. What do these relative risk estimates mean for the absolute risk of haemorrhagic stroke in the female population? The risk of haemorrhagic stroke attributable to OC use is not increased in younger women (under 35 years); however, it is increased in older women. From the WHO study it can be estimated that the excess risk of haemorrhagic stroke in Europe is 2 per 100,000 women-years for use of low oestrogen-dose OCs and 8 per 100,000 women-years for use of higher oestrogen-dose OCs [41].

Thromboembolic Stroke

Thromboembolic (ischaemic) stroke occurs more frequently in women of reproductive age than haemorrhagic stroke. Previous studies showed that the risk of thromboembolic stroke was often increased in OC users compared with nonusers (see Table 6). Under the early studies that investigated the risk of thromboembolic stroke associated with OC use, there was one large study which included 140 patients. In this study, a ninefold increased relative risk for OC use compared with nonuse was found [43]. Other smaller studies also found evidence for a clearly increased relative risk of ischaemic stroke when using OCs (see Table 6).

Among the recently conducted studies, most [12, 34, 38, 40, 42] found an increased risk of thromboembolic stroke for OC use. Another study found no increased risk [39]. In the WHO study, the Transnational study and a population-based Danish case-control study, the risk of thromboembolic stroke was about threefold increased in OC-users compared with nonusers [12, 40]. Modern oral contraceptives with less than 50 μg oestrogen content showed numerically lower risk estimates than higher-dose oestrogen OCs. In two of the case-control studies, there was no significant difference in risk between OCs containing traditional progestagens and those containing modern progestagens (gestoden and desogestrel) [12, 40], whereas another study showed a lower relative risk for preparations with the newer progestagens [42].

Table 7. Relative risk (odds ratio) of ischaemic stroke in current OC users in comparison with nonusers. Influence of the marker "Blood Pressure Check"

	WHO (Europe) [40]	Transnational Study [12] *
No blood pressure check	3.9 (1.8-8.3)	4.6 (2.2-9.5)
Cases/Controls	26/42	52/164
Blood pressure check done	2.3 (1.1-4.6)	2.1 (1.3-3.4)
Cases/Controls	23/45	92/396

* Calculations by LAJ Heinemann based on the method used by WHO [40]

Cardiovascular risk factors appear to play also a role for the risk of thromboembolic stroke in OC users. This was seen in the Transnational Study when the risk of stroke was analysed according to whether a blood pressure check was performed prior to the prescription of OCs (which may be used as a marker for the attention to cardiovascular risk factors) (Table 7): a higher risk of thromboembolic stroke was observed for OC users without blood pressure check compared with OC users who had a blood pressure check prior to prescription. Only a small difference was, however, found in the WHO study between the two groups.

According to calculations from the Transnational Study, about three thromboembolic strokes per 100,000 women and year may be attributable to OC use in the Middle-European female population under 45 years of age [12]. Insufficient screening for cardiovascular risk factors prior to prescription of OCs may contribute to this risk. The risk may therefore be further reduced if women with important cardiovascular risk factors, such as high blood pressure and smoking, are either not prescribed OCs or receive appropriate management of their cardiovascular risk factors prior to prescription of OCs [12, 40]. Actually, the differences in clinical practice (higher prevalence of women with blood pressure check prior to OC prescription) and risk factors (lower smoking prevalence in OC users) might be one reason for lower risk estimates for stroke in recent US studies than in European ones.

Venous Thromboembolism

Early studies also reported a remarkably increased relative risk of venous thromboembolism (VTE) associated with OC use (see Table 8). In an earlier review article, the median of the relative risk estimates from case-control studies ranged between four and eight, whereas it was lower in cohort studies where the median was between 2 and 4 [17]. In about 10% of the analysed case-control and cohort studies in the early 1980s, the risk estimate exceeded an eightfold increase [17, 44]. Table 9 provides an overview about relative risk estimates for VTE associated with OC use. Based on these results, an increased risk of idiopathic VTEs associated with OC use has been established for decades. It has been repeatedly discussed whether the risk of VTE also depends on the oestrogen dose of the OC.

Only the most recently performed large case-control studies also investigated the effect of newer progestagens (gestoden and desogestrel) on the VTE risk [45-52]. An overview of the results of these studies is presented in Table 9. In the first of these recently published studies, the suspicion was raised that pills with the newer proges-

Table 8. Relative risk (odds ratio) of VTE in relation to current OC use (compared with nonuse). (Table modified and supplemented after M. Thorogood [6])

Author, Year	Study Type	No. of Cases	Relative Risk for OC Users
RCGP, 1967 [105]	CC	24	2
Inman, 1968 [84]	CC	26	8
Vessey, 1969 [85]	CC	84	6
Sartwell, 1969 [106]	CC	129	4
Vessey, 1970 [107]	CC	30	3.8
Bottinger, 1971 [108]	CC	84	11
Green, 1972 [109]	CC	60	6
BCDSP, 1973 [110]	CC	43	11
Petitti, 1978 [111]	CC	17	7.7
Maguire, 1979 [112]	CC	45	5
Porter, 1985 [113]	CO	9	3
Vessey, 1986 [64]	CO	29	7.2
Helmrich, 1987 [114]	CC	61	8
WHO, 1988 [115]	CC	88	2.9
Thorogood, 1992 [116]	CC	60	2
Vandenbroucke, 1994 [117]	CC	155	3.8
WHO, 1995 [118]	CC	433	4.2
Spitzer, 1996 [46]	CC	471	4.0

CC Case-Control-Study; *CO* Cohort Study

Table 9. Relative risk (odds ratio) of VTE for users of 3rd generation OCs compared with users of 2nd generation Ocs

Author, Year	Study Type	Relative Risk (Odds Ratio)
Jick, 1995 [47]	CC	2.2 (1.1—4.4)
Bloemenkamp, 1995 [48]	CC	2.2 (0.9—5.4)
WHO, 1996 [45]	CC	2.6 (1.6—4.2)
Spitzer, 1996 [46]	CC	1.5 (1.1—2.1)
Farmer, 1997 [49]	CO/CC	1.3 (0.7—2.4)
Lidegaard, 1997 [51]	CC	No significant difference in risk for more than 1 year of use
Suissa, 1997 [52]	CC	No significant difference in risk for first time users
Farmer, 1998 [50]	CC	0.77 (0.4—1.6) #

CC Case-Control-Study; *CO* Cohort Study
Unadjusted odds ratio

tagens gestoden and desogestrel (so-called "third generation" OCs) have a 1.5- to 2.5-fold increased risk of VTE compared with OCs with traditional progestagens (levonorgestrel) which were called "second generation OCs" [45-48]. Other more recently conducted studies, some of which have not been fully published yet, failed to show a differential effect of progestagens on the VTE risk in first time OC users [52], after more than 1 year of duration of OC use [51] or did not find an increased risk at all [49, 50]. Under these most recently conducted studies there was a case-control study from Denmark that included all Danish women suffering from VTE. This study is particularly important since it is representative of all cases in a country [51].

The results of these recently published studies [45-48] which showed an increased VTE risk associated with third generation OCs led to regulatory activities in

1995/1996, particularly in Germany and in the UK. The study results and regulatory activities were discussed intensively and controversially also in the lay press which led to insecurity among physicians and pill users and very often to a sudden interruption of the OC use (so-called "pill scare"). A controversial scientific discussion followed as to whether the slightly increased risk of VTEs associated with third generation OCs was due to residual confounding and bias inherent in these studies and also whether the reported relative risk (odds ratio) was of clinical relevance. This discussion also raised the question of the limits of epidemiologic research, in this case, in the context of relatively rare drug-related risks [8, 11, 53]. A similar discussion about the limits of epidemiologic research and the interpretation of small risks in cancer epidemiology was recently led by famous epidemiologists in the scientific journal "Science" [54]. Because of the intensive scientific debate triggered by regulatory activities, we will discuss the effect of bias and confounding in the recent VTE studies more extensively in the following paragraphs.

Bias and Confounding

Observational studies have the common problem that they are prone to bias (systematic error in the study results) or confounding (the apparently increased risk is in reality due to a third factor that was not properly taken care of in the analysis). Moreover, in pharmacoepidemiological studies, in contrast to classical case-control and cohort studies dealing with other risk factors, such as environmental risk factors, the indication for the drug therapy must be seriously considered. One can assume that the prescription behaviour (physician) as well as the reasons for taking a drug (patient) are influenced by previously known drug risks and, more-over, by the marketing of the drug. The prescription of drugs to groups with different baseline risks, for instance, can lead to systematic error (bias) in studies of drug safety. Therefore, in the interpretation of such studies, one should carefully consider all possibilities for bias and confounding before accepting the study results and also discuss the biological and pharmacological (toxicological) plausibility of the study results.

In considering opportunities for bias in the estimation of the risk of VTE associated with different generation pills, one needs to take into account that clinical symptoms of deep venous thrombosis may vary considerably, a fact which is well known to clinicians. Moreover, symptoms of VTE are often not impressive that is they may neither lead to the attention of the patient nor the treating doctor. Clear symptoms of VTE of moderate and severe degree which will lead to further diagnostic work-up were estimated to occur in less than 50% of all venous thromboses [55, 56]. In other words, 50% of VTEs may not be detected, unless there are reasons for an increased attention to only mild symptoms such as risk factors for VTE or possibly OC use. Moreover, the misclassification rate of VTEs is fairly high and is estimated to range between 30% and 50% [57-60]. As a consequence of the great variability of VTE symptoms, VTEs are often not documented because neither the patient nor the consulted physician may feel it necessary to follow up mild or unspecific VTE symptoms in a patient. If, however, a patient receives further diagnostic work-up for mild and unspecific symptoms because there was a specific reason for such increased attention, this could result in a systematic error of the calculated risk estimate (so-called "unmasking bias").

Representation of Reality in Observational Studies

One should remember that case-control studies in females are only a substitute for the investigation of the entire female population. The question is then: How good is the female population represented in these studies? Do the number and distribution of cases in the study population reflect sufficiently well all women with VTE in the entire population regarding for instance all degrees of severity of VTEs? If cases are considered to be representative for the entire population, one should examine whether the same also applies for the controls. For example, is the exposure of the controls with respect to different generations of OCs representative for the exposure in the entire female population? The problem is that the ideal, namely the perfect representation of reality in the study population, can hardly ever be achieved. With respect to the unequal VTE risk increase observed under different generation OCs, the following question was therefore raised: could it be that women with second generation OCs underwent less often an intensive search for thrombosis in the case of unspecific or mild symptoms of VTE as compared with women using third generation OCs? If this were the case, there would be an unequal (differential) selection of cases between users of different generation pills, i.e. the studies would show a biased picture of reality (Fig. 1).

In case-control studies with cases representative for the entire population the controls should be equally representative. Most of the recently published case-control studies of the VTE risk associated with OC use used hospitalised patients as controls, some studies recruited additionally population or GP-based controls. A more detailed analysis of the results of these studies showed that comparisons with population controls led to lower risk estimates for third generation OCs than comparisons with hospital controls [45, 46]. The different risk estimates when comparing cases with different control groups leads to the often discussed question which control group is "valid" or more appropriate for the respective study.

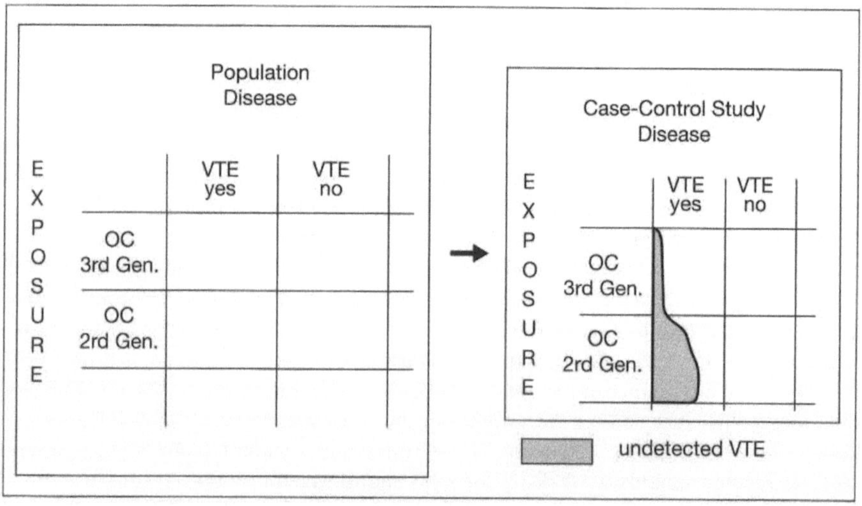

Fig. 1. Representation of a population in a case-control-study. Possible problem of distortion by more unrecognized VTE cases in users of 2nd generation OCs

Time Trends in the Risk of VTE

It is often observed that drugs exhibit an apparently higher risk of adverse events in the first time after market introduction as compared to periods when they have already been available for longer time periods. If one investigates the VTE risk estimates for OC use versus nonuse for time trends, one can see that the estimates of the relative risk ranged between 6 and 11 in the late 1960s and early 1970s, where the majority of pills still had a relatively high content of oestrogens. In the 1980s, the relative risk of VTE associated with OC use decreased to about four. In the mid 1980s, the relative risk increased again to about 5-8 [61], after many new OCs had been introduced in the 1970s which contained lower doses of oestrogens. Later the estimates decreased again to about two to four. Following the market introduction of OCs with newer progestagens (gestoden, desogestrel, norgestimate) in the mid-1980s, the risk estimates ranged between three and four in the studies.

Just for illustration, Fig. 2 shows schematically some relative risk estimates for VTE associated with OC use from different studies over the course of time: As an example for the risk of OCs with high dose oestrogen content (>50 μg oestrogen), the results of the Royal College General Practitioner (RCGP) cohort study are depicted for 1974 [62] and 1978 [63]. The risk estimates from the studies of Vessey 1986 [64] and Jick 1995 [47] likely illustrate risk estimates for OCs with low-dose oestrogen content, since these studies were performed at a time where low-dose oestrogens were dominant. In the lower part of Fig. 2, the declining risk for third generation OCs can be seen using the odds ratios from the UK-based GPRD Study [47] and the Transnational Study [46]. Possible reasons for the declining trend in the risk estimates could either be changes in the study designs or changes in the cohort of OC users or both.

The declining trend of the VTE risk for different pill types over time appears to be associated with the duration of time since market introduction of the respective pill. One may assume that women who did not suffer pill-related complaints or side effects will continue to use the same pill for years, whereas women who experience side effects or complications will either stop using the pill at all or switch to a more "modern" brand. A methodological problem will result, if one compares the risk in two user cohorts at one point in time, where one cohort is still on the peak of its risk (as for example users of OCs with newer progestagens at the beginning of the 1990s), whereas the other user cohort (for example, OCs with levonorgestrel at the beginning of the 1990s) already shows a declining risk towards the remaining baseline risk (Fig. 3). This phenomenon is also called "healthy user effect" and was demonstrated with the data of the Transnational Study [65]. In such a situation, a comparison between drugs may lead to results which are neither biologically nor pharmacologically plausible. For example, the Transnational Study showed that in the age group of women (22-44 years of age), who could have used either traditional or newer pills for a longer time period, the VTE risk for OCs containing norgestimate compared with that for levonorgestrel-containing OCs was twofold increased, although the biologically active substance of norgestimate is broadly identical with levonorgestrel itself [65]. As a second example, one may consider the VTE risk of desogestrel when given in combination with different doses of oestrogens: While the combination of desogestrel with 30 μg oestrogen showed a 1.5-fold increased relative risk compared with levonorgestrel-containing OCs, the relative risk was 2.8-fold increased for desogestrel in combination with 20 μg oestrogen (introduced 10 years later) in comparison with levonorgestrel-containing OCs. This, however, does not appear to be biologically plausible [65].

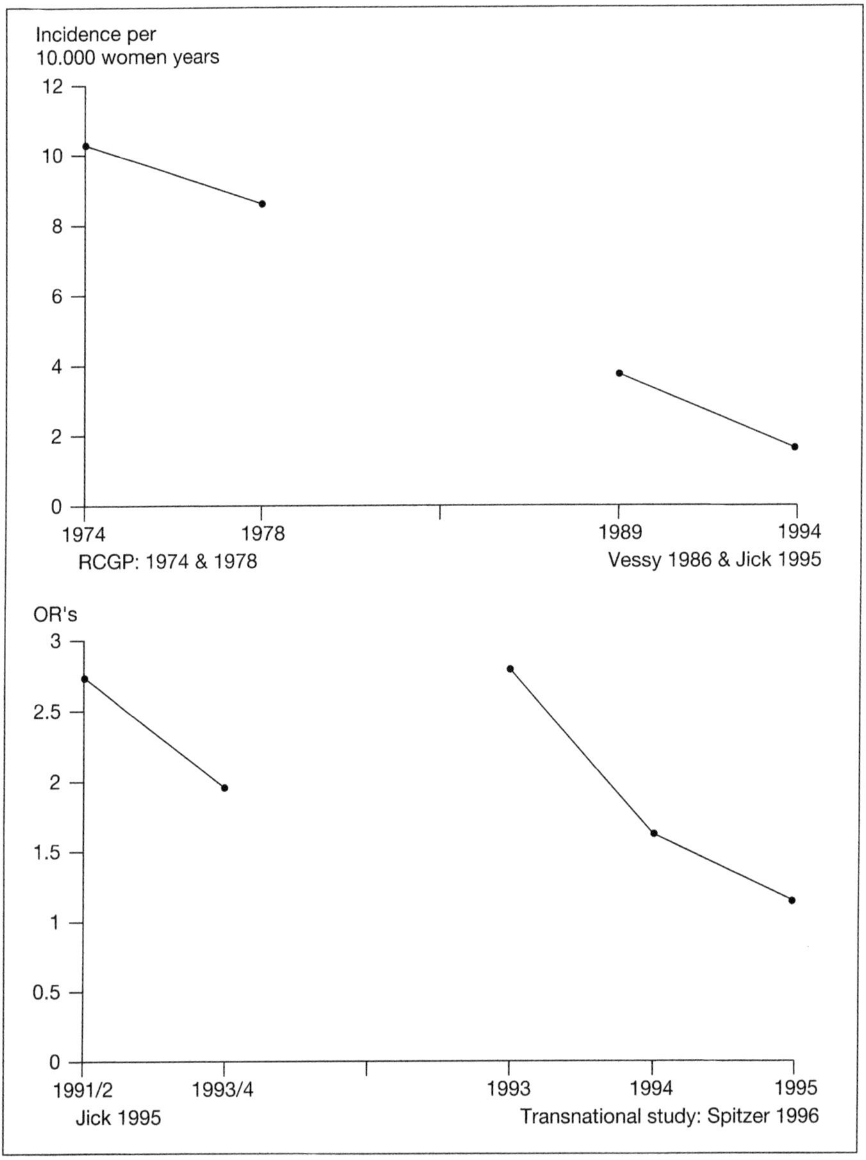

Fig. 2a, b. Development of the risk of thrombosis over time. *a* Decrease of OC-related incidence of VTE (per 10,000 women-years); 1974/78 RCGP (OCs with >50 μg oestrogen) [62, 63]; Vessey1986 [64]/ Jick 1995 [47]. *b* Decrease of the relative risk (OR) of VTE associated with 3rd generation vs. 2nd generation OCs; Boston Collaborative Drug Surveillance Program Study (Jick 1995 [47]), Transnational Study (Spitzer1996 [46])

Opportunities for Bias in the VTE Studies

The two first large case-control studies, the WHO Study and the Transnational Study, lacked information about various potential confounders or did not consider them sufficiently in the analysis [45, 46]. In this context, the following potential confounders shall be mentioned here: genetic predisposition for VTE (to be determined from blood samples); family history of VTE; previous VTE not treated in hospital; lifetime history of OC use to analyse switching patterns; OC prescription behaviour; OC use patterns of excluded cases; duration of availability of different OCs on the respective markets, and others. Furthermore, information was missing on certain variables which are important for the diagnosis of VTE: severity of the initial symptoms, diagnostic and referral behaviour.

Information about the genetic background risk in cases and controls was missing in almost all of the studies, since most of the studies did not collect information about a family history of VTE or take a blood sample. From clinical research it is known that patients with VTE have in 40% some genetic risk [66], whereas the genetic risk for VTE in the general population is around 3-5% [66]. This missing information may result in "residual confounding" that could partly explain an increased VTE risk for OC users, if an association between OC use and genetic background risk could be empirically shown.

Apart from the possibility of "residual confounding" due to insufficient information in the various studies, the statistical analysis of the data was also raised as a problem: a re-analysis of the VTE risk for first ever-users of OCs based on data from the Transnational Study showed that when the variable 'duration of OC use' was taken into

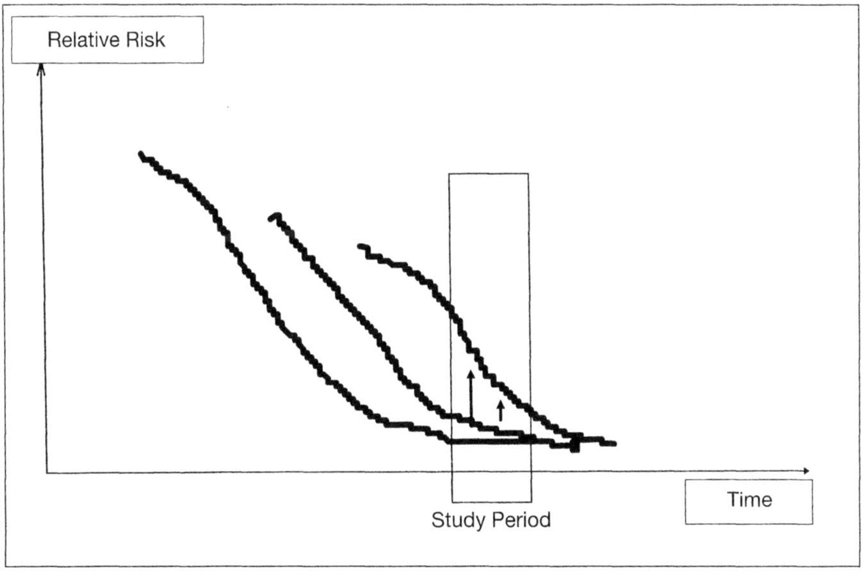

Fig. 3. Schematic representation of the decrease in VTE risk after introduction of three OC generations into the market. Observed risk differences in the study period (box) also reflect different phases in the hazard functions of the three generations

account in the analysis, the differential VTE risk for older (levonorgestrel) and newer progestagen-containing OCs (desogestrel, gestoden) disappeared [52]. This analysis suggests that apart from age (matching or adjustment for exact age seems to be important in VTE studies) also the duration of OC use may act as an important confounder (particularly for the risk of VTE and less so for myocardial infarction and stroke which has been shown in the Danish studies) [26, 42].

Besides the already mentioned possibilities for bias, some studies suggest that further forms of bias may have played a role and could possibly explain the unexpected difference in VTE risk between OCs with traditional and recently introduced progestagens:

- *Prescribing Bias.* Several published analyses showed that pills with newer progestagens (desogestrel, gestoden) that were thought to be safer because of their marketing were preferentially prescribed to women with a higher baseline risk for VTE as for example to pill starters [67-70], to women in higher age groups [49, 69, 71-73], to women with a personal history of VTE [68, 69, 72] or a family history of VTE [67, 68], to women with obesity [49, 68], or chronic inflammatory diseases [69], or clinical venous signs [69] or a combination of risk factors [68, 72, 74]. However, information on prescribing practice was not gathered in the recent OC studies.
- *Diagnostic Bias.* It is likely that OC-using women with a higher baseline risk for VTE were more carefully monitored for the occurrence of VTE by their physicians. In case of trace symptoms, these women had a greater chance of being referred for further diagnostic tests and of receiving a definite diagnosis of VTE [68]. If these women were more likely to be prescribed pills that had been introduced into the market only recently (for example, desogestrel- and gestoden-containing pills – see prescribing bias), then more attention would be paid to mild symptoms and signs of VTE in users of third generation pills. This would lead to a preferential inclusion of VTE cases with mild (trace) symptoms who had been users of third generation OCs. Unfortunately, no study collected information about the severity of the initial symptoms, and, therefore, the statistical analysis could not adjust for this problem.
- *Healthy User Bias.* This form of bias has already been mentioned under time trends for VTE risk. Women who experience any kind of problem with an older generation pill, will usually switch to a newer brand, if they do not stop using the pill at all, whereas women who are healthy and do not suffer complaints from the pill will likely continue using the same pill. The longer an OC is on the market, the more women with pill problems or possibly even an increased risk of VTE will disappear from the user cohort. As for other drugs, it has been shown for OCs that the risk of unexpected adverse drug reactions diminishes over time. If we compare OCs with modern progestagens which were introduced in the 1980s with traditional OCs which were introduced in the 1970s, we are comparing women who are still very much on the peak of their risk with women with an already reduced risk. This has been shown for the Danish and the Transnational Studies [11, 51, 65, 73]. If one does not take into account the duration of use when comparing new with traditional OCs, increased and sometimes implausible risk estimates for the newly introduced OCs will result [65].
- *Causal Association.* If one disregards for a moment the considerations about bias and residual confounding as a possible explanation for the unequal VTE risk of different progestagens and takes the 1.5- to 2.5-fold increase in risk for newer

progestagens in comparison with traditional progestagens at face value – is it likely to be causal? Before one can accept causality for an observed association, a number of criteria should be met which have been formalised by Bradford Hill some of which we will discuss in this context [9]:

- The *Strength of the Association.* A relative risk of less than two which comes as an unexpected or new result of an observational study and does not follow a prior biologic hypothesis represents a "weak" association only which in the opinion of many epidemiologists cannot be used to substantiate causality [54]. The well-known epidemiologist Samuel Shapiro elaborated on this point: "Relative risks of low magnitude (say, less than 2) are virtually beyond the resolving power of the epidemiologic microscope: we can seldom demonstrably eliminate all sources of bias, and we can never exclude the possibility of unidentified and uncontrolled confounding" [75]. Robert Temple from the Food and Drug Administration, USA, also requested for such situation a relative risk of at least 3 or 4 [54].
- *Consistency of the Results.* A causal relationship is also supported by the consistency of a result across several studies which should ideally be performed by different investigators in different settings applying different methods. If one considers the first four published case-control studies only [45-48], a relatively consistent result of the association between the risk of VTE and OCs containing newer progestagens was observed. However, the then following studies and a re-analysis of one of the first four studies failed to show a differential risk for second versus third generation OCs [49-52]. Moreover, there was little consistency in the risk estimates neither across countries or study regions nor across different control groups which has already been discussed [45, 46, 76].
- *Dose-Response Relation.* A further criterion for causality is evidence of a dose-response relationship or a biological gradient. With respect to oestrogens and the risk of VTE, it has been reported that higher doses of oestrogens are associated with a higher VTE risk than lower doses of oestrogens [6, 62, 63, 77]. This biological gradient between oestrogen dose and VTE risk was, however, not observed in some of the studies that showed a higher VTE risk for newer progestagens than for older ones. On the contrary, an inverse dose-response relationship was observed in some studies [45-47] in that some low-dose oestrogen-containing OCs had a higher risk of VTE than pills with high-dose oestrogen content which is biologically implausible. This biologically implausible inverse relation has already been discussed in the context of the healthy user effect, the different points in time of market introduction of the various OCs and the resulting time trends of the risk estimates [45-47, 76, 78].
- *Biological Plausibility.* Another important criterion in support of causality of an observed association is the biological plausibility of the finding. The reported unexpected finding of a higher VTE risk for third generation OCs in comparison with second generation OCs is not sufficiently supported by laboratory research (haemostaseology), yet. There is no convincing biological concept as to how gestoden or desogestrel could lead to a higher thrombotic risk than OCs containing more traditional progestagens. Recently, Rosing et al. published data which point to a higher acquired APC resistance under third generation OCs as a possible explanation [79]. However, this result was challenged, since their study presented several methodological problems: The authors used a new test the clinical

relevance of which has not yet been sufficiently validated for VTE. Another larger study based on a random sample of the population and a conventional and validated APC test, showed no difference in APC resistance between different pill generations, but the well-known phenomenon that the APC resistance is generally higher in OC users than in nonusers [80]. It is expected that in the near future many studies in basic research will be launched to investigate the stability and validity of the new Rosing test and to study the role of acquired APC resistance and other genetic factors in the aetiology of VTE. As long as these results are not available, the observation of the Rosing study should be interpreted with great caution, and it is to early to use the current results as evidence for the biological plausibility of a "differential VTE risk" of different types of progestagens.

Conclusions Regarding the Risk of VTE Associated with OCs

The risk of VTE associated with OC use appears to have declined in the course of the past decades. The very small excess risk of VTEs observed for third-generation OCs compared with second-generation OCs in some [45-48], but not in all studies [49-52] is possibly an artefact due to limitations in the design of the initial studies. Various possibilities for bias and residual confounding in these studies have been discussed. The differential risk observed for OCs with different progestagens does not meet important criteria which are generally used in epidemiologic research to provide evidence for a causal relationship. Currently, some studies analyse time trends of the incidence and mortality from VTE with respect to the time of market introduction of third generation OCs in different countries. An analysis of VTE mortality in seven European countries showed no evidence for an "epidemic" of fatal VTE events since the introduction of OCs with modern progestagens [81]. Based on the contradictory results of different studies and the discussed possibilities for bias and confounding, the currently available evidence is not sufficient to conclude that third generation OCs carry a higher risk of VTE than second generation OCs. VTEs associated with the use of oral contraceptives are, in general, very rare events that are counterbalanced by the numerous public health benefits of OCs which result from their reliable contraceptive action.

Risk and Benefit: An Example of Quantification

If one compares the well-known contraceptive and noncontraceptive benefits of OC use (see Table 10) with the potential risks of OC use, as was done by Vessey in 1989 [82], the positive balance is impressive.

For the purpose of this crude comparison, the beneficial aspects of OC use, as estimated from the literature and given in Table 10, were used. The contraceptive benefit was arbitrarily determined to be "0.9" that is a 10% chance of failure of oral contraceptives. The "event rates" for the beneficial and harmful events were estimated from a German hospital discharge statistics of the 20- to 44-year-old female population for the end of the 1980s [83]. Only first events were counted and expressed as incidence rates per 100,000 women and year in this age group. The rates for OC users were

Table 10. Contraceptive and noncontraceptive benefits of OC use estimated from the literature

	Reduction (%)
Contraceptive Benefits	
Pregnancy	>90
Deaths at birth	>90
Abortions (spontaneous/induced)	>90
Extrauterinal Pregnancy	>90
Noncontraceptive Benefits	
Cycle disturbances	25-50
Anaemia	25
Pelvic inflammation	50
Uterus tumours	50
Ovarial tumours	50
Benign mammal tumours	25-50

calculated as the product of these incidence rates in the female population aged 20-44 years and the relative risk of these events under OCs estimated from the literature. Table 11 shows the difference between OC users and nonusers for the different events per 100,000 women-years. The negative sign means that 20- to 44-year-old women without OC use have more events than women in the same age group using OCs.

One can see in Table 10 that the contraceptive benefits of OCs quantitatively prevail. OCs also have a number of noncontraceptive benefits of which the public appears to be less aware. Obviously, the contraceptive and noncontraceptive benefits of OCs numerically far outweigh the risks of OC use. It is quite clear, however, that such a crude comparison of numbers for beneficial and risk events is not the final answer. These events may have a quite different individual and public health impact which renders a simple numerical comparison inadequate. For a quantitative comparison, the events need to be standardised to one or several common endpoints such as quality of life or mortality. Such a final model is, however, currently not available. The manifold and quantitatively frequent beneficial effects of OCs in comparison with the rare risks of use have led to a clear, positive benefit-risk-evaluation for OCs both in science and in medical practice.

Table 11. Positive and negative events associated with OC use: an attempt of a schematic balance (figures give absolute difference in the number of events per 100,000 women-years in comparison with nonusers)

Positive:	Less	Negative	More
Induced abortions	-1800	Venous thromboembolism	+24
Spontaneous abortions	-486	Myocardial infarction	+3
Ectopic pregnancies	-72	Thromboembolic stroke	+14
Dysmenorrhoe	-160	Haemorrhagic stroke	+0.6
Anaemia	-6	Benign liver tumours	+1
Pelvic inflammation	-225	Liver cancer	+0.1
Benign mammal tumours	-27	Mammal cancer	+5
Benign Ovarial tumours	-70		
Ovarial carcinoma	-1		
Endometrial Carcinoma	-4		

(Based on incidence estimates from a German hospital discharge statistics of the 20- to 44-year-old female population)

Conclusions

1. Incidence and mortality of cardiovascular diseases are extremely low in women of reproductive age.
2. Cardiovascular risks measured in epidemiological studies have declined over the past 20 years. The decrease in cardiovascular risks for OCs is at least partly due to the changed composition of the OC preparations.
3. The observed reduction of cardiovascular risks under OCs is likely to be also an effect of the increased attention of physicians and pill users to cardiovascular risk factors and appropriate management of these risk factors prior to prescribing OCs. If risk factors are detected and women adequately counselled before prescribing OCs, the risk of cardiovascular complications of modern OCs is extremely low.
4. For young women under 35 years of age without cardiovascular risk factors (smoking, hypertension, diabetes) who are current users of OCs the increase in risk for myocardial infarction is negligible, also if they have used OCs in the past or for longer time periods. There is need for further research to clarify whether newer progestagens (gestoden and desogestrel) reduce the risk of myocardial infarction and to study possible physiological mechanisms for such an effect.
5. The risk of cerebral haemorrhage increases with age and is increased in women with hypertension and cigarette smoking. Women under 35 years of age who do not have these risk factors and use OCs do not seem to have an increased risk of developing a cerebral haemorrhage, even those with long-lasting or past use.
6. The risk of thromboembolic (ischaemic) stroke also depends to a great extent on the risk factors age, hypertension and cigarette smoking. In women who do not smoke and have no increased blood pressure the risk of ischaemic stroke is increased about 1.5- to 2-fold (in European more than in US studies), independent of the duration of OC use or past use. It has been estimated that in Europe in women under the age of 45 three cases of ischaemic stroke per 100,000 women per year might be associated with OC use. However, this estimate also includes women where cardiovascular risk factors were not sufficiently checked prior to prescribing OCs.
7. In women using OCs, the relative risk of VTE is increased about 3- to 4-fold compared with women not using OCs. The risk is likely to be highest in the first year of use and declines with the duration of use. Further investigations are needed to evaluate the VTE risk in relation to the duration of pill use, pill switching patterns and a genetic predisposition for VTE.
8. In spite of the intensive scientific debate about the VTE risk for so-called "second and third generation pills", there is no clear evidence that pills containing newer progestagens (gestoden and desogestrel) have a different cardiovascular risk than pills with traditional progestagens such as levonorgestrel.
9. The benefits of pill use outweigh by far the risks. Benefit and risk aspects of OC use should not be considered in isolation. Medical counselling of the individual woman should take into account all aspects of benefit and risk and evaluate these aspects in the context of the individual woman as the basis for an "informed choice" on OC use.

References

1. World Health Organization (1997) WHO Scientific Group Meeting on Cardiovascular Disease and Steroid Hormone Contraceptives. Summary of Conclusions. Weekly Epidemiological Record 48:361-363
2. Diczfalusy E (1997) The contraceptive revolution. Parthenon Publishing, New York
3. World Health Organization (1997) Progress in human reproduction research. WHO Progress 42
4. Jordan WM (1961) Pulmonary embolism (letter). Lancet 2ii:1146-1147
5. Lorentz IT (1962) Parietal lesion and "Enavid" (letter). BMJ 2:1191
6. Thorogood M (1993) Oral contraceptives and cardiovascular disease: an epidemiologic Overview. Pharmacoepidemiology and Drug Safety 2:3-16
7. Heinemann LAJ (1998) Venous thrombosis and oral contraceptives: point of view of an epidemiologist. In: Speroff L (ed): New insights in gynecology and obstetrics. Carnforth, Parthenon Publishing, New York, pp 286-291
8. Heinemann LAJ (1997) Möglichkeiten und Grenzen der Epidemiologie.Steroidhormone und venöse Thrombosen? Gynäkologe 30:296-304
9. Bradford Hill A (1971) Statistical evidence and inference: Principles of Medical Statistics. Oxford University Press, New York 309-323
10. Strom BL (1994) When should one perform pharmacoepidemiology studies? In: Strom BL (ed): Pharmacoepidemiology. John Wiley & Sons, Chichester, New York, pp 61-63
11. Heinemann LAJ (1996) Background to epidemiology of the recent pill scare. Proceeding of the joint symposium on oral contraceptives and venous thromboembolism, In: Cohen J (ed): Oral Contraceptives and Cardiovascular Disease. Parthenon Publishing, New York, pp 19-32
12. Heinemann LAJ, Lewis MA, Thorogood M, et al (1997) Case-control study of oral contraceptives and risk of thromboembolic stroke: results from international study on oral contraceptives and health of young women. BMJ 315:1502-1504
13. Lewis MA, Heinemann LAJ, Spitzer WO, MacRae KD, Bruppacher R (1997) The use of oral contraceptives and the occurrence of acute myocardial infarction in young women. Results from the Transnational Study on Oral Contraceptives and the Health of Young Women. Contraception 56:129-140
14. Barth W, Löwel H, Lewis MA, et al (1996) Coronary heart disease mortality, morbidity, and case fatality in five East and West German cities 1985-1989. J Clin Epidemiol 49:1277-1284
15. Weber I, Abel M, Altenhofen L, Bächer K, et al (1990) Dringliche Gesundheitsprobleme in der Bevölkerung in der Bundesrepublik Deutschland. Nomos Verlagsgesellschaft, Baden-Baden 409:446-449
16. Neumann H-G (1985) Zur Bewertung von Mitteilungen über Nebenwirkungen hormonaler Kontrazeptiva. Zeitschrift für ärztliche Fortbildung 79:1033-1036
17. Heinemann LAJ (1989) Epidemiological assessment of cardiovascular effects of hormonal contraception, In: Michal F (ed): Safety requirements for contraceptive steroids. Cambridge University Press, Cambridge, New York, pp 113-125
18. Slone D, Shapiro S, Kaufman DW, Rosenberg L, Miettinen OS, Stolley PD (1981) Risk of myocardial infarction in relation to current and discontinued use of oral contraceptives. New Engl J Med 305:420-424
19. La Vecchia C, Franceschi S, Decarli A, Pampallona S, Tognoni G (1987) Risk factors for myocardial infarction in young women. Am J Epidemiol 125:832-843
20. Sidney S, Petitti DB, Quesenberry CPJ, Klatsky AL, Ziel HK, Wolf S (1996) Myocardial infarction in users of low-dose oral contraceptives. Obstetrics and Gynecology 88:939-944
21. Rosenberg L, Palmer JR, Lesko SM, Shapiro S (1990) Oral contraceptive use and the risk of myocardial infarction. Am J Epidemiol 131:1009-1016
22. Thorogood M, Mann J, Murphy M, Vessey M (1991) Is oral contraceptive use still associated with an increased risk of fatal myocardial infarction? Report of a case-control study. Br J Obstet Gynaecol 98:1245-1253
23. Lewis MA, Spitzer WO, Heinemann LAJ, et al (1996) Third generation oral contraceptives and risk of myocardial infarction: an international case-control study. BMJ 312:88-90
24. Jick H, Jick SS, Myers MW, Vasilakis C (1996) Risk of acute myocardial infarction and low-dose combined oral contraceptives. Lancet 347:627-628
25. WHO Collaborative Study of Cardiovascular Disease and Steroid Hormone Contraception (1997) Acute myocardial infarction and combined oral contraceptives: results of an international multicentre case-control-study. Lancet 349:1202-1209

26. Lidegaard O, Edström B (1997) Myocardial infarction, cerebral thrombosis and oral contraceptives. Two case-control studies. Posterabstrakt FIGO Weltkongress August
27. Bergink EW, Kloosterboer HJ (1985) Structural requirements for optimal receptor binding of contraceptive progestogens. Adv Contracept 1:256-257
28. Victor A, Weiner E, Johansson EDB (1977) Relation between sex hormone binding globulin and d-norgestrel levels in plasma. Acta Endocrinologica 86:430-436
29. Lipworth L, Adami H-O, Trichopoulos D, Carlstrom K, Mantzoros C (1996) Serum steroid hormone levels, sex-hormone-binding globulin, and body mass index in the etiology of postmenopausal breast cancer. Epidemiology 7:96-100
30. Kjaer A, Lebech A-M, Borggaard B, et al (1989) Lipid metabolism and coagulation of two contraceptives: correlation to serum concentrations of levonorgestrel and gestodene. Contraception 40:665-673
31. Collins JA (1995) Progestins and lipoproteins: the implications for clinical practice. Journal SOGC [Suppl.] 12-18
32. Engel H-J, Engel E, Lichtlen PR (1983) Coronary atherosclerosis and myocardial infarction in young women - role of oral contraceptives. Eur Heart J 4:1-6
33. Vessey MP, Lawless M, Yeates D (1984) Oral contraceptives and stroke: findings in a large prospective study. BMJ 289:530-531
34. Thorogood M, Mann J, Murphy M, Vessey M (1992) Fatal stroke and use of oral contraceptives: Findings from a case-control study. Am J Epidemiol 136:35-45
35. Hannaford PC, Croft PR, Kay CR (1994) Oral contraception and stroke. Evidence from the Royal College of General Practitioner's Oral Contraception Study. Stroke 25:935-942
36. Petitti DB, Wingerd J (1978) Use of oral contraceptives, cigarette smoking, and risk of subarachnoid haemorrhage. Lancet ii:234-236
37. Collaborative Group for the Study of Stroke in Young Women (1975) Oral contraceptives and stroke in young women. Associated risk factors. JAMA 231:718-722
38. Lidegaard O (1993) Oral contraception and risk of a cerebral thromboembolic attack: results of a case-control study. BMJ 306:956-963
39. Petitti DB, Sidney S, Bernstein A, Wolf S, Quesenberry C, Ziel HK (1996) Stroke in users of low-dose oral contraceptives. New Engl J Med 335:8-15
40. WHO Collaborative Study of Cardiovascular Disease and Steroid Hormone Contraception (1996) Ischaemic stroke and combined oral contraceptives: results of an international, multicentre, case-control study. Lancet 348:498-505
41. WHO Collaborative Study of Cardiovascular Disease and Steroid Hormone Contraception (1996) Haemorrhagic stroke, overall stroke risk, and combined oral contraceptives: results of an international, multicentre, case-control study. Lancet 348:505-510
42. Lidegaard O, Kreiner S (1997) Cerebral thromboembolism and oral contraceptives: A case-control study. (Abstract no. 297) in 13th International Conference on Pharmacoepidemiology, Orlando, Fl. August.
43. Collaborative Group for the Study of Stroke in Young Women (1973) Oral contraception and increased risk of cerebral ischemia or thrombosis. New Engl J Med 288:871-878
44. Realini JP, Goldzieher JW (1985) Oral contraceptives and cardiovascular disease: a critique of the epidemiologic studies. Am J Obstet Gynecol 152:729-798
45. WHO Collaborative Study of Cardiovascular Disease and Steroid Hormone Contraception (1995) Effect of different progestagens in low oestrogen oral contraceptives on venous thromboembolic disease. Lancet 346:1582-1588
46. Spitzer WO, Lewis MA, Heinemann LAJ, Thorogood M, MacRae KD, Transnational Research Group on Oral Contraceptives and the Health of Young Women (1996) Third generation oral contraceptives and risk of venous thromboembolic disorders: an international case-control study. BMJ 312:83-88
47. Jick H, Jick SS, Gurevich V, Myers MW, Vasilakis C (1995) Risk of idiopathic cardiovascular death and nonfatal venous thromboembolism in women using oral contraceptives with differing progestagen components. Lancet 346:1589-1593
48. Bloemenkamp KWM, Rosendaal FR, Helmerhorst FM, Büller HR, Vandenbroucke JP (1995) Enhancement by factor V Leiden mutation of risk of deep vein thrombosis associated with oral contraceptives containing a third-generation progestagen. Lancet 346:1593-1596

49. Farmer RDT, Lawrenson RA, Thompson CR, Kennedy JG, Hambleton IR (1997) Population-based study of risk of venous thromboembolism associated with various oral contraceptives. Lancet 349:83-88
50. Farmer RDT, Todd J-C, Lewis MA, MacRae KD, Williams TJ (1998) The risks of venous thromboembolic disease among German women using oral contraceptives: A database study. Contraception 57: 67-70
51. Lidegaard O, Edström B (1997) Oral contraceptives (OC) and venous thromboembolism: a case-control study. Eur J Contracept Reproduct Health Care 2:73
52. Suissa S, Blais L, Spitzer WO, Cusson J, Lewis M, Heinemann L (1997) First-time use of newer oral contraceptives and the risk of venous thromboembolism. Contraception 56:141-146
53. Heinemann LAJ (1996) Haben Ovulationshemmer der 3. Generation ein neues Risikoprofil? Deutsche Medizinische Wochenschrift 121:1037-1039
54. Taubes G (1995) Epidemiology faces its limits. Science 269:164-169
55. Fobbe F, Koppenhagen K (1995) Diagnostik der symptomatischen und asymptomatischen venösen Thrombose. Hämostaseologie 15:148-155
56. Geerts WH, Code KI, Jay RM, Chen E, Szalai JP (1994) A prospective study of venous thromboembolism after major trauma. New Engl J Med 331:1601-1606
57. Grossmann K (1979) Die Diagnostik venöser Erkrankung der Extremitäten mit apparativen Methoden. Zeitschrift für ärztliche Fortbildung 73:13-17
58. Heinemann LAJ, Heine H (1981) Angiologie in der Ärztlichen Praxis. Fischer Verlag, Jena, pp 235
59. Bergqvist DB, Bergentz S-E (1990) Diagnosis of deep vein thrombosis. World J Surg 14:679-687
60. Nielsen HK, Fasting H, Husted SE (1990) Venous thromboembolism. The emperor's new clothes or a silent menace? Nordisk Medicin 105:139-143
61. Lidegaard O (1996) Oral contraceptives and venous thrombosis: an epidemiological review. Eur J Contraception Pbl Health Care 1:13-20
62. Royal College of General Practitioners (1974) Oral contraceptives and health. Pitman Medical Publishing, Turnbridge Wells
63. Royal College of General Practitioners's Oral Contraception Study (1978) Oral contraceptives, venous thrombosis, and varicose veins. J Royal Coll Gen Pract 28:393-399
64. Vessey M, Mant D, Smith A, Yeates D (1986) Oral contraceptives and venous thromboembolism: Findings in a large prospective study. BMJ 292:526
65. Lewis MA, Heinemann LAJ, MacRae KD, Bruppacher R, Spitzer WO, Transnational Research Group on Oral Contraceptives and the Health of Young Women (1996) The increased risk of venous thromboembolism and the use of third generation progestagens: role of bias in observational research. Contraception 54:5-13
66. Bauersachs R, Lindhoff-Last E, Ehrly AM, Kuhl H (1996) Die Bedeutung der hereditären Thrombophilie für das Thromboserisiko unter der oralen Kontrazeption. Zentralblatt für Gynäkologie 118:262-270
67. Lidegaard O (1997) The influence of thrombotic risk factors when oral contraceptives are prescribed: A control-only study. Acta Obstet Gynecol Scand 76:252-260
68. Heinemann LAJ, Lewis MA, Assmann A, Gravens L, Guggenmoos-Holzmann I (1996) Could preferential prescribing and referral behaviour of physicians explain the elevated thrombosis risk found to be associated with third generation oral contraceptives? Pharmacoepidemiology and Drug Safety 5:285-294
69. Jamin C, Mouzon Jd (1996) Selective prescribing of third generation oral contraceptives (OCs). Contraception 54:55-56
70. WHO Collaborative Study of Cardiovascular Disease and Steroid Hormone Contraception (1996) Ischaemic stroke and combined oral contraceptives: result of an international, multicentre, case-control study. Lancet 348:498-505
71. Lis Y, Spitzer WO, Mann RD, et al (1993) A concurrent cohort study of oral contraceptive users from the VAMP Research Bank. Pharmacoepidemiology and Drug Safety 2:51-63
72. Herings RMC, Boer Ad, Urquhart J, Leufkens HGM (1996) Non-causal explanations for the increased risk of venous thromboembolism among users of third-generation oral contraceptives. Pharmacoepidemiology and Drug Safety 5:88
73. Farmer RDT, Lawrenson R (1996) Utilization patterns of oral contraceptives in UK General Practice. Contraception 53:211-215

74. Van Lunsen HW (1996) Recent oral contraceptive use patterns in four European countries: evidence for selective prescribing of oral contraceptives containing third-generation progestogens. Eur J Contracept Reproduct Health Care 1:39-45
75. Shapiro S (1994) Meta-analysis/ Shmeta-analysis. Am J Epidemiol 40:771-778
Spitzer WO (1997) The 1995 pill scare revisited: anatomy of a non-epidemic. Human Reproduction 12:2347-2357
77. Gerstman BB, Piper JM, Tomita DK, Ferguson WJ, Stadel BV, Lundin FE (1991) Oral contraceptive estrogen dose and the risk of deep venous thromboembolic disease. Am J Epidemiol 133:32-37
78. Farmer R (1996) Letter to the editor. Results of AAH Meditel Study. Lancet 347:259
79. Rosing J, Tans G, Nicolaes GAF, et al (1997) Oral contraceptives and venous thrombosis: different sensitivities to activated protein C in women using second- and third- generation oral contraceptives. Br J Haematol 97:233-238
80. Schramm W, Heinemann LA (1997) Oral contraceptives and venous thromboembolism: acquired APC resistance? Br J Haematol 98:491-492
81. Farmer RDT, Newson RB, MacRae K, Lawrenson RA, Tyrer F (1997) Mortality from venous thromboembolism among young women in Europe: no evidence for any effect of third generation oral contraceptives. J Epidemiol Commun Health 51:630-635
82. Vessey MP (1989) Lessons learnt from epidemiology, in Michal F (ed): Safety requirements for contraceptive steroids. Cambridge University Press, Cambridge, New York, pp 148-156
83. Ministerium für Gesundheitswesen: Institut für Medizinische Statistik und Datenverarbeitung (ed): Das Gesundheitswesen der DDR. Berlin 1987-1990
84. Inman WHW, Vessey MP (1968) Investigation of deaths from pulmonary, coronary, and cerebral thrombosis and embolism in women of child-bearing age. BMJ 2:193-199
85. Vessey MP, Doll R (1969) Investigation of relation between use of oral contraceptives and thromboembolic disease. A further report. BMJ 2:651-657
86. Mann JI, Thorogood M, Water WE, Powell C (1975) Oral contraceptives and myocardial infarction in young women: A further report. BMJ 2:631-632
87. Mann JI, Doll R, Thorogood M, Vessey MP, Waters WE (1976) Risk factors for myocardial infarction in young women. Br J Preventive and Social Med 30:94-100
88. Mann JI, Inman WHW (1975) Oral contraceptives and death from myocardial infarction. BMJ 2:245-248
89. Jick H, Dinan B, Rothman KJ (1978) Oral contraceptives and non-fatal myocardial infarction. JAMA 239:1403-1406
90. Shapiro S, Slone D, Rosenberg L, Kaufman DW, Stolley PD, Miettinen OS (1979) Oral contraceptive use in relation to myocardial infarction. Lancet i:743-747
91. Rosenberg L, Hennekens CH, Rosner B, Belanger C, Rothman KJ, Speizer FE (1980) Oral contraceptive use in relation to non-fatal myocardial infarction. Am J Epidemiol 111:59-66
92. Krueger DE, Ellenberg SS, Bloom S, et al (1980) Fatal myocardial infarction and the role of oral contraceptives. Am J Epidemiol 125:832-843
93. Ramcharan S, Pelligrin FA, Ray R, Hsu J-P (1981) The Walnut Creek Contraceptive Study, in Anonymous Center for Population Research Monograph. Washington, NIH; pp 564
94. Adam SA, Thorogood M, Mann JI (1981) Oral contraception and myocardial infarction revisited: The effects of new preparations and prescribing patterns. Br J Obstet Gynaecol 88:838-845
95. Mant D, Villard-Mackintosh L, Vessey MP, Yeates D (1987) Myocardial infarction and angina pectoris in young women. J Epidemiol Commun Health 41:215-219
96. Croft P, Hannaford PC (1989) Risk factors for acute myocardial infarction in women: evidence from the Royal College of General Practitioner's oral contraception study. BMJ 298:165-168
97. Talbott E, Kuller LH, Detre K, et al (1989) Reproductive history of women dying of sudden cardiac death: A case-control study. Int J Epidemiol 18:589-594
98. D'Avanzo B, La Vecchia C, Negri E, Parazzini F, Franceschi S (1994) Oral contraceptive use and risk of myocardial infarction: an Italian case-control study. J Epidemiol Community Health 48:324-325
99. Jick H, Porter J, Rothman KJ (1978) Oral contraceptives and non-fatal stroke in healthy young women. Ann Intern Med 88:58-60
100. Chang KK, Chow LP, Rider RV (1986) Oral contraceptives and stroke: A preliminary report on an epidemiologic study in Taiwan, China. Int J Gynaecol Obstet 24:421-430
101. Oleckno WA (1986) Selected factors and stroke in young adults, 15-40 years of age. J R Soc Health 3:102-107

102. Alvarez J, Matias-Guiu J, Sumalla J, et al (1989) Ischemic stroke in young adults. I. Analysis of the etiological subgroups. Acta Neurol Scand 80:28-34
103. Carolei A, Marini C, De Matteis G (1996) History of migraine and risk of cerebral ischaemia in young adults. Lancet 347:1503-1506
104. Haapaniemi H, Hillbom M, Juvela S (1997) Lifestyle-associated risk factors for acute brain infarction among persons of working age. Stroke 28:26-30
105. Royal College of General Practitioners (1967) Oral contraception and thromboembolic disease. J Royal Coll Gen Practitioners 13:267-279
106. Sartwell PE, Masi AT, Arthes FG, Greene GR, Smith HE (1969) Thromboembolism and oral contraceptives: An epidemiologic case-control study. Am J Epidemiol 90:365-380
107. Vessey MP, Doll R, Fairbairn AS, Glober G (1970) Postoperative thromboembolism and the use of oral contraceptives. BMJ 3:123-126
108. Bottiger LE, Westerholm B (1971) Oral contraceptives and thromboembolic disease. Acta Medica Scandinavia 190:455-463
109. Green GR, Sartwell PE (1972) Oral contraceptive use in patients with thromboembolism following surgery, trauma or infection. Am J Public Health 69:680-685
110. Boston Collaborative Drug Surveillance Program (1973) Oral contraceptives and venous thromboembolic disease, surgically confirmed gall bladder disease, and breast tumours. Lancet i:1399-1404
111. Petitti DB, Wingerd J, Pellegrin F, Ramcharan S (1978) Oral contraceptives, smoking and other factors in relation to risk of venous thromboembolic disease. Am J Epidemiol 108:480-485
112. Maguire MG, Tonascia J, Sartwell PE, Stolley PD, Tockman MS (1979) Increased risk of thrombosis due to oral contraceptives: A further report. Am J Epidemiol 110:188-195
113. Porter JB, Hunter JR, Jick H, Stergachis A (1985) Oral contraceptives and nonfatal vascular disease. Obstet Gynecol 66:1-4
114. Helmrich SP, Rosenberg L, Kaufman DW, Strom B, Shapiro S (1987) Venous thromboembolism in relation to oral contraceptive use. Obstet Gynecol 69:91-95
115. WHO Collaborative Study of Cardiovascular Disease and Steroid Hormone Contraception (1988) Cardiovascular disease and use of oral contraceptives. Bulletin of the World Health Organization 67:417-423
116. Thorogood M, Mann J, Murphy M, Vessey M (1992) Risk factors for fatal venous thromboembolism in young women: A case-control study. Int J Epidemiol 21:48-52
117. Vandenbroucke JP, Koster T, Briet E, Reitsma PH, Bertina RM, Rosendaal FR (1994) Increased risk of venous thrombosis on oral-contraceptive users who are carriers of factor V Leiden mutation. Lancet 344:1453-1457
118. WHO Collaborative Study of Cardiovascular Disease and Steroid Hormone Contraception (1995) Venous thromboembolic disease and combined oral contraceptives: results of international multicentre case-control study. Lancet 346:1575-1582

6 Injectable Contraceptives

Catherine d'Arcangues, Rachel C. Snow

Introduction

An estimated 16 million women throughout the world are currently relying on injectable steroids for contraception. The choice of injectable methods includes products effective for 3 months, 2 months, or 1 month (Table 1). Although little known in Europe, these methods represent the third most prevalent form of reversible contraception worldwide. Trend estimates suggest that this number is rising, due to the reassuring World Health Organization (WHO) data regarding cancer risk, and the recent approval of the 3-monthly injectable depo medroxy-progesterone acetate (DMPA, or Depo-Provera) by the United States Federal Drug Administration (USFDA).

DMPA was developed in 1954 by the Upjohn Company for treatment of endometriosis and habitual or threatened abortions. In the early 1960s it was noted that women receiving DMPA for premature labor subsequently had a marked delay in return of fertility following delivery. This observation led to the development of DMPA as a fertility-regulating agent. In the mid-1960s, Upjohn requested a contraceptive product license for DMPA in many countries, and received approval to market it as a contraceptive in most of them. Administered as a dose of 150 mg DMPA in 1 ml aqueous suspension, the injection is given every 90 days deep into the gluteal or deltoid muscles, and one injection inhibits ovulation for at least 14 weeks. It is estimated that 13 million women are currently using DMPA, and the method is marketed in more than 90 countries worldwide.

As the 3-monthly injectable DMPA was promoted and brought to market by Upjohn, several alternative injectable contraceptive formulations were developed and underwent partial clinical evaluation. Few of these products gained widespread use other than norethisterone enanthate (NET-EN), which is given as an oily preparation intramuscularly at a dose of 200 mg every 60 days. Current users of NET-EN total approximately 1 million. The principal distinctions between DMPA and NET-EN are their durations of effectiveness and the incidence of drug-induced amenorrhea, and little else typically determines prescriptive practice. Nonetheless, given slight differences in the steroid derivation of the two drugs, experience of different side-effects with the two methods (e.g., weight gain or hirsutism), cannot be ruled out; however, most comparative data show few clinical differences other than duration of action.

The development of monthly, combined injectables actually preceded development of DMPA, with the first formulation tested in 1963 (Siegel 1963). Numerous products underwent partial development, clinical evaluation (and registration) in select countries. In the 1970s, motivated by interest in ensuring availability of an injectable that would not cause the disruption of menstrual bleeding commonly associated with

Table 1. Formulation, Injection Schedule, and Availability of Injectable Contraceptives

Formulation	Developer	Brand Name/ Manufacturer	Injection Schedule	Availability
Progestin only: 150 mg depot medroxy-progesterone acetate (DMPA)	The Upjohn Company	Depo-Provera/Upjohn Megestron/Organon	Every 3 months, 12 weeks, or 90 days	Registered in over 100 countries; available in both public and private sectors.
Progestin only: 200 mg norethindrone (norethisterone) enanthate (NET EN)	Schering AG	Noristerat[a]/Schering AG Doryxus/ Richter Gedeon Ltd.	Every 2 months[b]	Registered in over 60 countries; available in both public and private sectors.
Progestin + estrogen: 25 mg DMPA + 5 mg estradiol cypionate	Upjohn, WHO	Cyclofem/Aplicaciónes Farmaceuticas (Mexico), Upjohn (US) Cyclo Geston/PT Tunggal, PT Triyasa Nagamas Farma (Indonesia)	Every month	Registered in 18 countries; available in both public and private sectors.
Progestin + estrogen: 50 mg NET EN + 5 mg estradiol valerate	WHO	Mesigyna, Norigynon Schering AG	Every month	Registered in 35 countries.
Progestin + estrogen: 150 mg dihydroxy-progesterone acetophenide + 10 mg estradiol enanthate	Squibb Pharma-ceutical Company	Perlutan, Topasel, Agurin Horprotal, Uno-Ciclol/ Various manufacturers in Latin America	Every month	Available in pharmacies in many Latin American countries and Spain; generally not available in public family planning programs.
Half-dose: 75 mg dihydroxy-progesterone acetophenide + 5 mg estradiol enanthate		Anafertin, Yectames/ Various manufacturers in Latin America	Every month	Latin America
Progestin + estrogen: 250 mg 17α-hydroxy-progesterone caproate + 5 mg estradiol valerate	Chinese researchers; Squibb Pharmaceutical Company	Chinese Injectable No. 1	Every month, 2 injections in first month	China

[a] Called Norigest in Pakistan
[b] Alternative, less effective schedule: every 2 months for 6 months and then every 3 months
Sources: Population Reports (1995), WHO (unpub.)

DMPA and NET-EN, the Task Force on Long-acting Systemic Agents for Fertility Regulation, Special Programme of Research, Development and Research Training in Human Reproduction (HRP), WHO, undertook a review of all available combined, monthly preparations. They decided to optimize the dosage and the progestogen/ estrogen ratio of two combination formulations, Cyclofem and Mesigyna, and to oversee their clinical evaluation.

Cyclofem consists of 25 mg depot medroxyprogesterone acetate plus 5 mg estradiol cypionate, in a microcrystalline suspension in a 0.5-ml aqueous solution. Mesigyna consists of 50 mg norethisterone enanthate plus 5 mg estradiol valerate in a 1.0-ml oily solution of castor oil and benzyl benzoate, 60:40. Both preparations are given by deep, intramuscular injection into the gluteal or deltoid muscles. The first injection is given during the first 5 days after the onset of menses, or before the sixth week postpartum among women not breast-feeding. The second, and subsequent injections, are given 30±3 days from the last injection. It is estimated that approximately 1.5-2 million women currently use once-a-month injectables, mainly in Latin America and China.

Two additional monthly, combined injectable methods warrant mention. Deladroxate (commercially labelled as Perlutan, Topasel, Agurin, Horprotal and Uno-Ciclo in various countries), is a combination of 150 mg dihydroxyprogesterone acetophenide and 10 mg estradiol enanthate, and is available in many Latin American countries and Spain. The method is highly effective, without a single pregnancy reported in large clinical trials (Koetsawang 1994). Although available since the 1960s, the method has not been studied as extensively as Cyclofem or Mesigyna. The original manufacturer withdrew support due to toxicological concerns with dihydroxyprogesterone acetophenide, and clinical evaluations continue to be published. A recent dose-finding trial compared the standard available dose of 150/10 with a lower dose of 90/6, and concluded the lower dose was equally effective (Coutinho et al. 1997).

Chinese Injectable No. 1, consisting of 250 mg 17-hydroxyprogesterone caproate and 5 mg estradiol valerate in an oily solution, is widely available in China. A comparative phase-III trial of Chinese Injection No.1, Cyclofem, and Mesigyna was conducted in China in collaboration with the WHO in the late 1980s (Sang, Shao, Ge et al. 1995). The monthly injection schedule (30±3 days) of Chinese Injecatble No. 1 was aborted when it was noted that this schedule was associated with an unacceptably high failure rate. Thereafter, the injection schedule was modified to a different schedule currently in use in China. Two initial injections are administered 10 days apart, and then subsequent injections are administered either 10-12 days following the next menstrual bleed, or 28 days following the last injection if no bleeding has occurred. The modified injection schedule is associated with a failure rate of 0.8 pregnancies per 100 woman-years (Sang, Shao, Ge et al. 1995). Informal reports suggest that use of this injection is declining in China, as alternative methods are promoted by the State Family Planning Commission. The method is also found in neighboring countries, such as Myanmar and Cambodia, but is perceived to have a high failure rate (Sadana, forthcoming), possibly due to difficulties maintaining the injection schedule required for optimal effectiveness.

Pharmacokinetic and Pharmacodynamic Features

Following a first injection of DMPA, MPA levels are at maximum concentration within the first three weeks (5-22 days) post-injection, at 15-26 nmol/l, decreasing to <1.0 nmol/l in the majority of women by 90-190 days post-injection (Garza-Flores

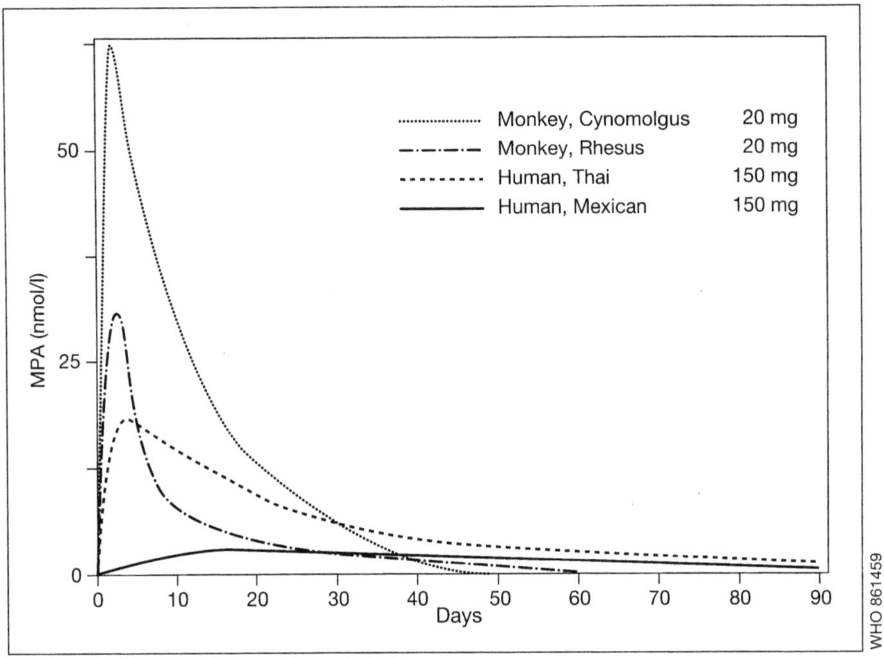

Fig. 1. MPA levels in the circulation of the rhesus and cynomolgus monkeys after a single dose of 20 mg DMPA and in Mexican and Thai women after a single dose of 150 mg DMPA.

1994) (Fig. 1). NET-EN levels fall more rapidly than MPA, falling below detectable levels in most women within 46-110 days after injection.

Ethnic variations in the pharmacokinetic pattern with DMPA have been reported from multi-center trials in different regions (Garza-Flores et al. 1994; Fotherby et al. 1980). A particularly rapid absorption and metabolism of DMPA has been noted among Thais, with high Cmax values followed by rapid elimination half-lives (Garza-Flores 1994). A comparatively slower absorption of DMPA has been observed among Mexicans, with blood levels an order of magnitude lower than some Thai women, and measurable concentrations of MPA observed 6 months after injection (Garza-Flores et al. 1994); limited available data from other ethnic groups suggest pharmacokinetic values between these two extremes.

Pharmacokinetic and dynamic studies of the monthly injectables Cyclofem and Mesigyna were conducted in Stockholm (Aedo et al. 1985). Among users of Cyclofem the mean Cmax of medroxyprogesterone acetate was 2.9(2.4-3.7) nmol/l decreasing to 0.72(0.46-1.1) nmol/l 30 days after the last injection. Among users of Mesigyna, the mean maximum norethisterone levels were 10.1(6.4-15.8) nmol/l decreasing to 1.7(1.2-2.3) nmol/l 30 days after the last injection. From the schematic representation of the pharmacokinetic and pharmacodynamic profile of these preparations (Fig. 2), the biphasic nature of the steroid profile can be seen. Following the first injection a "combined phase" is characterized by a rise in progestogen and estrogen levels; when the estrogen level decreases approximately 2 weeks later, there is a "progestogen-dominated" second phase.

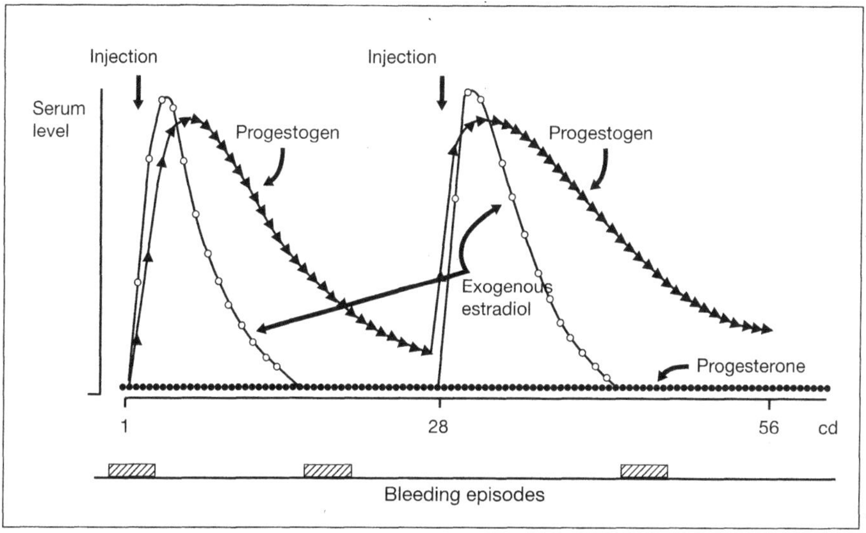

Fig. 2. Idealized pharmacokinetic/pharmacodynamic profile of a typical estrogen/progestogen monthly injectable contraceptive. Adapted from: Fraser and Diczfalusy, 1980

A prospective pharmacokinetic study of 17 Chinese women was designed to evaluate whether there was any measurable month-to-month accumulation of NET in the body during use of Mesigyna. NET concentrations in serum and saliva were measured after the 1st, 6th, and 12th monthly injection The mean peak concentrations of NET were 8.1 ng/ml, 6.6 ng/ml and 5.7 ng/ml, and the AUC's1-28 were 96.6 ng/ml-1/day, 84.6 ng/ml-1/day and 77.3 ng/ml-1/day, respectively. These data affirm that there is no accumulation of NET over 6 months or 12 months of treatment with Mesigyna (Sang 1994). Unpublished data on the pharmacokinetics of Cyclofem indicate a measurable month-to-month accumulation of MPA that continues for up to 6 months, and then levels off (Sang Guo-Wei, unpublished). Both studies were conducted in Chinese women, and no similar data have been collected elsewhere. The latter observation is consistent with evidence from efficacy trials (discussed below), that the few pregnancies recorded with Cyclofem have occurred in the first several months of use.

Effectiveness

Current formulations of injectable contraceptives are highly effective. One injection of DMPA inhibits ovulation for 14 weeks, suppressing both FSH and LH. Cervical mucus is thickened, decreasing sperm penetration, the endometrium is atrophied with inactive glands, and there is decreased tubal motility. Pregnancies due to method failure are consistently low, with cumulative life-table rates of 0-0.1 percent at 12 months.

NET-EN is also highly effective. When given at 60-day intervals, the cumulative life-table rates are 0.4% at 12 months, and 0.4% at 24 months.

Likewise, cumulative life-table pregnancy rates with Cyclofem and Mesigyna are between 0.0 and 0.2 at 12 months (WHO 1988b). In large, multi-center trials coordinated by the WHO, including more than 9000 women, all of the 13 pregnancies which occurred took place during the first few injection cycles, and no pregnancy occurred after the sixth injection (Koetsawang 1994).

Return of Ovulation

The return of ovulation following discontinuation of DMPA occurs approximately 5 months after the expected effect of the last injection, but the variance extends over several months. In a study of 14 women in Mexico with a duration of treatment lasting 1.2 to 5.0 years, the return of ovulation was 5.5 ± 1.9 months ($x \pm sd$) after the expected effect of the last injection (Garza-Flores et al. 1985). The time to return of ovulation did not appear to vary with the duration of use, or with body mass index.

In the majority of women, ovulation does not occur as long as plasma levels of MPA are above 100 pg/ml (Ortiz et al. 1977). The return of ovulation occurs promptly thereafter, and individual variations in the return of ovulation appear to coincide largely with differences in metabolic clearance. In a pharmacodynamic study among Thai women, it was found that after a single dose of MPA (150 mg), eight subjects had varying times to return of ovulation (20-21 weeks in one subject, at sometime between 25 weeks and 33 weeks among four subjects, and not before 33 weeks in three subjects). However, the variance in the return of ovulation coincided with plasma concentrations of MPA. Seven of eight women had a return of ovulation only when MPA levels were no longer detectable; in one subject, ovulation occurred in the presence of very low, but detectable, levels of MPA (Lan et al. 1984).

It should be noted, however, that a small comparative study of ovarian function following DMPA injection in India and Sweden reported that Indian women had a return of luteal function in the presence of higher doses (MPA>600 pg/ml) (Fotherby 1980).

When DMPA and NET-EN have been compared in the same population, with a common method for detecting ovulation, the 2-month injectable noresthisterone enanthate (NET-EN) has a comparatively shorter time for the return of ovulation, relative to DMPA (Garza-Flores et al. 1985). The comparative study among 24 Mexican women reported a more rapid re-establishment of menses following NET-EN than after DMPA, and an earlier return of ovulation (Fig. 3).

Data on the return of ovulation following use of Cyclofem and Mesigyna are limited, but available data indicate that it is more rapid than after use of DMPA or NET-EN. Three separate studies evaluated the return of ovulation after a Cyclofem treatment interval of three injections. In the second cycle after treatment, the authors reported that 55%, 88% and 71% of women, respectively, had ovulatory cycles (Fotherby et al. 1982; Aedo et al. 1985; WHO 1988b). In two similar studies following three injections of Mesigyna, 86% and 67% of women were ovulatory in the second cycle posttreatment (Aedo et al 1985; WHO 1988b). In a separate study among women who had used monthly injectables for 2 years, 60% of Cyclofem users, and 55% of Mesigyna users, ovulated at least once in the 90 days following treatment (see Bassol and Garza-Flores 1994).

In a small study (n=7) following the use of Delodrexate (in a 150/10 combination) for 1-2 years, ovulation returned within 60-90 days among all seven women. Among 16 women evaluated after at least 2 years of Delodrexate use, all returned to spontaneous ovulation 12-42 weeks after treatment (see Bassol and Garza-Flores 1994).

Return of Fertility

The return of fertility after DMPA use coincides with data on the return of ovulation: approximately 5 months. The largest prospective study followed 796 Thai users of DMPA who stopped using the method to have a planned pregnancy, and reported a median time to conception of 5.5 months after the expected effect of the last injection (Pardthaisong 1984). The same study included 427 women who stopped using oral contraceptives, and 125 women who had an IUD removed. The median time to conception after these methods was 3 months, and 4.5 months, respectively. An earlier life table analysis of 135 Thai women aged 18-37 years, who had discontinued DMPA, showed a cumulative pregnancy rate of 76.8% at 12 months (McDaniel and Pardthaisong 1973). When confined to 80 women, 18-25 years of age, the cumulative pregnancy rate was slightly higher (78.4%) at 12 months.

Among 69 Indian women discontinuing DMPA in order to plan a pregnancy, the cumulative conception rate at 12 months was 72.5% (ICMR, 1986), a value only slightly lower than that observed for DMPA among Thai women (McDaniel and Pardtheisong 1973).

Studies of the return of fertility after NET-EN suggest values closer to DMPA. A prospective follow-up of 69 women who had used NET-EN for a minimum of six

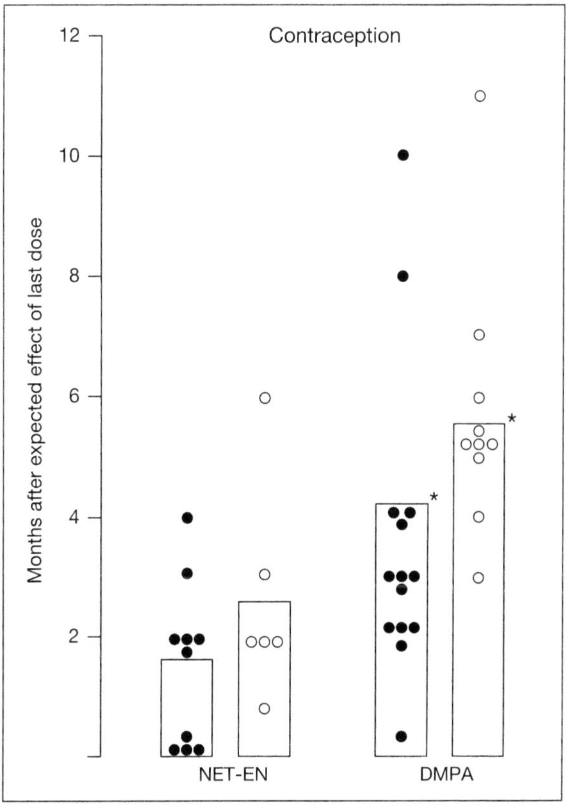

Fig. 3. Return to menstruation (dark circles) and return to ovulation (clear circles) after norethisterone enanthate (NET-EN) or depo-medroxyprogesterone acetate (DMPA), *$p<0.001$ when the two injectables were compared.
Ref: Garza-Flores et al. 1985

Fig. 4a. Cumulative conception rates in subjects who discontinued the method due to amenorrhoea. Ref: Saxena et al. 1986

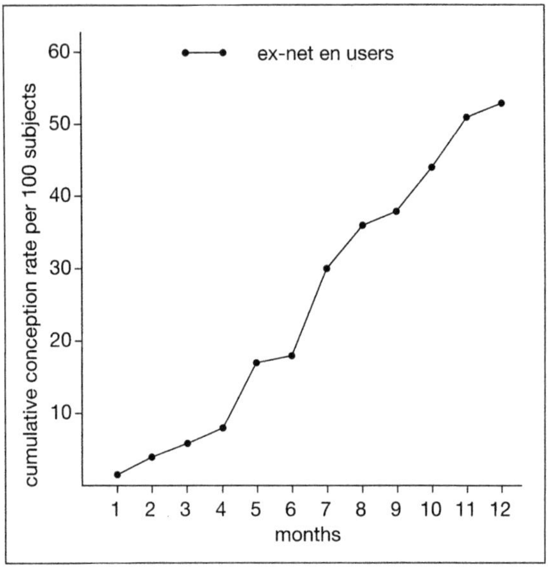

Fig. 4b. Cumulative conception rates in subjects who discontinued the method due to excessive bleeding.
Ref: Saxena et al. 1986

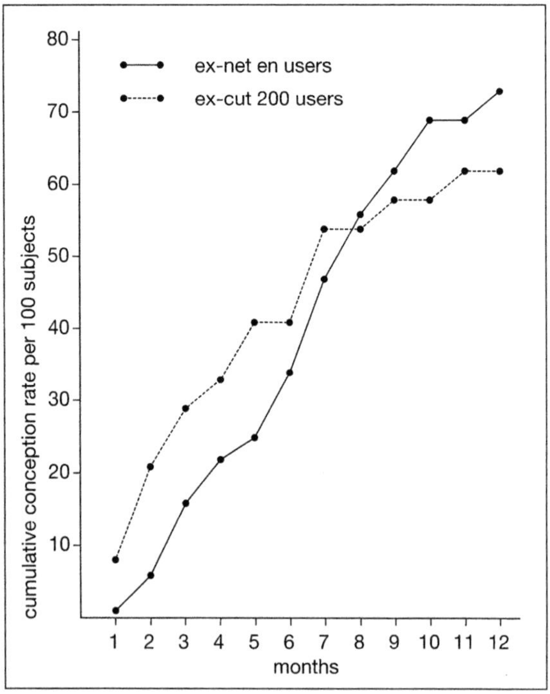

months reported a cumulative conception rate of 72.5 percent at 12 months (ICMR, 1986). However, the median time to conception was 7.8 months, longer than might be expected from data on the return of ovulation (i.e., 2.6 months) reported among Mexican women (Garza-Flores et al. 1985).

Individual and regional variations in the time to return of fertility after DMPA and NET-EN use are noteworthy; variances on the mean time until return of fertility are wide, and regional reports differ significantly. A retrospective review of clinical data on 363 Australian women suggested a mean interval from the end of the effective dose of DMPA to conception of 10.8 months (sd 9.7 months, median 9.2 months) (Fraser and Dennerstein, 1994), an interval twice as long as that reported from Thailand (Pardtheisong 1973). Regional differences may reflect underlying differences in the fecundability of different population groups (due to infection or cohort effects), differences in client motivation to conceive, or more fundamental differences in pharmacokinetics.

A study at the ICMR in India reported large differences in the cumulative pregnancy rates of ex-NET-EN users, when dividing them by bleeding experience while using the methods (ICMR 1986). Women discontinuing because of amenorrhea had a significantly slower cumulative conception rate over the ensuing 12 months (Fig. 4), relative to women who discontinued because of excessive bleeding. The 12-month conception rate for women discontinuing due to amenorrhea was 51%, compared with 73.5% among women who discontinued due to excessive bleeding.

The return of fertility following monthly injectables is considerably shorter than that observed for the progestogen-only injectables. Bahamondes et al (1997) reported observations on 70 Latin American women who had used between 1 and 19 injections of Cyclofem and discontinued to become pregnant. More than 50% were pregnant at 6 months, and the cumulative pregnancy rate was 82.9% at 12 months (Fig. 5). Return

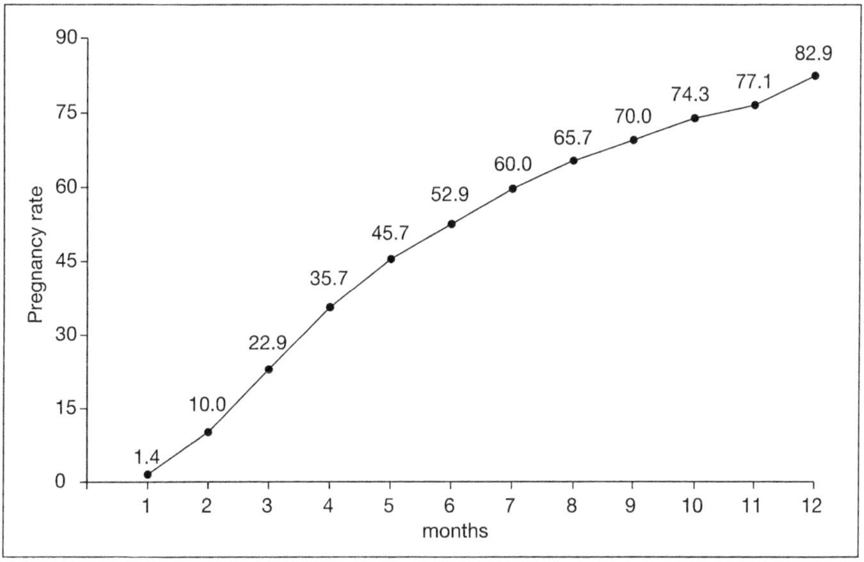

Fig. 5. Cumulative pregnancy rate up to 12 months after discontinuation of Cyclofem.
Ref: Bahamondes et al, Contraception 1997; 55:307-10

Table 2. Proportions (%) of Women Experiencing Different Types of Bleeding Patterns

Group	Days	Number of Diaries	Amenorrhea	Infrequent Bleeding	Frequent Bleeding	Irregular Bleeding	Prolonged Bleeding	Variations from Regular Patterns (total)	Regular Pattern
Untreated	1-90	3893	1.3	3.4	0.2	4.5	2.6	9.7	90.3
	91-180	3893	1.5	2.9	0.3	4.8	2.3	9.2	90.8
	181-270	3893	1.3	2.8	0.1	5.4	2.6	9.9	90.1
	271-360	3893	1.6	3.1	0.3	8.6	4.3	14.9	85.1
Cyclofem	1-90	1001	0.1	0.1	22.3	39.6	20.8	57.0	43.0
	91-180	885	0.2	3.4	3.3	23.5	13.3	36.8	63.2
	181-270	802	1.1	5.4	2.8	25.4	9.4	38.7	61.3
	271-360	730	2.3	3.7	6.5	13.6	10.1	30.0	70.0
Mesigyna	1-90	1000	0.2	0.1	29.6	34.6	16.2	52.8	47.2
	91-180	860	0.6	2.2	5.5	25.2	11.1	37.2	62.8
	181-270	766	1.3	2.9	4.9	24.8	12.6	36.7	63.3
	271-360	713	2.0	5.0	6.2	14.6	12.7	31.6	68.4
DMPA	1-90	509	10.6	15.7	17.7	46.0	43.4	91.0	9.0
	91-180	406	23.9	25.8	10.5	35.7	27.7	93.1	6.9
	181-270	311	37.0	24.8	8.3	27.7	17.3	93.6	6.4
	271-360	241	38.6	27.8	6.6	17.9	16.5	91.7	8.3

Ref.: Fraser IS. Contraception 1994; 49:399-420

of fertility was not related to a woman's age, weight, or the number of Cyclofem injections. Among 19 women discontinuing use of Mesigyna to become pregnant, the cumulative pregnancy rate at 3 months was 100% (Sang, 1983). Keifer et al. reported that among 17 subjects who discontinued use of Delodrexate (150/10) to become pregnant, all conceived between 3 months and 36 months (see Bassol and Garza-Flores 1994).

Women's Experience of the Methods

Irregularities in Vaginal Bleeding

The main side effect that women experience with injectable contraceptives is a disruption of their regular menstrual pattern. This is particularly the case with progestogen-only contraceptives, which induce an unpredictable pattern with episodes of prolonged and heavy bleeding, mostly during the first months of use. With DMPA, long periods of amenorrhea become increasingly frequent with continued use.

To illustrate these irregularities, the analysis of menstrual diaries from first year users of Cyclofem, Mesigyna and DMPA is shown in Table 2, in comparison with those of women using no method of contraception (Fraser 1994). During the first 3 months of DMPA use, close to half of the users experience irregular and prolonged bleeding. With continued use, these patterns become less frequent, while an increasing number of women experience infrequent bleeding or even complete amenorrhea. A similar trend is noted with the use of NET-EN, although the incidence of amenorrhea is not as high with this method.

As noted above, monthly combined injectables were developed to offer an alternative to women who could not tolerate such irregularities in their bleeding pattern. Following the first injection of these methods, both estrogen and progestogen levels rise. When the estrogen level decreases, i.e., approximately 2 weeks later (depending on the estrogen ester), a bleeding episode occurs which reflects this estrogen withdrawal. With monthly administration of the preparation, this phenomenon recurs on a monthly basis, giving the woman the experience of a first short cycle followed by regular monthly cycles. Data from multicenter studies (Table 2) (Fraser 1994) show that, with Cyclofem and Mesigyna, indeed two-thirds of the women will experience a regular monthly bleeding episode once the bleeding pattern is established. One-third will experience irregular or prolonged bleeding.

It has been shown that even with progestin-only methods, the amount of blood loss is not a problem. In fact, the volume of blood loss is decreased compared with that measured during the natural untreated cycle, and anemia is not a significant risk associated with use of these methods. However, women do not tolerate the irregularity and unpredictability in vaginal bleeding which these methods induce.

Many women regard regular menses as the "pulse" of their reproductive health, indicative of their fertility and pregnancy status, and they associate an irregular menstrual pattern with ill-health. In addition, their menstrual pattern has sexual, socio-cultural, economic and sometimes religious implications, which make it an important factor affecting their everyday lives. It is, thus, not surprising that women

Table 3. A survey of different approaches to management of menstrual disturbances in women using injectable contraceptives (Fraser, 1994)

Regimens used for the management of prolonged or frequent light bleeding during use of injectable contraceptives	Regimens used for the management of prolonged amenorrhea occuring with injectable contraceptives
1. Counselling only: widely used in most centres	1. Counselling only: almost all centres (ideally with abdominal and vaginal examination although this may not be easy in some cultures)
2. Medical, including vaginal examination: If indicated; most centres.	2. Urinary or serum pregnancy test: in selected cases
3. Early repeat contraceptive injection: several centres give next injection earlier than 90 days when troublesome bleeding occurs in DMPA users. One entre tries oral MPA 5 mg daily for 14 days in obese patients and if this works gives next DMPA injection early	3. One or two short courses of "oestrogen": if greatly prolonged amenorrhea and patient unduly concerned 3.1 Combined oral contraceptive pill for one "cycle", i.e. 21 days 3.2 Ethinyl oestradiol 20-50 µg daily for 10-21 days 3.3 Premarin (conjugated equine oestrogens) 2.5 mg daily for 10 days 3.4 Progynova (oestradiol valerate) 1 mg daily for 10-14 days 3.5 Oestradiol cyplonate 5 mg by intramuscular injection
4. One or more short courses of: "oestrogen": sometimes advised 4.1 Various combined oral contraceptive pills given in different regimes: for example: 4.1.1 One tablet daily for 14-21 days 4.1.2 Two-three tablets daily until bleeding stops then one daily for further 14 days. 4.2 Ethinyl oestradiol 50 µg daily for 7-21 days 4.3 Premarin (conjugated equine oestrogens) 1.25-5 mg daily for 7-21 days 4.4 Stilboestrol 0.5 to 1 mg daily for 5-21 days 4.5 Oestradiol cypionate 5 mg by intramuscular injection 4.6 These treatments were usually only advised for one treatment course	4. Cyclical supplement oral oestrogen: Any one of above regimens (3.1 to 3.4) daily for 5-21 days out of each month; previously used in several centres but no longer used as a routine in any centres. Still used very occasionally in individual cases in a few centres.
5. Supplements and placebos: 5.1 Iron supplements, usually oral 5.2 Vitamins C and K, multivitamin preparations 5.3 Calcium tablets 5.4 Diazepam 2 to 5 mg daily 5.5 Bed rest	
6. Diagnostic curretage: for further investigation of persistent bleeding. Very rarely needed and most clinicians had never needed to use it. More often mentioned when women were over age 35 to 40 or were very long-term users of injectable contraceptives.	

do not easily tolerate disruptions of their menstrual patterns, and that menstrual disturbances are the main medical reason why women discontinue the use of injectable contraceptives (d'Arcangues et al. 1992).

Various modalities are used by clinicians to alleviate the problem of menstrual disturbances, but few of those have been tested in placebo-controlled clinical trials. In 1983, Fraser published a survey of known practices adopted in 20 countries worldwide for the management of menstrual disturbances in women using injectable contraceptives. These findings are still valid, and the mere variety of approaches (summarized in Table 3) testifies to the lack of consensus, and of firm data available.

One placebo-controlled randomized clinical trial (WHO 1996b) was conducted to compare the effects of a 14-day treatment with either 50 μg ethinyl estradiol daily or 2.5 mg estrone sulfate daily, on DMPA-induced prolonged bleeding. Treatment with ethinyl estradiol was successful in stopping the bleeding episode in 93% of cases, compared with estrone sulfate and placebo, which had success rates of 76% and 74%, respectively. However, immediately after treatment, women given ethinyl estradiol had less bleeding but a more unpredictable pattern than the other two groups. Thus, treatment of DMPA-induced prolonged bleeding with ethinyl estradiol had a short-term effect, but no beneficial effect on the acceptability of DMPA as a contraceptive method, and treatment with estrone sulfate was no different from placebo.

Amenorrhea itself is not well tolerated by some women as it gives them doubt about their fertility and their pregnancy status (Guzman-Garcia et al. 1997). A study (Piya-Anant 1998) was conducted among amenorrheic DMPA users to test the effect of switching to the monthly injectable Cyclofem. It showed that this approach will induce vaginal bleeding in 80% of women within 6 months. This approach has the benefits that a woman continues with a similar mode of contraception (i.e., injection), while the steroid load is actually reduced [3 x 25 mg vs 150 mg of DMPA for 3 months]; the traditional approach would have been to add supplemental oral estrogen to DMPA treatment (refer to Table 3).

Phase-I studies clearly demonstrated that the efficacy of once-a-month injectables was dependent on the estrogen/progestogen ratio (Garza-Flores et al. 1991). In particular, ovulation was no longer inhibited if the dose of estrogen was increased. Thus, it is not recommended to treat vaginal bleeding disturbances experienced by users of combined injectables with steroid hormones. Non-steroidal agents may be helpful, although their effectiveness has not been tested in controlled clinical trials.

Changes in Body Weight

A majority of women using DMPA gain body weight while using the method. Product information provided by the Upjohn Company (manufacturer of DMPA) describes average weight gain of 2.5 kg after 1 year of use (Product Information 1994). An early collaborative study of DMPA use among 3857 women in the USA reported a mean weight gain of approximately 2.3 kg after 1 year, 3.7 kg after 2 years, and 6.3 kg after 4 years (Schwallie and Assenzo 1973). Another early trial among 138 women in Calcutta reported mean weight gains above 4.0 kg at 1 year, and above 6.0 kg at 2 years (Mukherjee et al. 1980). A more recent WHO multicentre phase-III clinical trial of DMPA reported a mean weight gain of 1.5 kg per year (WHO 1986).

A study of NET-EN users after 1 year of use reported an average weight gain of 5.0 kg among 20% of clients, and an average weight loss of 5 kg among 15% (Howard et al. 1985).

Slight increases in body weight have been reported with use of both Mesigyna and Cyclofem in phase-III trials (Koetsawang 1994). In a 3-year clinical trial of Mesigyna, one-third of clients gained 3-8 kgs (Kesseru et al. 1994). In a multi-country study of Cyclofem from Indonesia, Jamaica, Thailand, and Tunisia, cumulative 12-month discontinuation rates for weight gain were only 4% in Thailand, and from less than 1.0% to 2.5% in the other three research sites (Hall et WHO 1994).

Women's Perspectives

The principal patient complaint with DMPA and NET-EN is disruption of menstrual bleeding. DMPA has the highest discontinuation rate among modern, highly-effective contraceptives, and dissatisfaction with changes in menstrual bleeding is the most common method-related reason for discontinuation (d'Arcangues et al. 1992); this observation holds across different countries and ethnic groups.

Pretreatment counseling regarding expected side-effects with DMPA increases continuation rates (possibly by increasing tolerance for abnormal bleeding). A recent pre-DMPA counseling intervention trial in China reported 12-month discontinuation rates of only 11%, compared with 42% without counseling (Lei et al. 1996).

While Cyclofem and Mesigyna provide better menstrual cycle control than DMPA, abnormal bleeding is still the main drug-related complaint with these methods, and the principal reason for discontinuation.

Headaches, mood changes and decreased libido have each been documented in association with DMPA use, but with wide variations in the frequency of reporting across different studies. A retrospective study of 363 women using DMPA in Australia reported sexual difficulties (loss of interest, dry vagina, dyspareunia), to be the third most important method-related side effect leading to discontinuation (after bleeding and headaches), and the principal complaint cited by women (43%) continuing with the method (Fraser and Dennerstein 1994).

In a large clinical trial in Egypt, 10 percent of continuers, and 24 percent of women discontinuing Cyclofem and Mesigyna (and 10 percent of those continuing) reported daily headaches (Hassan et al. 1994). In the same study 91 percent of continuers, and 91 percent of discontinuers reported no changes in libido with Cyclofem or Mesigyna.

Qualitative data on women's attitudes to injectable contraceptives underscore users' appreciation of the high method effectiveness, the possibility of using these methods secretly (the lack of paraphernalia), and the chance to use these methods for discrete intervals of protection (Guzman-Garcia 1997; Snow et al. 1997; Bledsoe et al. 1994). Women's discontent over the disruption of menstrual bleeding associated with these methods is a significant limitation; additional perceived negative attributes include the failure to have a rapid and predictable return of fertility after discontinuation, the lack of protection provided against STDs, the potential for provider abuse, and the lack of user-controlled reversibility within the injection interval (Guzman-Garcia et al. 1997; Snow et al. 1997).

Clinical Eligibility and Safety

Medical Eligibility Criteria

Current knowledge on injectable contraceptives justifies the use of these methods by many women. However, use is contraindicated for women with specific illnesses or conditions, and there are important differences in the suitability of progestogen-only preparations and combined methods. In 1994 and 1995, WHO convened two meetings of experts to review the medical eligibility criteria of the most widely used contraceptive methods. Their recommendations were published the following year (WHO 1996a) and those relevant to injectable contraception are summarized in Table 4.

The basis for the WHO recommendations was: (a) indirect evidence or theoretical concern based on studies on suitable animal models, laboratory studies on humans, or analogous situations; (b) evidence derived from effects of the contraceptive method on women without the condition; and (c) evidence based on direct studies or observations of the contraceptive method on women with the condition. For combined injectables, there is little epidemiological data on their long-term effects as they have been introduced only recently. Thus, until such data become available, their suitability in the presence of severe pathologies was assessed conservatively, by analogy with combined oral contraceptive preparations.

Conditions affecting eligibility for the use of each contraceptive method were classified under one of the following four categories:

1. A condition for which there is no restriction for the use of the contraceptive method
2. A condition where the advantages of using the method generally outweigh the theoretical or proven risks
3. A condition where the theoretical or proven risks usually outweigh the advantages of using the method
4. A condition which represents an unacceptable health risk if the contraceptive method is used

These eligibility criteria were reviewed both to consider the initiation of use of a contraceptive method and also its continuation in case a medical condition develops during use of the method. When the criteria for these two situations differ and lead to different classification, these are indicated under "I" for initiation and "C" for continuation.

Cancer

DMPA exerts a protective effect against the risk of endometrial cancer. A collaborative hospital-based case-control study in 11 countries, coordinated by the WHO, reported an overall relative risk of 0.2 (95% confidence interval 0.1–0.8) (WHO 1991b). This protective effect appears similar, or even greater, than that associated with combined oral contraceptives, and the protective effect continues for at least 8 years after discontinuation of DMPA.

There is no epidemiological evidence of an association between DMPA use and the risk of ovarian cancer (Lumbiganon 1994), or between DMPA use and the risk of cervical cancer (La Vecchia 1994).

Table 4. WHO Eligibility Classification for use of progestin only (DMPA and NET-EN) and combined injectable contraceptives by key health condition. Ref: WHO 1996a

		DMPA & NET-EN	Combined injectables
Age	• menarche to 16 years	2	1
	• 16-40 years	1	1
	• ≥ 40 years	1	1
Obesity		1	1
Smoking	• age < 35 years	1	2
	• age ≥ 35 years, light	1	2
	• age ≥ 35 years, heavy (> 20 cigarettes/day)	1	3
Parity	• any	1	1
Pregnancy		4	4
History of pre-eclampsia		1	1
Past ectopic pregnancy		1	1
Breast feeding	• < 6 weeks post-partum	3	4
	• 6 weeks to 6 month post-partum	1	3
	• ≥ 6 months post-partum	1	2
Post partum (in non-breast-feeding women)	• < 21 days	1	3
	• ≥ 21 days	1	1
Post abortion	(first trimester, second trimester, post-septic abortion)	1	1
Vaginal bleeding patterns		I C	I C
	• irregular pattern without heavy bleeding	1 2	1 1
	• with heavy or prolonged bleeding (including regular patterns)	2 2	1 1
Unexplained vaginal bleeding (suspicious for serious underlying condition) - before evaluation		4 2	3 2
Severe dysmenorrhea		1	1
Breast disease	• undiagnosed mass	2	2
	• benign brest disease	1	1
	• family history of breast cancer	4	4
	• cancer – past and no evidence of current disease (5 years disease-free interval)	3	3
Cervical intraepithelial neoplasia (CIN)		2	2
Cervical cancer (awaiting treatment)		2	2
Cervical ectropion		1	1
Benign ovarian tumours		1	1
Endometrial, ovarian cancer		1	1
Uterine fibroids		1	1
Endometriosis		1	1
Trophoblast disease (benign or malignant)		1	1
Prior pelvic surgery		1	1
Pelvic inflammatory disease (current or past, with or without subsequent pregnancy)		1	1
STDs (at increased risk, current or recent disease)		1	1
HIV/AIDS (high risk of HIV, HIV positive, AIDS)		1	1
Hypertension	• history of - (where blood presure cannot be evaluated)	2	3
	• mild (140-159/90-99)	2	2
	• moderate (160-179/100-109)	2	3
	• severe (180+/110+)	3	4
	• vascular disease	3	4

Table 4. Continued

		DMPA & NET-EN	Combined injectables
Deep Venous Thrombosis (DVT)/Pulmonary Embolism (PE)	• history of DVT/PE	1	4
	• current DVT/PE	1	4
	• major surgery with prolonged immobilization	1	4
	• major surgery without prolonged immobilization	1	2
	• minor surgery without immobilization	1	1
Superficial venous thrombosis	• varicose veins	1	1
	• superficial thrombophlebitis	1	2
Ischemic heart disease (current or history of -)		3	4
Stroke (history of cerebro-vascular accident)		3	4
Known hyperlipidemias		2	2/3
Valvular heart disease	• uncomplicated	1	2
	• complicated (pulmonary hypertension, risk of atrial fibrillation, history of sub-acute bacterial endocarditis)	1	4
Headaches		I C	
	• mild	1 1	1
	• severe: recurrent, including migraine:		
	without focal neurologic symptomes	2 2	2
	with focal neurologic symptoms	2 3	4
Diabetes	• hx of gestational disease	1	1
	• non-vascular disease, non insulin dependent	2	2
	• nephropathy/retinopathy/neuropathy	3	3/4
	• other vascular disease or diabetes of > 20 years' duration	3	3/4
Biliary tract disease (current or treated, asymptomatic)		1	2
History of cholestasis	• pregnancy-related	1	2
	• past combined oral contraceptive-related	2	2
Viral Hepatitis	• active	3	3/4
	• carrier	1	1
Cirrhosis	• mild (compensated)	2	2
	• severe (decompensated)	3	3
Liver Tumours	• benign (adenoma)	3	3
	• malignant (hepatoma)	3	3/4
Thyroid disease	• (simple goitre, hypothyroidism, hyperthyroidism)	1	1
Sickle cell disease		1	2
Iron deficiency anemia		1	1
Thalassemia		1	2
Epilepsy		1	1
Schistosomiasis (any stage)		1	1
Malaria		1	1
Tuberculosis		1	1
Drug interactions	• commonly used drugs with affect liver enzymes		
	- antibiotics (griseofulvin, rifampicin)	2	3
	- anticonvulsants (phenytoin, carbamazeptine, barbiturates, primadone)	2	3
	• other antibiotics (excluding griseofulvin and rifampicin)	1	1

Several recent publications have contributed substantially to our understanding of the breast cancer risk associated with use of DMPA. A study coordinated by the WHO in Kenya, Thailand, and Mexico (WHO 1991a), and a second conducted in New Zealand (Paul et al. 1989) have provided convincing evidence that there is no overall risk of breast cancer with DMPA. However, both studies reported a small elevated relative risk in certain sub-groups. Current or recent use of DMPA, and women less than age 35 years at the time of cancer diagnosis, each showed a slight increased risk of breast cancer.

As both of the above studies shared similar designs and methodologies, yet each alone lacked the statistical power to adequately substantiate and interpret the observed risk for these sub-groups, data from the two studies were combined for a pooled analysis (Skegg et al. 1995). The conclusion of the pooled analysis was that current or recent use of DMPA was the key factor associated with the increased risk observed in both sub-groups, and women who had started using DMPA within the previous 5 years were estimated to have a relative risk of 2.0 (95% confidence interval,1.5-2.8). It was concluded that the increased risk previously observed for women diagnosed under the age of 35 years was probably due to the fact that younger women were more likely to have used DMPA recently.

Limited epidemiological data are available regarding the cancer risk associated with monthly, combined injectables. In a small retrospective study reviewing contraceptive histories of 267 women with breast cancer, and 1520 controls, the relative risk of breast cancer among users of monthly injectables was 0.83 (95% CI 0.46-1.5) (Asham 1990).

While early reports from Chile suggested an increased risk of invasive cervical cancer with monthly injectable use, further data from both Chile and Mexico did not support such an association. A further study in Latin America noted that users of injectable contraceptives (55% monthly, 43% 3-monthly) tended to have fewer sexual partners and initiated sexual life at a later age than non-users. Adjusting for these factors, the overall relative risk of cervical cancer among women who had used injectables was 0.8 (95% CI 0.5-1.2). However, women who had used injectables for at least 5 years had a relative risk of 2.4 (95% CI 1.0-5.7) (Herrero et al. 1990). These data are not conclusive, but underscore the need for further study.

Chronic parenteral toxicity studies of Cyclofem for 24 months in monkeys reported Cyclofem was nontoxic, hormonally active, and noncarcinogenic at all doses including 50 times the human dose (Cooksen 1994).

Metabolic Effects

DMPA and NET-EN have minimal effects on most metabolic parameters. Lipid changes are minor and without clinical significance. Following a first injection of DMPA, there is a decline in fasting triglyceride and cholesterol levels, with a rapid return to pretreatment levels at the end of the injection interval (Amatayakul et al. 1980). Most studies of DMPA and NET-EN find slightly higher levels of LDL-cholesterol and lower levels of HDL-cholesterol. In a multi-center study, 50 women who had used DMPA for 3-9 years were compared with 120 users of IUDs. Findings differed among centers, but consistently noted unfavorable changes of moderate magnitude (WHO 1993). No significant changes in liver metabolism have been observed (Fotherby 1980;

Amatayakul et al. 1980), nor are there any measurable effects on blood pressure or coagulation factors.

Likewise, most studies of monthly, combined injectables find minimal metabolic effects. Multi-center studies of lipid effects (UNDP/UNFPA/WHO/World Bank 1997) indicate slight changes without clinical significance, and the observed changes revert to baseline promptly after method discontinuation. The observed changes in lipids were biphasic: during the combined phase, HDL cholesterol and apolipoprotein A were increased, while LDL cholesterol and apolipoprotein B were decreased. In the second "progestogen-dominated" phase of the injection interval, these trends reversed.

No significant effects on blood pressure, blood coagulation or liver function have been found with use of monthly, combined injectables. In a multi-country study of liver function among users of Mesigyna and Cyclofem, the WHO found that both injectables caused a small increase in bilirubin, but values remained within the normal range. A small reduction in alkaline phosphatase was also within the normal clinical range, and there were no measurable changes in liver enzymes (UNDP/UNFPA/WHO/World Bank 1998).

Changes in Glucose Dynamics

DMPA use is associated with a significant, albeit small, shift in the insulin response curve to an oral glucose challenge (Spellacy 1974; Vermeulen and Thiery 1974). There is a significant rise in both glucose and insulin values in response to glucose challenge, and an increase in the insulin to glucose ratio, suggesting mild insulin resistance. Clinicians agree that these changes do not indicate a risk of inducing diabetes in normal women, but the method is contra-indicated for women with diabetes.

Data on the association between Cyclofem or Mesigyna and carbohydrate metabolism indicate only minor changes in glucose tolerance, with minimal changes in insulin response to an oral glucose challenge. These changes were numerically larger with Mesigyna, but were judged to be of no clinical significance for either injectable (UNDP/UNFPA/WHO/World Bank 1998).

Exposure in Utero

Despite the high efficacy of progestin-only injectables, exposure of infants to these drugs in utero occurs, when the first injection is inadvertently given in very early pregnancy. A large number of studies have investigated the effect of exposure to DMPA, while few data are available on NET-EN. Exposure to DMPA was not found to increase teratogenicity (Katz 1985). Follow-up of children over the 17 years following exposure failed to show an effect on long-term health and development (Jaffe 1990), intellectual development (Jaffe 1988), or on the sex-dimorphic behaviors of aggressiveness, assertiveness and physical activity (Jaffe 1989).

As Cyclofem and Mesigyna are both relatively new, as well as very effective methods, there are very few reports available on infants exposed to these drugs in utero. In the few cases that are documented (WHO 1988a; EFCS 1993), all pregnancies ended with the birth of full-term healthy infants after exposure to one or three injections of a combined injectable. Follow-up beyond the time of birth is not available.

Exposure of Breast-Fed Infants

Transmission of steroidal hormones through breast milk is variable. MPA levels in breast milk are close to maternal plasma levels and are still detectable 12 weeks after DMPA injection. In contrast, NET levels in breast milk are about one-third of maternal plasma levels and are rarely detectable beyond 8 weeks (Koetsawang 1982). DMPA use during lactation does not appear to affect milk volume and has only minimal effects on milk composition (WHO 1988a). It is estimated that breast-fed infants receive 0.25 µg/kg/day 3-4 weeks after injection, and that this level falls progressively to 0.08 µg/kg/day when the next injection is due (Johansson and Odlind 1987).

Exposure to DMPA through breast milk was not found to affect the adrenal and gonadal functions of infants (Virutamasen 1996), nor their growth and development (WHO 1994a; 1994b). Follow-up of exposed children into early adulthood also failed to show any adverse effect on long-term growth and development (Pardthaisong 1992).

Combined hormonal contraceptive methods are not recommended during breast-feeding in view of the well-documented deleterious effect of combined pills on milk output and composition, duration of lactation and infant growth (Croxatto 1983; Diaz 1983; WHO 1984). Consequently, no report is available on the effect of combined injectables on lactation and on the growth of breast-fed infants.

Emerging Questions: Bone Density, HIV Transmission

DMPA Effects on Bone Mineral Density

In 1991, a study from New Zealand reported that women who had used DMPA for at least 5 years showed significantly lower bone densities in both the femoral neck and the lumbar spine than premenopausal controls (Cundy et al. 1991). The study was criticized for failing to control for smoking or prior oral-pill use, but it raised concerns about the impact of long-term DMPA use on bone density, and hence, fracture rates.

DMPA suppresses follicular estrogen production, and estrogen maintains bone density by slowing bone resorption. Studies of circulating estrogen among DMPA users suggest that, on average, estrogen levels are above those found among postmenopausal women (Cundy et al. 1991; Mishell et al. 1972). However, given that amenorrheic athletes with estrogen levels between 30 pg/ml and 40 pg/ml (levels comparable to those observed among DMPA users), have lower lumbar bone densities than eumenorrheic athletes (Marcus et al. 1985; Snead et al. 1992), more research on the long-term impact of DMPA on bone integrity is warranted.

A subsequent follow-up report from New Zealand suggests that the bone-density loss among DMPA users is reversed after discontinuation of the method (Cundy 1994). A recent study in Thailand found no measurable differences in bone density between 50 DMPA users (who had been using the method for at least 3 years) and 50

IUD users (Taneepanichskul 1997). Measuring bone density at the distal and ultradistal forearm by dual energy X-ray absorptiometry (DEXA), the authors found mean bone mineral densities at the distal forearm were 0.48±0.05 g/cm^2 in both groups, while bone mineral densities at the ultradistal forearm were 0.38±0.06 g/cm^2 among DMPA users, and 0.4±0.05 g/cm^2 among IUD users. These recent data are reassuring, but long-term prospective data in different populations are needed to characterize the impact of DMPA on bone densities.

No data are currently available on the possible impact of monthly, combined injectables on bone mineral density.

DMPA Effects on Vaginal Transmission of HIV

A study in 1996 reported that rhesus monkeys given subcutaneous progesterone implants, and subsequently exposed vaginally to the simian immunodeficiency virus (SIV), showed enhanced vaginal transmission of SIV, 7.7-fold over placebo implants (Marx et al. 1996). Progesterone treatment thinned the vaginal mucosal epithelium, a plausible mechanism for the observed effect.

The implications of this observation for humans are not clear. Available epidemiological data have largely suggested no measurable association between DMPA use and risk of becoming HIV infected. Ever use of DMPA bore no association to HIV infection in studies from Rwanda (Allen 1991), Tanzania (Kapiga 1994) or Kenya (Mati 1995). Two studies of current use of DMPA bore no association to HIV infection in Kenya (Mati 1995) or Thailand (Siraprapasiri 1991), yet a third study in Thailand reported a risk associated with DMPA (Rehle 1992). A prospective follow-up to the Rehle study reported a persistent increased risk of HIV sero-conversion among prostitutes using DMPA, compared with no method, or other methods (1995).

There is no available data on the association between NET-EN and risk of HIV infection. The WHO and United Nations Programme on AIDS (UNAIDs) continue to recommend that women who believe themselves at risk of HIV infection should be encouraged to use female or male condoms; further studies on possible interaction of progestin-only contraceptives and HIV transmission are ongoing.

Due to the fact that combined, monthly injectable contraceptives contain estrogens, they can be expected to cause no thinning of the vaginal mucosa. However, there are no available epidemiological data on the association of combined, monthly injectables and HIV transmission.

Injectable Contraceptives under Development

Steroidal Preparations

A number of approaches are being used in the development of new injectable formulations. These aim at controlling the release of the active compound in order to avoid the peak serum level which follows the injection, and to extend the duration of action. Such improved pharmacokinetic profile would, in principle, allow a lower dose to provide the same efficacy, while minimizing the side effects of the contraceptive preparation.

Monolithic microspheres

Over the past few years, the Instituto Nacional de la Nutricion Salvador Zubiran and Applicaciones Farmaceuticas, both in Mexico, have developed a new method of synthesizing microspheres of steroids. The method uses a pulsating jet of melted drug to form microspheres, which are then annealed and sieved to obtain the desired range of particle size. These are then formulated to provide stable and long-lasting aqueous suspensions.

This technology is being explored for the development of testosterone microspheres which would have 60-90 days duration of action and could be used as androgen replacement or for male contraception. The technology is also being investigated with progesterone in order to develop a two-monthly injectable contraceptive for lactating women.

The most advanced preparation based on this technology is a combined injectable contraceptive containing 250 mg of progesterone and 5 mg of estradiol. It was tested in 30 women for a single cycle and appeared to block ovulation for a month. Work is continuing on reproducibility of the microspheres, and on the evaluation of the impact of multiple injections on vaginal bleeding patterns. This method is being extended to mixtures of natural steroids and cholesterol, as preliminary data suggest that such microspheres provide an even more favorable pharmacokinetic profile. Finally, the application of this technology to synthetic steroids such as levonorgestrel-cholesterol, MPA or nestorone is under investigation.

Steroid Esters

In the mid-1970s HRP/WHO, in collaboration with the National Institute of Child Health and Human Development (NICHD, USA), established a program for the synthesis of new long-acting progestogens and androgens (Crabbe 1983). The approach chosen was to develop esters of known steroids, which would act as prodrugs and be converted to an active contraceptive agent by enzymatic hydrolysis in vivo.

Chemists from 12 countries worldwide synthesized 230 ester oximes and esters of norethisterone and levonorgestrel and 72 esters of testosterone. After purification and formulation, these compounds were tested in rodents, and in sub-human primates for the most promising ones. From these biological studies, it emerged that levonorgestrel esters were usually longer acting than the norethisterone esters; aqueous suspensions were generally better than oily solutions; and the duration of action of the longest acting agents was highly dependent on the crystal size of their aqueous suspensions.

After clinical testing, two compounds were selected for further development: levonorgestrel butanoate and testosterone buciclate. Levonorgestrel butanoate is being formulated as a three-monthly injectable contraceptive for women, and testosterone buciclate as a three-monthly injectable for male hormone-replacement therapy. The combination of both compounds is being considered as an injectable contraceptive for men, the inhibition of gonadotrophin secretion and suppression of spermatogenesis affected mainly by the progestogen, while the testosterone is provided primarily for androgen replacement.

Microsphere Formulations

The use of biodegradable poly- (lactide-co-glycolide) matrixes has been investigated for the delivery of natural and synthetic steroids as injectables. Investigators at Biotek, Inc. used this approach with progesterone, achieving sufficiently high loading of drug in the polymer to enable delivery of adequate amounts of progesterone for approximately 90 days in vitro and at least 77 days in rabbits. However, this work was stopped when safety issues were raised concerning the solvent used in the process. The same technology was investigated with testosterone and with synthetic steroids (norethisterone, levonorgestrel, norgestimate, nestorone), but these projects were abandoned because of additional concerns over reproducibility and cost.

Immunocontraceptives

Immunocontraceptives (Stevens et al. 1997) are based on the principle of using the body's own defense mechanisms to provide protection against pregnancy. Thus, they present a totally new approach to contraception. They have many potential advantages, including:
- Freedom from menstrual, systemic, metabolic and endocrine side effects
- Suitability for either men or women, depending on the target antigen
- No interference with sexual response or activity
- Sustained, reversible duration of action
- Use during all stages of a man's or woman's reproductive life
- Confidentiality of use
- Low manufacturing and storage costs
- Ease of distribution and administration within the health-care infrastructure.

A number of different targets are being used: hCG was chosen as the target for some formulations, because the hormone is usually only produced in women when fertilization and pregnancy occur, and it should not interfere with ovulation or the production of sex steroid hormones. Some of these preparations have reached the stage of clinical testing. Other immunocontraceptives are being developed that will exert their anti-fertility effect prior to fertilization. These preparations are intended for use by both men and women. They include immunocontraceptives directed against hypothalamic and pituitary hormones which are intended to inhibit ovulation and spermatogenesis, and immunocontraceptives directed against the mature ovum and spermatozoon which are intended to interfere with gamete interaction and fertilization. Some of the anti-hormone immunocontraceptives have reached the stage of initial assessment in clinical trials, but the anti-gamete immunocontraceptives are at an earlier stage of development.

hCG Immunocontraceptives

The most advanced immunocontraceptives are those based on hCG. Three main types have been developed to the stage of clinical testing:
- hCG beta subunit conjugated to tetanus toxoid (hCG-TT)

- hCG beta subunit – ovine LH alpha subunit heterodimer conjugated to tetanus toxoid and diphtheria toxoid (HSD-TT-DT)
- hCG beta subunit C-terminal 37 residue synthetic peptide conjugated to diphtheria toxoid (CTP-DT).

All three preparations have been tested in phase-I (safety) clinical trials; they generated antibody levels estimated to provide protection against pregnancy in fertile women and no health hazards were noted. The HSD-TT-DT preparation was tested in a phase-II (efficacy) clinical trial and this study demonstrated that an hCG immunocontraceptive can be effective in preventing pregnancy.

However, none of these preparations will be suitable for general use. Their immunogenicity needs to be improved so that they can be effective in virtually all recipients, and their duration of action should be such that a single application can convey protection for at least 6 months. Thus, the objective of current research is to determine a more effective adjuvant than was used in the HSD immunogen already tested. The CTP-DT prototype was also abandoned, and a new product was developed that utilizes DT conjugates of two peptide segments of hCG: the original CTP portion (residues 109-145) and an analogue of a second peptide representing the amino acid 38-57 region. The resultant combined immunogen is more potent in inducing hCG reactive antibodies and these antibodies are much more effective in the bioneutralization of hCG in vitro and in vivo. In addition, biodegradable microsphere and emulsion technologies provide new opportunities for the sustained delivery of these preparations.

GnRH and FSH Immunocontraceptives

The immunological inhibition of gonadotropin releasing hormone (GnRH) is being investigated to achieve contraception in men. GnRH inhibition by antibodies has been shown to result in gonadal atrophy and sterility; however, this state of physiological castration also results in feminizing effects. To overcome these problems, sufficient androgen supplementation needs to be given to restore libido and secondary sex characteristics, but not to restore spermatogenesis and fertility. The validity of this approach remains to be demonstrated.

Investigators in India and Germany (CONRAD report 1996) have shown that immunization of non-human primates with native FSH led to reversible inhibition of spermatogenesis and subsequent infertility. However, it is unclear whether, in men, the inhibition of FSH will cause the arrest of spermatogenesis. Another approach uses the FSH receptor, and recombinant peptides of the extra-cellular domain of the FSH receptor are being tested for their immunogenicity, and their ability to inhibit fertility alone and in combination with an FSH vaccine.

Sperm and Ovum Immunocontraceptives

Both sperm and ovum immunocontraceptives are currently being developed as methods to be used by women to prevent fertilization. Sperm antigens suitable for immunocontraception include sperm enzymes and sperm membrane glycoproteins.

The most promising enzyme is the sperm-specific isoenzyme of lactic dehydrogenase (LDH-C4) and preliminary studies in female baboons using recombinant and chemically-synthesized LDH-C4 peptide antigens have shown varying degrees of anti-fertility efficacy. A number of glycoproteins have also shown anti-fertility effects when used in in vitro systems or to immunize experimental animals. However, none of these antigens has reached the stage of clinical testing in humans.

The most well-studied ovum-associated antigens are the zona pellucida (ZP) glycoproteins. However, while animal studies confirmed that immunization with ZP proteins induced pronounced anti-fertility effects, this was accompanied by disturbances in ovarian function. Thus, current research aims at isolating specific peptide antigens, particularly from the primary sperm receptor ZP3, or to develop recombinant ZP proteins, to achieve a safe method. Another approach under investigation is the use of specific antigens in the oolemma, which may have the advantage of being restricted to the peri-ovulatory stage of oocyte development. In any event, the feasibility of developing a safe, effective and reversible ovum-based immunocontraceptive remains to be established.

Future Prospects

As a totally new approach to fertility regulation, immunocontraceptives will present new clinical challenges in order to ensure their safe delivery in family planning services, including monitoring the time to effect, maintenance of effect, and reversibility in individual users. Researchers are addressing these points by improving the formulations in order to reduce inter-individual variability, and by developing a means of inducing reversibility at will. The practicality of these methods remains to be confirmed.

Conclusion

Injectable contraceptives are a significant and growing share of worldwide contraceptive use. They offer many positive attributes, including a high measure of safety, high method effectiveness, the chance to avoid a daily pill, no interruption of coitus, different options for the length of effectiveness, and the chance for a woman to contracept without knowledge of her partner or family. For many women, these attributes are clearly very important, as indicated by the high method use worldwide.

At the same time, injectable methods have been a focus of concern by feminists for many years, due largely to the fact that these methods can be used covertly, and they cannot be discontinued or reversed until the drug has passed from the body. More recent concerns include the fact that these methods fail to protect women or men from sexually transmitted diseases, or the lethal threat of HIV.

The challenge for clinicians and family planning practitioners is to promote and prescribe contraceptive methods that are appropriate to the health risks, as well as the social needs and preferences, of the individual client. Current injectable methods offer safe and effective options for women not at risk of STDs or HIV; they can also provide an important component of dual protection for women wishing to combine a highly effective long-acting method with barrier protection.

An injectable mode of delivery for contraception has proven appeal for many women and, most likely, for men as well. Continuing research efforts to ensure the safety of available methods is very much warranted, particularly regarding the impact of progestogen-only methods on the risk of vaginal HIV transmission, and the long-term integrity of bone. Continuing research efforts to develop new, long-acting injectable contraceptives is to be encouraged if new products will offer measurable reductions in unwanted side-effects associated with current methods, particularly the disturbances to menstrual bleeding, and the delayed return of fertility.

References

d'Arcangues C, Odlind V, Fraser I (1992) Dysfunctional uterine bleeding induced by exogenous hormones. In: N.J. Alexander, C. d'Arcangues (eds) Steroid hormones and uterine bleeding. Washington, AAAS Press, pp 81-105

Aedo AR, Landgren BM, Johannisson E et al. (1985) Pharmacokinetic and pharmacodynamic investigations with monthly injectable contraceptive preparation. Contraception 31:453-469

Allen S, Lindan C, Serufilira A et al. (1991) Human immunodeficiency virus infection in urban Rwanda. JAMA 266:1657-63

Amatayakul K, Sivassomboon B, Singkamani R (1980) Effects of medroxyprogesterone acetate on serum lipids, protein, glucose tolerance and liver function in Thai women. Contraception 21:283-298

Ashman JAM (1990) Monthly injectable contraceptives and breast cancer (Master of Science thesis). University of Washington, WA, USA

Bahamondes L, Lavín P, Ojeda G et al. (1997) Return of fertility after discontinuation of the one-a-month injectable contraceptive cyclofem. Contraception 55:307-310

Bledsoe CH, Hill AG, D'Alessandro P et al. (1994) Forthcoming. local cultural interpretations of western contraceptive technologies in rural Gambia. Population and Development Review, March

Cookson KM (1994) The parenteral toxicity of Cyclofem. Contraception 49:335-345

Coutinho E M, Spinola P, Barbosa I et al. (1997) Multicenter, double-blind, comparative clinical study on the efficacy and acceptability of a monthly injectable contraceptive combination of 150 mg dihydroxyprogesterone acetophenide and 10 mg estradiol enanthate compared to a monthly injectable contraceptive combination of 90 mg dihydroxyprogesterone acetophenide and 6 mg estradiol enanthate. Contraception 1997; 55:175-181

Crabbé P, Archer S, Benagiano G, Diczfalusy E, Djerassi C, Fried J, Higuchi T (1983) Long-acting contraceptive agents: design of the WHO Chemical Synthesis Programme. Steroids 41:243-253

Croxatto HB, Diaz S, Peralta O et al. (1983) Fertility regulation in nursing women: IV. long-term influence of a low-dose combined oral contraceptive initiated at day 30 postpartum upon lactation and infant growth. Contraception 27:13-25

Cundy, T et al. (1991) Bone density in women receiving depot medroxyprogesterone acetate for contraception. BMJ 303:13-16

Cundy T, Cornish, J, Evans MC, Roberts H, Reid, IR (1994) Recovery of bone density in women who stop using medroxyprogesterone acetate. BMJ 308:247-248

Cushman LF, Kalmuss D, Davidson AR et al. (1996) Beliefs about Depo-Provera among three groups of contraceptors. Adv Contracept 12:43-52

Diaz S, Peralta O, Juez G et al. (1983) Fertility regulation in nursing women: III. short-term influence of a low-dose combined oral contraceptive upon lactation and infant growth. Contraception 27:1-11

Egyptian Fertility Care Society (1993) A comparative clinical trial of two once-a-month injectable contraceptives (Cyclofem and Mesigyna). Final report (unpublished)

Fotherby K, Benagiano G, Toppoyada HK et al. (1982) A preliminary pharmacological trial of the monthly injectable contraceptive, Cycloprovera. Contraception 25:261-272

Fotherby K, Saxena BN, Shrimanker K et al. (1980) A preliminary pharmacokinetic and pharmacodynamic evaluation of depot-medroxyprogesterone acetate and norethisterone oenanthate. Fertil Steril 34:131-139

Fraser IS (1983) A survey of different approaches to management of menstrual disturbances in women using injectable contraceptives. Contraception 28:385-397

Fraser IS (1994) Vaginal bleeding patterns in women using once-a-month injectable contraceptives. Contraception 49:399-420
Fraser IS, Dennerstein GJ (1994) Depo-Provera use in an Australian metropolitan practice. Med J Aust 160:553-556
Fraser IS, Diczfalusy E (1980) A perspective of steroidal contraception and abnormal bleeding: What are the prospects for improvement? In: Diczfalusy E, Fraser IS, Webb FTG (eds) Endometrial bleeding and steroidal contraception. Pitman Press Ltd, Bath, England, pp 384-413
Garza-Flores J, Cardenas S, Rodríguez V, Cravioto MC, Diaz-Sanchez V, Perez-Palacios G (1985) Return to ovulation following the use of long-acting injectable contraceptives: a comparative study. Contraception 31:361-366
Garza-Flores J, Guo-wei S, Hall P (1994) Population and delivery systems: variability in pharmacokinetics of long-acting injectable contraceptives. In: Snow R, Hall P (eds) Steroid contraceptives and women's response. Plenum Press, New York
Garza-Flores J, Hall PE, Perez-Palacios G (1991) Long-acting hormonal contraceptives for women. J Steroid Biochem Mol Biol 40:697-704
Guzman-Gracia S, Snow R, Aitken I (1997) Preferences for contraceptive attributes: voices of women in ciudad Juárez, Mexico. Int Family Planning Perspect 23:52-58
Hall PE (1987) Long-acting injectable formulations. In: Diczfalusy E, Bydgeman M (eds) Fertility regulation today and tomorrow - Raven Press, New York pp 119-141
Hall PE, WHO Task Force (1994) The introduction of cyclofem into national family planning programmes: experience from studies in Indonesia, Jamaica, Mexico, Thailand and Tunisia. Contraception 49:489-507
Hassan EO, El-Nahal N, El-Hussein M (1994) Acceptability of the once-a-month injectable contraceptive Cyclofem and Mesigyna in Egypt. Contraception 40 (5): 469-488
Herrero R, Brinton LA, Reeves WC et al. (1990) Injectable contraceptives and risk of invasive cervical cancer: evidence of an association. Int J Cancer 46:5-7
Howard G, Blair M, Fotherby K, Elder MG, Bye P (1985) Seven years clinical experience of the injectable contraceptive, norethisterone oenanthate. Br J Family Planning 11:9-16
ICMR Task Force on Hormonal Contraception (1986) Return of fertility following discontinuation of an injectable contraceptive - norethisterone oenanthate (net en) 200 mg dose. Contraception 34:573-582
Jaffe B, Hralap S, Baras M et al. (1988) Long-term effects of MPA on human progeny: intellectual development. Contraception 37:607-619
Jaffe B, Shye D, Harlap S et al. (1989) Aggression, physical activity levels and sex role identity in teenagers exposed in utero to MPA. Contraception 40:351-363
Jaffe B, Shye D, Harlap S et al. (1990) Health, growth and sexual development of teenagers exposed in utero to medroxyprogesterone acetate. Paediatr Perinat Epidemiol 4:184-195
Johansson E, Odlind V (1987) The passage of exogenous hormones into breast milk - possible effects. Int J Gynaecol Obstet 25 [Suppl]:111-114
Kapagi SH, Shao JF, Lwihula GK et al. (1994) Risk factors for HIV infection among women in Dar-es-Salaam, Tanzania. J Acquir Immune Defic Syndr 7:301-309
Katz Z, Lancet M, Skornik J et al. (1985) Teratogenicity of progestogens given during the first trimester of pregnancy. Obstet Gynecol 65:775-780
Kesserü EV, Aydinlik S, Etchepareborda JJ (1994) Multicentred, phase III clinical trial of norethisterone enanthate 50 mg plus estradiol valerate 5 mg as a monthly injectable contraceptive; final three-year report. Contraception 50:329-337
Koetsawang S (1994) Once-a-month injectable contraceptives: efficacy and reasons for discontinuation. Contraception 49:387-398
Koetsawang S, Nukulkarn P, Fotherby K et al. (1982) Transfer of contraceptive steroids in milk of women using long-acting gestagens. Contraception 25:321-331
La Veccia C (1994) Depot-medroxyprogesterone acetate, other injectable contraceptives, and cervical neoplasia. Contraception 49:223-230
Lan PT, Aedo AR, Landgren BM, Johannisson E, Diczfalusy E (1984) Return of ovulation following a single injection of Depo-Medroxy-Progesterone acetate: a pharmacokinetic and pharmacodynamic study. Contraception 29:1-18
Lei ZW, Wu SC, Garceau RJ et al. (1996) Effect of pretreatment counseling on discontinuation rates in chinese women given depo-medroxyprogesterone acetate for contraception. Contraception 53:357-361

Lumbiganon P (1994) Depot-medroxyprogesterone acetate (DMPA) and cancer of the endometrium and ovary. Contraception 49:203-209
Marcus T. et al. (1985) Menstrual function and bone mass in elite women distance runners. Ann Intern Med 102:158-164
Marx PA, Spira AI, Gettie A et al. (1996) Progesterone implants enhance SIV vaginal transmission and early virus load. Nat Med 2:1084-1089
Mati JKG, Hunter DJ, Maggwa BN et al. (1995) Contraceptive use and the risk of HIV infection in Nairobi, Kenya. Int J Obstet Gynaecol 48:61-67
McDaniel E, Pardthaisong, MA (1973) Depot-medroxyprogesterone acetate as a contraceptive agent: return of fertility after discontinuation of use. Contraception 8:407-414
Mishell DR et al. (1972) Estrogenic activity in women receiving an injectable progestogen for contraception. Am J Obstet Gynecol 113:372-376
Mukherjea M, Mukherjee P, Biswas R (1980) Long-term contraception with Depo-Provera: a clinical evaluation. Int J Fertil 25:122-126
Newton JR, D'Arcangues C, Hall PE (1994) 'Once-a-month' combined injectable contraceptives. J Obstet Gynaecol 14 [Suppl 1]
Ortiz A, Hiroi M, Stanczyk FZ, Goebelsmann U, Mishell DR (1977) Serum medoxyprogesterone acetate (MPA) concentrations and ovarian function following intramuscular injection of Depo-MPA. J Clin Endocrinol Metab 44:32-38
Pardthaisong, T (1984) Return of fertility after use of the injectable contraceptive Depo-Provera: updated data analysis. J Biosoc Sci 16:23-24
Pardthaisong T, Yenchit C, Gray R (1992) The long-term growth and development of children exposed to Depo-provera during pregnancy or lactation. Contraception 45:313-324
Paul C, Skegg DCG, Spears GFS (1989) Depot medroxyprogesterone (Depo-Provera) and risk of breast cancer. BMJ 299:759-762
Piya-Anant M, Koetsawang S, Patrasupapong N et al. (1998) Effectiveness of Cyclofem in the treatment of DMPA-induced amenorrhea. Contraception (in press)
Population Reports (1995) Series K, No.5, Baltimore, John Hopkins School of Public Health, Population Information Program
Product Information (1994) Depo-Provera Contraceptive Injection. MI:Upjohn Company, Kalamazoo
Rehle T, Brinkmann U, Siraprapasiri T et al. (1992) Risk factors of HIV-1 infection among female prostitutes in Khon Kaen, Northeast Thailand. Infection 20:328-331
Sang GW, Shao QX, Ge RS et al. (1995) A multicentred phase III comparative clinical trial of mesigyna, cyclofem and injectalbe No.1 given monthly by intramuscular injection to Chinese women. Contraception 51:167-183
Saxena BN, Datey S, Gupta S et al. (1986) ICMR task force on hormonal contraception: return of fertility following discontinuation of an injectable contraceptive – norethisterone Oenanthate (NET EN) 200 mg dose. Contraception 34:573-582
Schwallie PC, Assenzo, Jr. (1973) Contraceptive use-efficacy study utilizing medroxyprogesterone acetate administered as an intramuscular injection once every 90 days. Fertil Steril 24:331-339
Siegel I (1963) Conception control by long-acting progestogens: Preliminary report. Obstet Gynecol 21:666-668
Siraprapasiri T, Rehle T, Brinkmann UK, Coplan P, Aiemsukawat C, Ungchusak K (1992) Risk factors of HIV-1 infection among female prostitutes in Khon Kaen, Northeast Thailand. Infection. 20:328-331
Skegg DCG, Noonan EA, Paul C et al. (1995) Depot medroxyprogesterone acetate and breast cancer. A pooled analysis of the World Health Organization and New Zealand Studies. JAMA 273:799-804
Snead DB et al. (1992) Reproductive hormones and bone mineral density in women runners. J Appl Physiol 72:2149-2156
Snow R, García S, Kureshy N et al. (1997) Attributes of contraceptive technology: women's preferences in seven countries. Reprod Health Matters pp 36-48
Snow R, Hall P (eds.) (1994) Steroid contraceptives and women's response. Plenum Press, New York
Stevens VC, Griffin PD, Jones WR (1997) Immunocontraceptives: an update. Bio Drugs
Taneepanichskul S, Intaraprasert S, Theppisai U et al. (1997) Bone mineral density in long-term depot medroxyprogesterone acetate acceptors. Contraception 56:1-3
The CONRAD Program (1996) Annual Report
Thomas DB, Molina R, Cuevas HR et al. (1989) Monthly injectable steroid contraceptives and cervical carcinoma. Am J Epidemiol 130:237-247

Ungchusak K, Rehle T, Thammapornpilap P, Spiegelman D, Brinkmann U, Siraprapasiri T (1996) Determinants of HIV infection among female commercial sex workers in northeastern Thailand: results from a longitudinal study. J Acquir Immune Defic Syndr Hum Retrovirol 12:500-507

UNDP/UNFPA/WHO/World Bank Special Programme of Research, Development and Research Training in Human Reproduction. Annual Technical Report 1997

UNDP/UNFPA/WHO/World Bank, Special Programme of Research, Development and Research Training in Human Reproduction, Task Force on Long-Acting Systemic Agents for Fertility Regulation (1997) Comparative Study of the effects of two once-a-month injectable steroidal contraceptives (Mesigyna and Cyclofem) on Lipid and Lipoprotein metabolism. Contraception 56:193-207

UNDP/UNFPA/WHO/World Bank, Special Programme of Research, Development and Research Training in Human Reproduction, Task Force on Long-Acting Systemic Agents for Fertility Regulation 1998. Comparative Study of the effects of two once-a-month injectable steroidal contraceptives (Mesigyna and Cyclofem) on Glucose Metabolism and Liver Function. Contraception 57:71-81.

Virutamasen P, Leepipatpaiboon S, Kriengsinyot R et al. (1996) Pharmacodynamic effects of depot-medroxyprogesterone acetate (DMPA) administered to lactating women on their male infants. Contraception 54:153-157

World Health Organization, Special Programme of Research, Development and Research Training in Human Reproduction, Task Force on Oral Contraceptives (1984) Effects of hormonal contraceptives on milk volume and infant growth. Contraception 30:505-522

World Health Organization (1986) A multicentred phase III comparative clinical trial of depot-medroxyprogesterone acetate given three-monthly at doses of 100 mg or 150 mg: 1. Contraceptive efficacy and side effects. Contraception 34:223-236

World Health Organization, Special programme of research, development and research training in human reproduction. Task Force on long-acting systemic agents for fertility regulation (1987) A multicentred pharmacokinetic, pharmacodynamic study of once-a-month injectable contraceptives. I. Different doses of HRP112 and Depoprovera. Contraception 36:441-457

World Health Organization, Special Programme of Research, Development and Research Training in Human Reproduction, Task Force on Oral Contraceptives, Effects of hormonal contraceptives on breast milk composition and infant growth (1988a) Studies in Family Planning 19:361-369

World Health Organization, Special Programme of Research, Development and Research Training in Human Reproduction. Task Force on Long-acting Systemic Agents for Fertility Regulation (1988b) A multicentred phase III comparative study of two hormonal contraceptive preparations given once-a-month by intra-muscular injection: I. Contraceptive efficacy and side-effects. Contraception 37:1-20

World Health Organization Collaborative Study of Neoplasia and Steroid Contraceptives (1988c) Endometrial cancer and combined oral contraceptives. Int J Epidemiol 17:263-269

World Health Organization Collaborative Study of Neoplasia and Steroid Contraceptives (1991a) Breast cancer and depot-medroxyprogesterone acetate: a multinational study. Lancet 338:833-838

World Health Organization Collaborative Study of Neoplasia and Steroid Contraceptives (1991b) Depot-medroxyprogesterone acetate (DMPA) and risk of endometrial cancer. Int J Cancer 49:186-190

World Health Organization, Special Programme of Research, Development and Research Training in Human Reproduction, Task Force on Long-Acting Systemic Agents for Fertility Regulation (1993) A Multicentre Comparative Study of Serum Lipids and Apolipoproteins in Longterm Users of DMPA and a Control Group of IUD Users. 47:177-191

World Health Organization, Special Programme of Research, Development and Research Training in Human Reproduction. Task Force for Epidemiological Research on Reproductive Health (1994a) Progestogen-only contraceptives during lactation: I. Infant growth. Contraception 50:35-53

World Health Organization, Special Programme of Research, Development and Research Training in Human Reproduction. Task Force for Epidemiological Research on Reproductive Health (1994b) Progestogen-only contraceptives during lactation: II. Infant development. Contraception 50:55-68

World Health Organization, Family and Reproductive Health (1996a) Improving access to quality care in family planning. Medical eligibility criteria for contraceptive use. pp 143

World Health Organization, Special Programme of Research, Development and Research Training in Human Reproduction, Task Force on Long-acting Systemic Agents for Fertility Regulation (1996b) Clinical evaluation of the therapeutic effectiveness of ethinyl oestradiol and oestrone sulfate on prolonged bleeding in women using depot-medroxyprogesterone acetate (DMPA) for contraception. Human Reproduction 11[suppl 2]:1-13

7 Intrauterine Contraception: Past, Present, and Future

Horst Wagner

Background

The desire to prevent unwanted pregnancies reaches far back into human history. In pre-Christian civilisations, people were already searching for ways of avoiding conception or of intervening in the early stages to terminate accidental pregnancies. This applied, in particular, to women of high social status. Depending on how much they knew about anatomy and the functioning of the female reproductive organs, they used „barriers“ of different materials placed within and outside the uterus, resulting not infrequently in the woman's death from infection or perforation. Whereas early attempts at intrauterine contraception were intended to prevent the consequences of extra-marital sexual intercourse on the part of women of high social standing, it has now undergone crucial change. Embedded in an international "Women's Health Care" programme, its primary purpose nowadays is to prevent over-population in developing countries, as it is an inexpensive method of contraception and hence affordable even to developing countries. This is why the use of intrauterine contraceptive devices world-wide is more widespread than any other method except sterilisation, particularly in China.

In western industrialised countries, intrauterine contraception provides a genuine alternative to hormone-based methods, as it comes close to what people see as an ideal contraceptive. The reliability of intrauterine contraceptive devices (IUCD/IUD) is high, whereas side effects are few, its action is fully reversible when the device is removed, it is simple and relatively painless to insert and remains effective for up to five years irrespective of when intercourse takes place. The introduction of gestagen-releasing IUDs has blurred the distinction from hormone-based contraception. Modern intrauterine devices now function only as a carrier for contraceptive substances that become active inside the uterus, be they copper or gestagens. There are indications that it may even be possible to dispense with the frame in future, as there are ways of introducing contraceptive systems into the cavum uteri and fixing them there reversibly.

This chapter previously appeared in *Der Gynäkologe*, **31**, 5/98, 426-437.

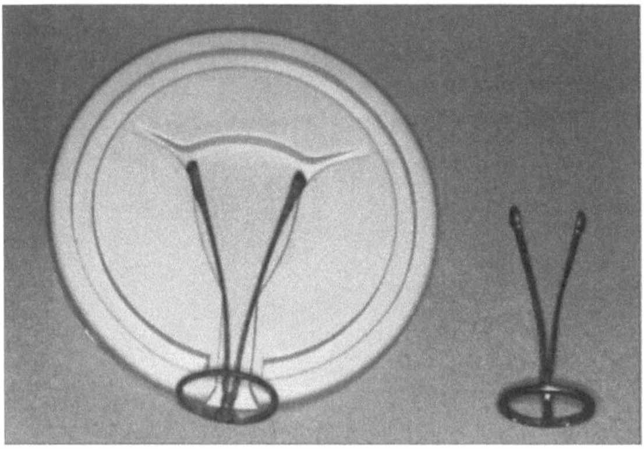

Fig. 1. Hollweg's dilation pessary. The model on the left shows a pessary inserted into the uterus to make the system more readily understood. The ring was positioned outside the uterus around the portio, while the dilated members were inside the uterine cavity. The device was available in different sizes

Introduction

Around the turn of the century, intrauterine pessaries were developed primarily for the treatment of dysmenorrhoea (by spreading the cervical canal). It was assumed that the major cause of dysmenorrhoea was an accumulation of menstrual blood in the cavity of the uterus due to tightness of the cervical os. By widening the cervix, it was hoped that the dysmenorrhoea would improve. It was not long before people realised that women with such a device in place did not become pregnant. The contraceptive effect was probably less due to local inflammatory reactions to the foreign body, i.e. the device itself, than to pelvic infection promoted by its uterovaginal positioning and its interference with the normal cervical protection against infection (Fig. 1). As might be expected in times before the discovery of antibiotics, morbidity and mortality were high among affected women.

The first person to invent intrauterine devices for purely contraceptive purposes was a German doctor called Richter [30]. His device was comprised of a loop of silk thread and came with an inserter in the form of a wooden rod (Fig. 2). In the thirties, Gräfenberg (probably working from Richter's ideas) developed the "Gräfenberg ring", arriving via the "Silk Thread Star" and the "Silk Thread Ring" at an annular metal coil made of gold, silver or argentan (also known as German silver or nickel silver, this is

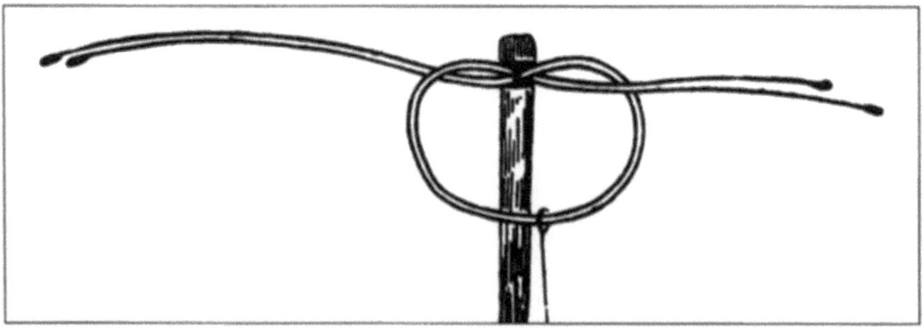

Fig. 2. Diagram of the silk thread pessary with wooden inserter, according to Richter [30]

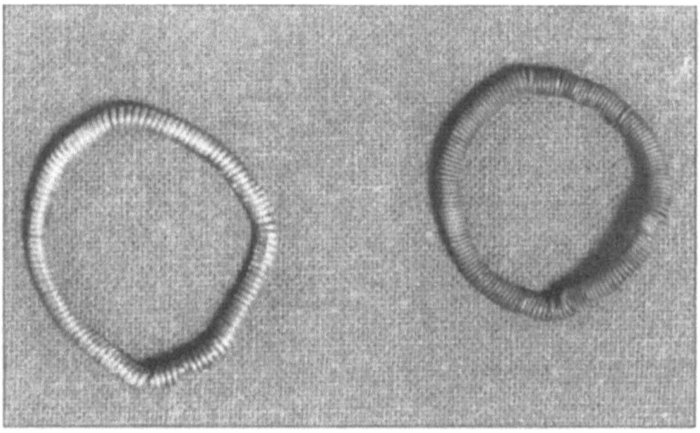

Fig. 3. Two original Gräfenberg rings. The one on the left is made of gold and was in place in the uterus for about 6 years. The one on the right is made of argentan and remained in situ for 31 years. The copper release rate of an argentan Gräfenberg ring was similar to that of a copper-T 200 after one year in situ. There is no weakening or fractionation of the wire coils on the ring. Copper alloys thus seem more suitable for long-term contraception in intrauterine devices (IUDs) than pure metallic copper.

an alloy of silvery appearance consisting of 45-67% copper, 10-26% nickel and 12-45% zinc). Studies proved that copper from the alloy was released inside the uterus [39]. Gräfenberg thus developed the first copper-releasing intrauterine pessary without knowing it (Fig. 3).

The Gräfenberg ring must be considered the first genuine IUCD, offering a high degree of reliability coupled with a very low number of undesirable effects. Gräfenberg selected his group of patients scrupulously and monitored them over a long follow-up period, with meticulous documentation of his results. The rate of pelvic inflammatory disease, for instance, was nil in his collective [22, 27]. Nevertheless, largely due to strong agitation by Gesenius, intrauterine contraception was outlawed by the German Society of Obstetrics and Gynaecology in the thirties, due to high associated morbidity. This did more than anything else to damage the image of intrauterine contraception in Germany [13].

It is not surprising, then, that the development of new devices for intrauterine contraception that set in after the Second World War took place abroad, especially in the U.S.A.; this was based in part on Gräfenberg's experience. The "Ota Ring" is an example (Fig. 4). In the age of plastics, the development of intrauterine contraceptives boomed, with varying degrees of reliability and adverse effects. The best results were

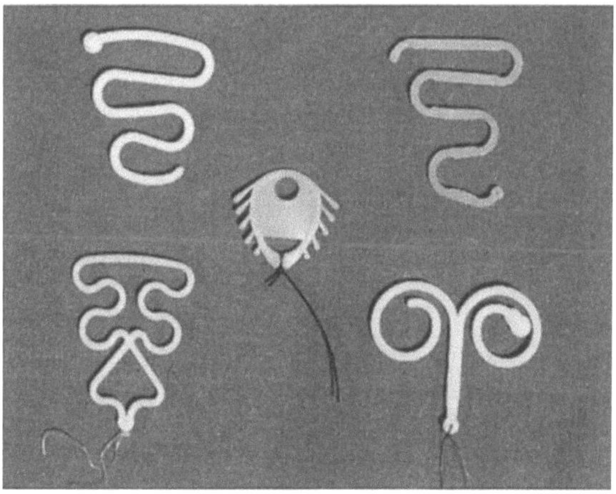

Fig. 4. Plastic intrauterine devices (IUDs). The original Lippes Loop is shown at the top left, an imitation of the Lippes Loop from the East on the top right, a Dalcon shield in the centre, a Dana Super at the bottom left of the kind that was in use especially in Eastern Europe and a Safe-T-Coil which was used world-wide like the Lippes Loop.

obtained with the Lippes Loop, which became very widespread and gave rise to the colloquial term "coil" for IUDs. The insertion technique was easy to learn and the device was inexpensive, so that it quickly became widely used in developing countries, where locally-made imitation products were often used to keep down costs.

Intrauterine devices were again discredited with the Dalcon Shield. Among women in the U.S.A. who did become pregnant while using this device, there was a very high rate of septic spontaneous abortion with some fatalities; this led to a virtual ban on the use of intrauterine devices by the FDA in the 1970s. The copper-bearing intrauterine devices developed in the intervening period by Zipper and Tatum (Copper 7, Copper T) were also hit by the ban – despite evidence of low side effects and high levels of contraceptive reliability [41].

Oddly, the high rate of sepsis in association with spontaneous abortion among users of the Dalcon Shield was observed only in the U.S.A. but not in the rest of the world. Nevertheless, the Dalcon Shield controversy again discredited intrauterine devices world-wide. Numerous global studies have now proved that the incidence of pelvic inflammatory disease is no higher in women using copper-bearing IUDs than in those using other methods such as oral contraception, while the reliability of copper-releasing intrauterine systems has almost caught up with that of hormone-based methods. Intrauterine devices are now permitted in the U.S.A. again.

Modern intrauterine contraceptives have little in common with older devices. Their effect is not achieved by the mechanical body; the plastic corpus acts merely as a carrier for active substances that prevent conception when released inside the uterus. To that effect, we now distinguish between those devices which have direct physical action on the cavity of the uterus itself and those which release active substances, mainly metallic copper and gestagen (particularly levonorgestrel, LNG). In future, it will be possible to anchor contraceptive agents in a suitable form directly to the endometrium inside the uterine cavity. Only then can we truly speak of intrauterine contraceptive systems (ICS).

Intrauterine Contraceptive Devices

Intrauterine devices whose simple presence inside the uterus leads to secondary change in the structure and function of the endometrium, thereby acting as a contraceptive without releasing substances of any kind, are also known as active agent-free, inert and non-medicated IUDs. The whole group can be termed simply as IUDs, because that is sufficient to distinguish them from copper IUDs and LNG IUDs.

IUDs are comprised of a plastic body varying in consistency and shape, or are made of stainless steel (Hall Ring). The plastic bodies must be neither too soft nor too hard (rigidity index). Plastic bodies that are too soft (low rigidity index), do not recover their original shape after being deformed during insertion. The result is high expulsion rates and reduced contraceptive reliability, although pain and bleeding rates are also very low. If the plastic body is too hard (high rigidity index), the expulsion rate is lower and reliability better, but insertion through the cervix is difficult and the pain and bleeding rates markedly higher. In practice, therefore, material components having a high and a low rigidity index (polyethylene and polypropylene respectively) are combined, and barium sulphate is added to enable the device to be identified in X-rays. A wide range of models of different geometries and sizes have been developed, giving rise to vehement debate about the most suitable shape to fill out the triangular slit inside the uterus while trying to do justice to the following assumptions:

The larger the area of the IUD in contact with the endometrium, the greater the contraceptive efficacy.

The larger the area of IUD and the greater the pressure on the endometrial surface (rigidity), the higher the pain and bleeding rate and the number of expulsions.

What was frequently forgotten is that the uterus is not a rigid structure, but one which changes in size and consistency in conjunction with the menstrual cycle and in which contractions may occur. The device that has proved most suitable in the age of plastics in respect of easy insertion, contraceptive reliability, the low rate of adverse effects and the length of time it can remain in situ is the widely-used Lippes Loop. Because it is so inexpensive, its use has spread widely, particularly in developing countries, where it has frequently been copied for reasons of cost. Where that was the case, the results were much less good, so it is essential to question whether the original or an imitation Lippes Loop was used when analysing publications.

The Lippes Loop was made of polyethylene and came in four sizes, A, B, C, and D. Size A was designed for the small uterus, and size D was the largest. In practice, this sizing was not appropriate because the thinking behind it was too mechanistic. In fact, it became apparent that the uterus itself needed to be of a suitable size and shape for intrauterine contraception. The reliability of the Lippes Loop was given as 3 to 4 on the Pearl Index, but it decreased considerably the longer the device remained in the uterus, particularly after five to six years. The Dalcon Shield was a more reliable

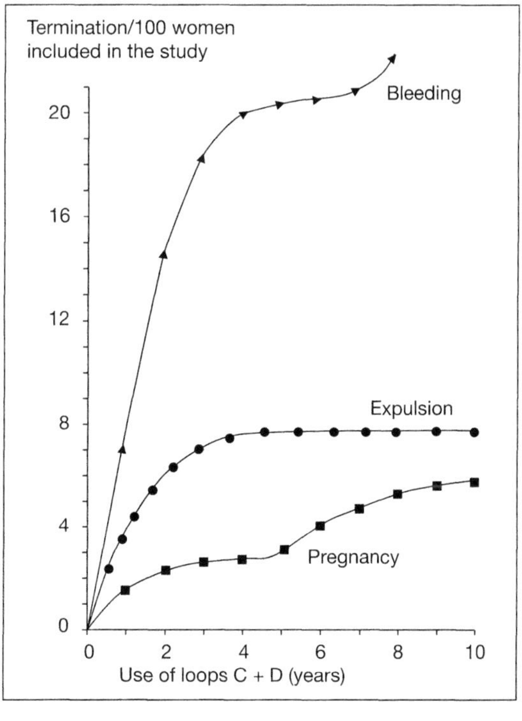

Fig. 5. Graph showing the incidence of bleeding, expulsion and unwanted pregnancies for the Lippes Loop C and D over a 10-year period [41]

contraceptive but carried a higher incidence of side effects [41]. Undesirable effects such as pain and expulsion of the device were accepted but not the marked increase in the quantity and duration of menstrual bleeding. This was a particular problem for women in the developing countries with anaemia, which was sometimes severe.

Originally, it was stated that the device could stay in place for ten years, but Lippes' own studies showed a rise in bleeding disorders and pregnancy rates after only five years (Fig. 5). Alteration of the loop's surface due to incrustation with polypeptides and salts, especially calcium salts, has been suggested as a possible cause.

The occurrence of ascending genito-urinary inflammation appeared to be favoured by the presence of a plastic intrauterine device. The risk of infection was calculated to be two to three times higher on average. For a long time, the string was blamed for the higher infection risk with plastic IUDs, particularly when it was a multi-filament tail like that of the Dalcon Shield. This theory has not been borne out by subsequent studies, however. It is more likely that mechanical irritation causes lesions on the surface of the endometrium, allowing bacteria to penetrate.

The mechanism of contraceptive action of plastic IUDs has never been definitively explained. The following theories are still under discussion:

- The device acts as a foreign body inside the uterine cavity, reacting non-specifically and resulting in invasion by lymphocytes, leukocytes, monocytes, plasma cells and macrophages, which are toxic to blastocysts.
- Implantation may be disrupted by chronic inflammation of the endometrium triggered by contamination of the IUD as it passes through the vagina, bringing bacteria with the mucus from the cervix into the uterine cavity, so that the blastocysts perish.
- The IUD causes premature decidual alteration of the endometrium. Implantation is not generally possible in the decidua. IUDs influence endocrine secretion, which reduces tubal motility.
- The IUD may influence sperm transport by inactivating the phagocytosis of sperm when in position in the uterus.
- The contraceptive effect of plastic IUDs still seems to be multifactorial, and our present knowledge covers only some of the factors [23, 25, 28, 38].

Contraception using plastic IUDs has never been and is still not significant. The Lippes Loop, the Dana Super, the Safe-T coil and the Dalcon Shield (Fig. 4) were all used in Western Europe and in Germany, but the Dalcon Shield controversy in the U.S.A. further reduced intrauterine contraception in Germany, while the Dana super and copies of the Lippes Loop continued to be used in some of the Eastern bloc countries. Another use was found for the Lippes Loop as an adhesion prophylactic after metroplastic surgery for uterus abnormalities, but as these operations are now performed almost exclusively by hysteroscopy, this indication has disappeared. Lippes Loop IUDs were also recommended as a treatment for Asherman's syndrome. In practice, however, they did not prove their usefulness of this rare disorder.

Copper-Bearing IUDs

Efforts to find the ideal structure for an IUD by modifying the geometry and size of plastic devices while keeping down the incidence of undesirable effects and ensuring ease of insertion even with a very tight cervical canal resulted in the development of the 7 and T shapes. With a Pearl Index of 20, however, the pregnancy rate with these models was too high. For this reason, research was directed towards substances effective as intrauterine contraceptives so that the pregnancy rate could be cut by adding them to the device at no detriment to user tolerance. This led to the discovery of copper's contraceptive action in animal experiments.

By winding the vertical section of the IUD with thin copper wires, contraception was greatly improved with no increase in the rate of undesirable side effects. Clinical studies provided evidence that contraceptive reliability increased in proportion to the surface area of copper and did not depend on the quantity or thickness of the copper wire. By contrast, the quantity of copper and thickness of the copper wire did have a crucial influence on the time such devices could safely remain in situ. Numerous studies eventually indicated that the surface area of copper needed to be between 300 and 400 square millimeters and that a copper wire thickness of 0.3 mm was sufficient to prevent fragmentation of the wire [41].

Longitudinal studies showed that the copper 7 IUD was not ideal because it had a relatively high expulsion rate and an increase in perforations by the free end of the horizontal and vertical members was observed in the endomyometrium and the cervix. Trial results with the T shape were better, but even here, cases of cervical perforation were described when vertical dislocation occurred. In addition, the copper surface area of 200 mm^2 proved to be insufficient to provide the desired contraceptive reliability and length of time in situ. The copper T 200 (Gyne T) was therefore superseded in Germany by the Nova-T, in which all the free ends are rounded and the copper wire has a silver core to prevent copper wire fragmentation. In the U.S.A., the Cu-T 220 C was developed with five copper sheaths on the vertical member and one each on the horizontal arms, and the Cu-T 380 A with one copper sheath on each of the horizontal arms and copper wire winding around the vertical leg. In this way, the copper surface was increased to an area of 220 mm^2 or 380 mm^2, respectively. A spherical thickening on all the free ends prevented perforation.

The multiload concept comprises IUDs with varying quantities of copper and lengths of the vertical leg. It differs from the T shape in that the horizontal arms have a horseshoe-shaped downward curve and 5 small protrusions on each side. The vertical leg comprises a copper coil winding with a surface area of between 250 mm^2 and 375 mm^2. It comes in two sizes, standard and short. Excellent experimental results and easy insertion have made the Multiload ML 375 to the most widely-used copper IUD in Germany. Mini versions of the IUD have not been successful because their expulsion rate is too high. Experience has shown that the uterine cavity has to have a constant size and shape to accommodate and "tolerate" an IUD [23, 41].

More recent developments are the Cu-Safe-T 300, which our own experience has shown to be especially suitable for use in young women who have never been pregnant, and the Medusa, which is encountered more frequently in the new federal states of Germany (Fig. 6). In concurrence with other authors, our own trials have shown that the best copper-release effect is achieved with copper wire winding. It offers the largest surface area with the smallest quantity of copper whilst allowing for maximum elasticity in the vertical limb of the device. The portions of the copper wire winding in contact with the plastic surface give off hardly any copper. The chemical release processes take place only on the open surface of the copper coils. To this extent, devices

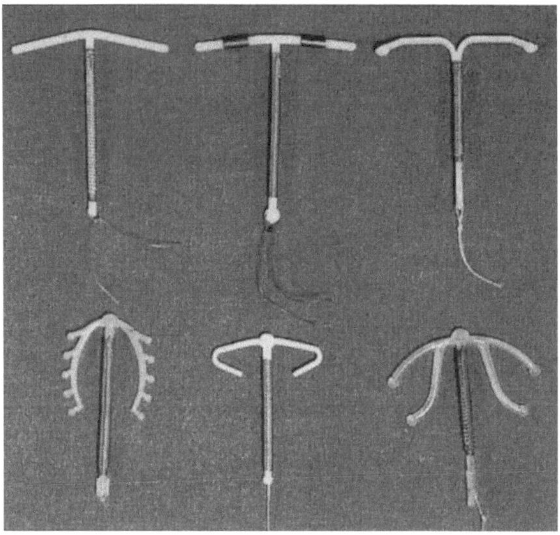

Fig. 6. Modern copper intrauterine devices (IUDs). Top row from left to right: copper-T 200, Copper-T 380, Nova-T. Bottom row from left to right: multiload ML 375 Cu, Cu-Safe 300 IUD and Medusa

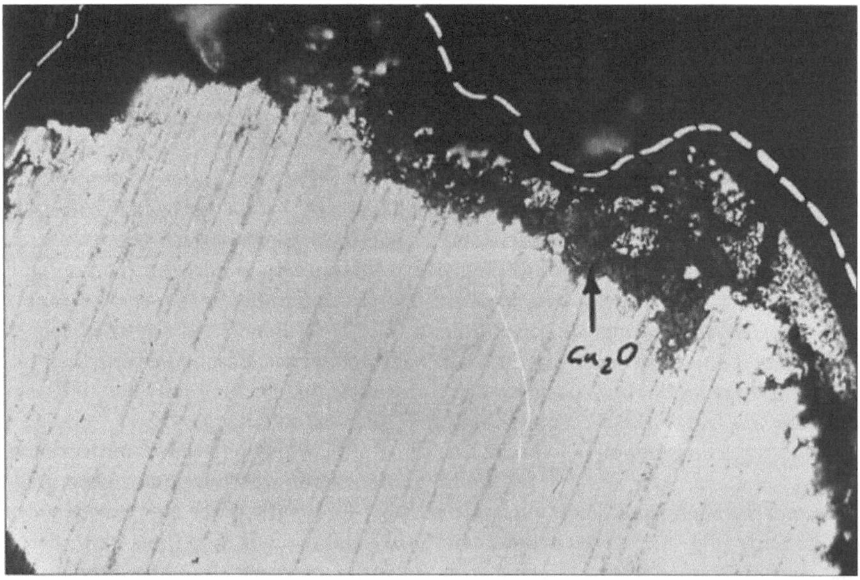

Fig. 7. Cross-section through the copper winding of a Cu-T 200 after approximately 1 year in the uterus. The light-coloured area corresponds to metallic copper, followed by a copper oxide layer and, above it, a dark, amorphous mucous layer with copper sulphate salts, calcium and peptides. The white dotted line marks the surface. The copper oxide is very friable and part of it crumbles away, so that the wire acquires an irregular cross-section which gradually thins down.

with copper sheaths have a much lower copper release rate in relation to the copper surface area.

In our experience, a silver core is not necessary to increase the stability of the copper wires and prevent copper breakage, as fragmentation is extremely rare and hence negligible in 0.3-mm thick pure copper wires. Moreover, metallographic examination has shown that tension can arise at the interface of the two metals, which may accelerate copper breakdown processes and impair stability.

Once inside the uterine cavity, copper radicals rapidly dissociate and accumulate in a high concentration in the surface secretions of the endometrium. An amorphous layer consisting of polypeptides, copper oxide, copper sulphate and other salts is formed on the surface of the copper (Fig. 7). The rate at which copper is given off is thus greatly reduced, but at the same time the period of release is prolonged. The quantity of copper does not influence the rate at which it is given off. After the device has been in place in the uterus for about three months, the daily rate is between 5 μg and 15 μg copper. According to our studies, copper IUDs with over 300mm2 of copper surface area can remain in situ for over 5 years without loss of efficacy. Copper concentrations measured on the surface and in the endometrium and cervical mucus are not sufficient in vivo to act as a bactericide, as was presumed for a time [41].

Biological Action of Copper on the Endometrium

Copper breaks up in endometrial secretions into copper radicals. A concentration gradient forms from the copper coils of the winding towards the periphery (Fig. 8), resulting in a non-specific foreign body reaction at the endometrial surface. This leads, in turn, to focal morphological and functional de-synchronisation of the endometrium that amounts to inhibition of implantation (Fig. 9). There is evidence of sperm phagocytosis in the presence of so many microphages and macrophages. Se-

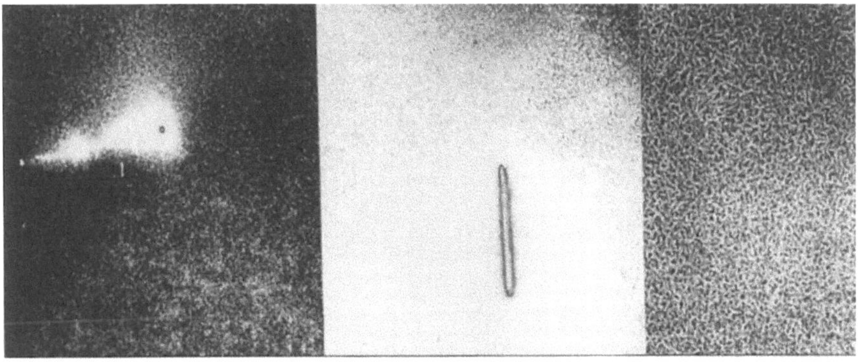

Fig. 8. Cell culture model to show copper dissociation in solution. The damage to the monolayer fibroblast coating distinctly shows up in the concentration gradient of copper dissociation. Top: pure fibroblast culture. Centre: fibroblast culture after insertion of a new Cu-T 200. The copper concentration is very high, the growth inhibition zone of the fibroblasts is very wide. Bottom: Cu-T 200 after one year in the uterus. The copper release rate is much lower, as is the breadth of dissociation; much smaller inhibition zone is recognisable.

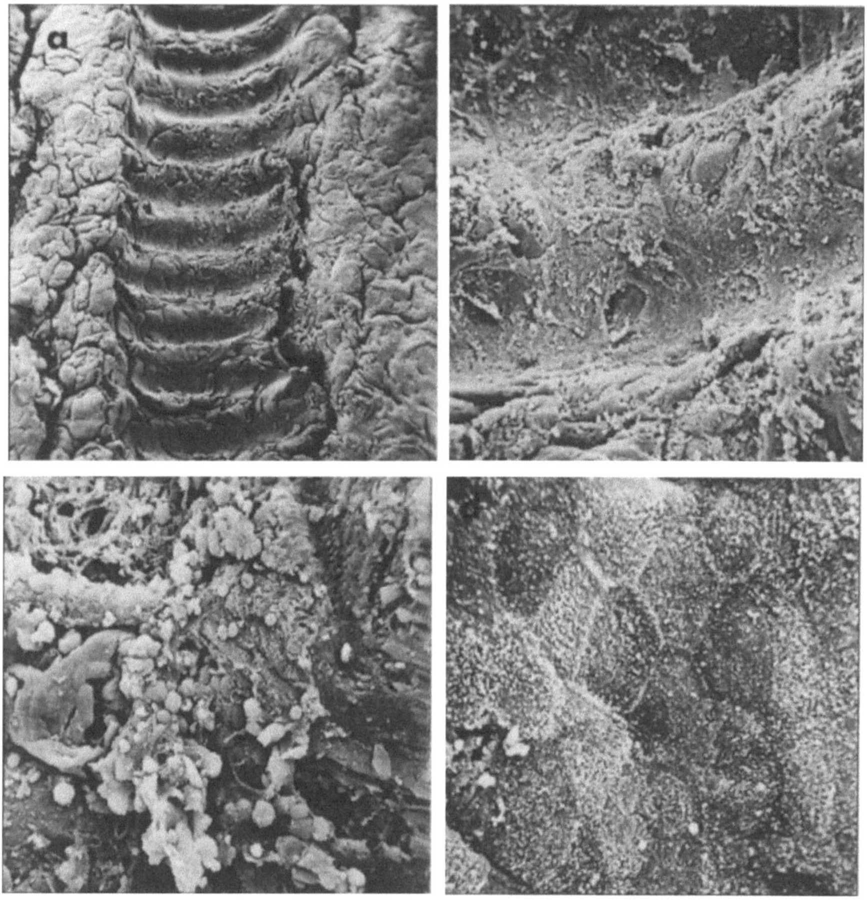

Fig. 9a-d. Scanning electron microscope photograph of the endometrial surface under the influence of a Cu-T 200. *a* Endometrial imprint of the copper bed; largely normal endometrium is seen outside the marginal zone. 20:1 enlargement. *b* In this even greater enlargement of an area of endometrium between two copper coils, accumulations of cells in mucus clefts are found after some time in situ (enlargement: 100:1). *c* Again, mainly micro and macrophages are found streaked with a network of fibrin-like material. (enlargement: 2000:1). *d* Surface of an endometrial cell beneath a copper coil. The flattened surface of the cell is clearly visible, with distinct intracellular boundaries and scant microvilli (enlargement: 500:1)

condary effects have also been identified to explain the undesirable effects during the first two or three cycles after insertion (Fig. 10). We now know enough about the intrauterine contraceptive action of copper to be sure that it is complex in nature, but more recent research such as post-coital testing has shown that conception is actually avoided by preventing sperm from penetrating beyond the uterine cavity by means of phagocytosis and enzymatic inactivation [16, 17, 18, 28, 34]. In post-coital use of the IUD, an effect due merely to the prevention of implantation cannot be ruled out.

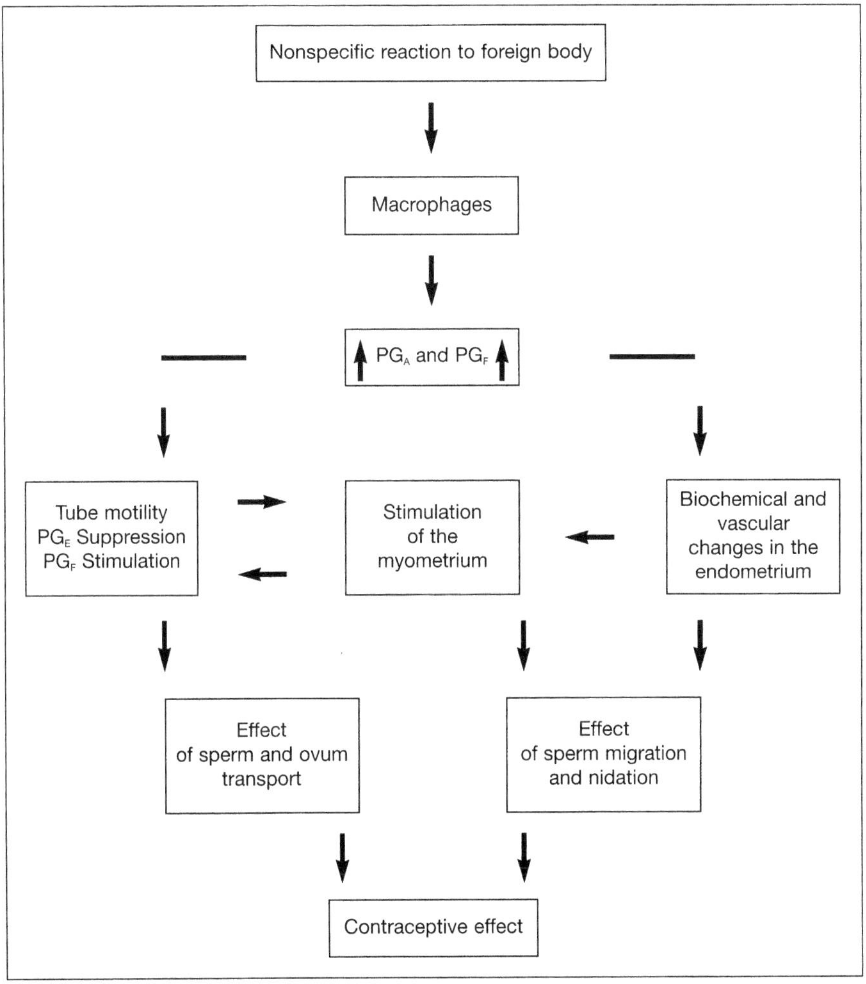

Fig. 10. Schematic showing contraceptive action of intrauterine (IU) copper with primary and secondary effects

Reliability

Copper IUDs provide reliable protection against unwanted pregnancy. The Pearl Index scores range between 0.5 and 2 depending on the type of device used.

Insertion

There are two main methods of IUD insertion. In the withdrawal method, the device is pulled into the inserter tube by its string, the inserter is then introduced through

Table 1. Insertion procedure for a copper intrauterine devices (IUD)

Take detailed patient history and obtain informed consent (in writing)
Examination
Speculum setting (native cytology etc.)
Disinfecting
Hook into portio
Determine length of probe (cavimetry)
Insertion of IUD
Shorten string
Verify correct positioning by ultrasound

the cervical canal into the uterine cavity, the device is ejected from the inserter by means of the plastic pusher rod, which is removed before the inserter is withdrawn (T devices). In the push-in method, the device is pushed through the cervical canal into the uterine cavity and the inserter is then withdrawn. The first method makes the passage through the cervix without dilatation easier, even if the canal is very tight. The second technique is simpler, but it requires a wider cervical canal.

Conditions for the insertion of IUDs and the insertion procedure itself are now standardised (Table 1). The size and shape of the intrauterine cavity should be known in advance. The geometry of the uterine slit can be identified with a cavimeter (cavimetry). It can be used, for instance, in the same way as a probe and introduced into the cervical canal. There are two dilator legs at the tip of the probe. The distance between them can be read on a scale so that the shape of the cervical canal can be identified as the probe is drawn back (Fig. 11). Any ultrasound equipment can display and measure the width and length of the slit of the uterine cavity. Cavimetry is particularly recommended before insertion of an IUD in very young nulligravida women. It is essential to hook into the portio before and extend the uterus during insertion. In principle, insertion can be performed at any time in the menstrual cycle, but the best and safest time is towards the end of the menses. After a pregnancy, insertion can take place either using one of the specially developed IUDs during the post-placental period or alternatively when the uterus has returned to its normal shape and size. It is urgently recommended that informed patient consent be obtained in writing well before the IUD is inserted. Forms for this purpose are available from pharmaceutical companies or wholesalers.

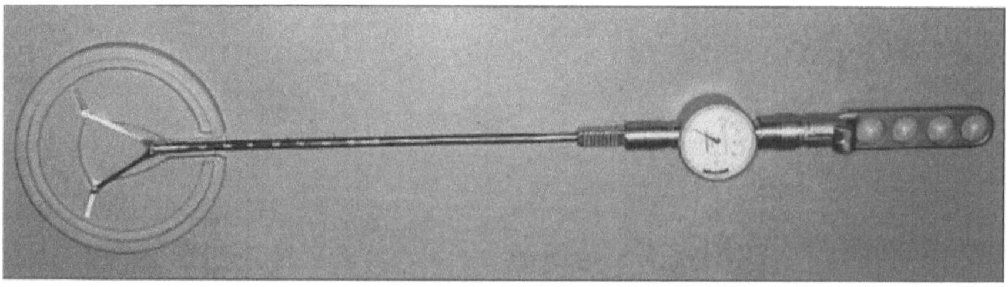

Fig. 11. Kurz cavimeter [20]. The cavimeter has the same dimensions as a normal uterine probe. When the tip is inserted to the fundus uteri, a hand lever dilates the two arms in a V-shape. The spacing between the two arms can then be read off a scale in centimetres. By pulling back the cavimeter, the transverse width of the cavity can be measured, e.g. centimeter by centimeter, so that a diagram of the whole cavity can be made. This model has been the most useful of all the different cavimeter developments throughout the world.

Dislocation, partial and complete expulsion, and partial and complete perforation do occur with copper-bearing IUDs, but steady improvements in the devices have made them very rare nowadays. Over 90% of perforations are of iatrogenic origin, usually caused inadvertently by a faulty insertion technique. Intracervical and complete expulsion often goes unnoticed by the user. Complete expulsion is mainly observed in women who use tampons for menstrual hygiene, because the IUD string was left too long. Contraceptive protection is obviously lost if this happens. If the IUD string is not visible in the cervical canal, or if there is no clear sonographic or X-ray evidence of the presence of the device in the uterus, the gynaecologist must rule out the possibility of complete expulsion or perforation (lost IUD). The safest way to do this is by a full abdomen X-ray in standing position. If the woman wishes to continue with intrauterine contraception after complete expulsion, it is advisable to recommend a different model and rule out any abnormalities of the uterine cavity before insertion. The safest method of checking the correct positioning of an IUD is to use ultrasound. The IUD is correctly positioned in the uterine cavity when the inferior pole of the vertical member lies no lower than the os uteri. A transabdominal ultrasound view of the uterus with a well filled urinary bladder still gives the best topographical assessment of an IUD.

Pain and menstrual disorders are fairly common during the first three menstrual cycles after insertion. We might describe them as a sort of adjustment to the IUD by the uterus. If they persist, further examination and diagnosis are required (to eliminate dislocation, perforation, infection). Heavier and longer periods, however, may continue for a considerable time. Despite a great deal of effort, no effective treatment has yet been found. In individual cases, there may be no alternative but to advise changing to a different method of contraception [36].

Pelvic inflammatory disease (PID) is now rare with modern copper-bearing IUDs. They do not protect against infection, but neither are they causally responsible for PID. Everything depends on the sexual behaviour of the woman herself and her partner. The risk of PID in the different age groups is no higher for IUD users than for those who use hormone-based contraception, as shown by our own experiments. If infection does occur in a woman using a copper-bearing IUD, however, it is usually more severe, so that removal of the device is recommended as soon as it is discovered, followed as early as possible by proper diagnosis and the appropriate treatment. Endoscopy has proved useful in confirming diagnosis and determining the severity of the infection, while high-dose intravenous broad-spectrum antibiotics in hospital are the treatment of choice [8]. The sooner PID is detected and treated, the less serious the post-inflammatory complications are likely to be. Women who use oral contraception have to have check-ups at six-monthly intervals to obtain their prescriptions; regular check-ups should be equally routine for IUD users (Table 2) [3, 4, 6, 10-12, 19, 31, 32].

Unwanted pregnancies with copper-bearing IUD in place are rare. Once pregnancy has set in, the IUD should be removed as soon as possible by the appropriate methods. As the intrauterine device quickly becomes overgrown with decidua and, hence, fixed to the wall of the uterus, retraction of the draw string into the cervical canal or even the uterine cavity may occur by the fourth or fifth week. If the string is no longer visible, the safest and least traumatic way of extracting the IUD is, in our experience, hysteroscopy. After the twelfth week, removal is seldom possible without trauma, and so the IUD should be left in place if the woman wishes to continue with the

Table 2. Indications for immediate gynaecological examination for Cu-intrauterine device (IUD) users and recommended 6-monthly routine check-ups

1. Immediate Examination in case of:
   Bleeding and/or pain
   Vaginocervical bacteriology
   Chlamydia
   Inflammation
   Expulsion, dislocation
   Menses more than 10 days overdue
2. Six-monthly check-ups in case of
   No symptoms
   History of gynaecological problems after insertion
   Speculum, native cytology
   Bacteriology findings if necessary
   Check string length
   Palpation
   Ultrasound scan (recommended)
   1-2 weeks after insertion
   3 months after insertion
   6 months after insertion
   etc.

pregnancy. As pregnancy progresses with the IUD still in the uterus, the risk of miscarriage, infection and premature labour increases, so that special ante-natal monitoring is required. No IUD or copper-specific birth defects have been observed in babies born after such pregnancies [2]. As in any other very early pregnancy, the possibility of ectopic pregnancy must be ruled out. There is no causal link between ectopic implantation and copper-bearing IUDs [9, 24, 42].

Copper allergies are extremely rare and have been described only in individual cases. Known allergies to heavy metals in patients' histories are mostly nickel allergies triggered by wearing costume jewellery [43].

Copper-bearing IUDs neither favour nor hinder the origination of genital carcinomas. For this reason, any symptoms in a user that seem to indicate genital cancer should be taken very seriously [5].

The string or strings attached to the device are there to help the woman and her doctor keep a check on its correct position in the uterus and make removal easier if necessary and do not facilitate either inflammation of the cervix or PID. After insertion of the device, the length of the string should be reduced to about 4 cm. It can even be cut off altogether outside the cervix, so that the end remains inside. Complete removal of the string before insertion is no problem, and the IUD can be inserted without it. It is not necessary for position checks, especially as most women are unable to feel it themselves anyway, and ultrasound scans are safer for position checks by the doctor, while modern techniques such as sonography or hysteroscopy are available to remove a stringless IUD [15]. If the string breaks off during an attempt at withdrawal, removal of the device by hysteroscopy is advisable as soon as possible for safety reasons.

X-ray diagnosis, magnetic resonance imaging (MRI) scans and spa treatments have no impact either on the reliability of the contraceptive method or on the woman's health as far as we know today. Short-wave therapy should be avoided, however, as the copper in the uterus may become considerably heated and trigger leucocytosis, the significance of which is not yet clear [14].

The morbidity and mortality risks associated with copper-bearing IUDs for reliable, popular and reversible contraception are low in comparison with other contra-

Table 3. Absolute and relative contraindications for the use of intrauterine devices (IUDs)

	Cu IUD	LNG IUD
Pregnancy	●●	●●
Suspected pregnancy	●●	●●
History of ectopic pregnancy	●	●
Abnormalities of the uterus	●●	●●
Hypoplasia of the uterus (uterine probe length <6 cm)	●	●
Hyperplasia of the uterus (uterine probe length >8 cm)	●	●
Abnormal position of the uterus	●	●
Pathological alteration of the uterus (e.g. myoma, adenomyosis)	●	●
History of adnexitis	●●	●●
Genital infection	●●	●●
Cervicitis	●●	●●
Cervical canal stenosis	●	●
Large lacerations of the cervix	●	●
Post-sectio / metroplasty	●	●
Dysmenorrhoea	●●	-
Hypermenorrhoea	●●	-
Recurrent irregular bleeding	●●	-
Tendency to haemorrhage	●●	●
Suspected genital carcinoma	●●	●●
Cu allergy	●●	-
Previous expulsion	●	●
History of breast cancer	-	●
Diabetes mellitus	-	-
Anticoagulant medication	●	-
Teenage nulligravida	●	●

●●, absolute, ●, relative; -, none

ceptive methods and pregnancy itself. This being so, correct indications, appropriate and skilful insertion, careful monitoring and good patient motivation, well-qualified doctors and scrupulous observation of exclusion criteria are essential (Table 3).

Intrauterine Contraception for Nulliparous Teenagers

The amendment of § 24 of the German Code of Social Law V means that women under 20 years of age can obtain contraceptives free of charge on prescription. The article explicitly names oral or hormonal contraceptives, IUDs (including insertion), which is paid for by the health funds for women with compulsory insurance, and anti-implantation drugs whose active principle takes effect before implantation of the fertilised ovum is complete so that they do not fall under the definition of agents for the termination of pregnancy according to § 218 of the Penal Code (Abortion). The long and bitter debate about whether or not to provide intrauterine contraception for very young nulligravidae has been virtually settled by these legal measures. According to the current view and our own experience of around 1200 IUD insertions for teenage nulligravidae, copper-bearing IUDs are suitable for such patients, subject to the appropriate menstrual pattern and size and shape of the uterine slit.

It is not sufficient simply to determine the length of the uterus before insertion, as the probe gives no indication of the transverse width and vertical length of the uterine cavity. In young women, the ratio of the portio to the corpus of the uterus is often less than 1:1 and not 1:3, as in the mature womb. T-models are therefore preferred for insertion in very young women, due to the tightness of the cervical canal, and our experience with the Cu-Safe-T 300 has been good. Nevertheless, it cannot be overstated that intrauterine contraception is not the method of choice for very young nulligravidae, and that it should only be considered at all by suitably qualified doctors experienced in the insertion technique. The contraceptive of choice for very young nulligravidae continues to be oral contraception [21, 35, 40].

Progestogen IUDs

Since the end of the sixties, a number of study groups have substituted progesterone for the copper in T-devices. In 1970, Progesteron-T went on the market in the U.S.A., followed in 1977 by Progestasert (Biograviplan) in Germany. The main advantage of Progestasert lies in reducing the menstrual blood loss; its drawbacks were bleeding disorders such as spotting, a high rate of ectopic pregnancy, the fact that it could stay in situ for only 12 months and its relatively high price. It was not long before it was taken off the market again in Germany.

Experimentation was going on concurrently with other progestogens. Levonorgestrel was favoured for its high gestagen potency. Whereas the transformation dose of progesterone was 200 mg per cycle, and 300-500 mg is required daily to suppress ovulation, the transformation dose for levonorgestrel is only about 2.5 mg per cycle and 0.05 mg per day for ovulation prevention. This made longer dwell times for the device possible by reducing the size of the depot required.

After experiments by the World Health Organization (WHO) to determine the dosage had been conducted in the U.S.A., an LNG-T was finally developed on the basis of the Nova-T. Its vertical member carries a plastic cylinder with a 52 mg. LNG depot instead of the copper wire winding. The daily release rate is 20 micrograms of LNG. The results of the WHO study were taken over by Leiras in Finland and further developed; by 1990 a marketable LNG device had at last been created and was introduced in the Nordic countries. In 1997, it was taken over by Schering for Germany too, and sold as

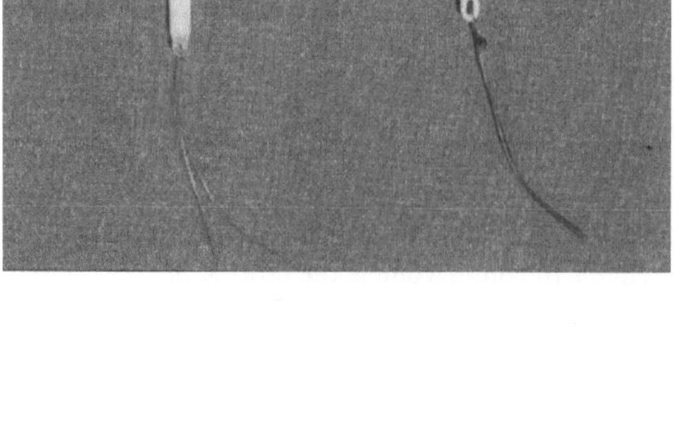

Fig. 12. Two gestagen releasing IUDs. Progestasert is shown on the left; on the right is the Mirena, an LNG IUD based on the Nova-T.

Table 4. Contraceptive effect of levonorgestrel (LNG) intrauterine device (IUD)

Cervix Factor	Increased viscosity, Reduction / prevention of sperm penetration (dose)
Endometrium	Non-specific foreign body reaction (slight) Secretory transformation ⇨ Atrophy
Tubes	Reduced motility (dose) (gestagen)
Endocrine system	Ovulation inhibition (partially via gonadotropin axis); Overall effect similar to that of "mini-pill"

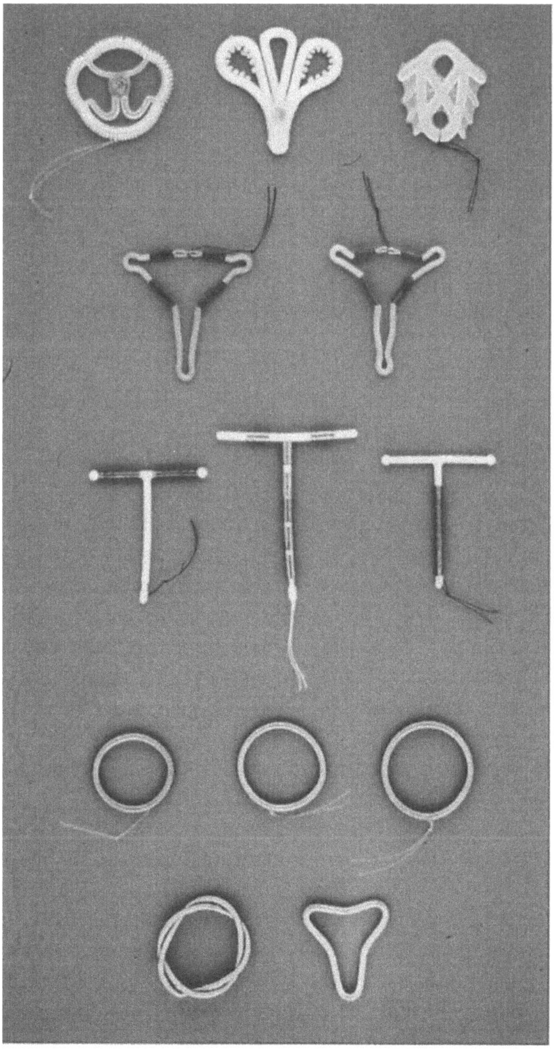

Fig. 13. Collection of Chinese IUDs, some of which are still used today. Some of them were developed by the Chinese themselves, others are imitations of Western models. Top row: left, a model following the OTA ring design; centre, the Canton flower with very flexible plastic fans that adjust to uterine motility; right, an imitation of the Dalcon Shield. Second row: Shanghai Cu V 200, made in different sizes. Third row (different T-shapes): centre, an imitation of the Copper-T 220 C. Fourth row: stainless steel coils based on the Hall ring, in various sizes. This is the most widely-used model in China. Bottom row: two more stainless steel IUDs; left, the Mahua ring made of two stainless steel intertwined coils.

"Mirena" (Fig. 12). An article by Odlind in this journal reports fully, so it is not necessary to go into detail at this point.

More research is needed into LNG's mechanism of contraceptive action. Nevertheless, it can be assumed that it is similar to that of the "mini-pill" (Table 4). Again, LNG devices have both good and bad points. The advantages are the reduction of the menstrual blood flow and the very low incidence of unwanted pregnancy, which rated almost zero on the Pearl Index. The downside during the first few cycles of use are bleeding disorders and dull aches that are just as bad as those with the copper IUD, a rate of amenorrhoea after a year of up to 20%, an insertion technique that is not without problems and the greatly increased difficulty of identification by either ultrasound or X-ray as well as the high price. In some study groups, the cumulative continuity rates for the Copper Nova T were higher than for the LNG Nova T [1, 7]. We shall have to wait for the results of long-term studies and our own results now that we have at last been able to gain experience in Germany. LNG IUDs are a welcome addition to the range of intrauterine contraception and are primarily suited to women who have completed their families but were previously unable to use copper-bearing IUDs due to hyper-menorrhoea, menorrhagia and metrorrhagia, yet refuse oral contraception. Such women need to be informed about the changes in menstrual bleeding, including amenorrhoea, before an LNG device is inserted. According to opinion polls in Germany, most women are willing to accept this kind of adverse effect.

The Future of Intrauterine Contraception

The significance of the IUD is bound to grow world-wide, as it is a reliable contraceptive with very low morbidity rates by comparison with other methods. Copper-bearing IUDs are the most inexpensive method of contraception, particularly when the manufacture of imitation devices in developing countries is taken into consideration. Insertion can be done by well-trained paramedical workers as well as by doctors (Fig. 13). Intrauterine contraception is currently the only practicable and affordable method of achieving world-wide, reliable and acceptable birth control in human terms [29].

In the United States and Western Europe, research is currently going on for new substances with intrauterine contraceptive action aimed in the long run to dispense with the IUD as a carrier. One example of this trend is Gyne-Fix, a copper-based intrauterine system (Cu-IUS) (Fig. 14). Copper sheaths of the type known from the Cu-T 220 C are threaded on a plastic string, the top end of which is anchored in the myometrium of the fundus by means of an astoundingly simple insertion technique. Similar intrauterine systems are conceivable using other active agents such as LNG (LNG-IUS) [37].

Experience with copper alloys has proved that it is possible to manufacture copper-bearing IUDs capable of remaining in place in the uterus for 30 years or more. If new developments like this are ever to reach the markets, it will be possible only with the scientific and financial resources of pharmaceutical companies. To that extent, further developments in intrauterine contraception will depend largely on the attitude of the pharmaceutical industry to the method itself and its market potential.

Efforts on the part of the European Union have ensured that IUDs will no longer be classified as medications but as medical products. In future, regulation of the IUD

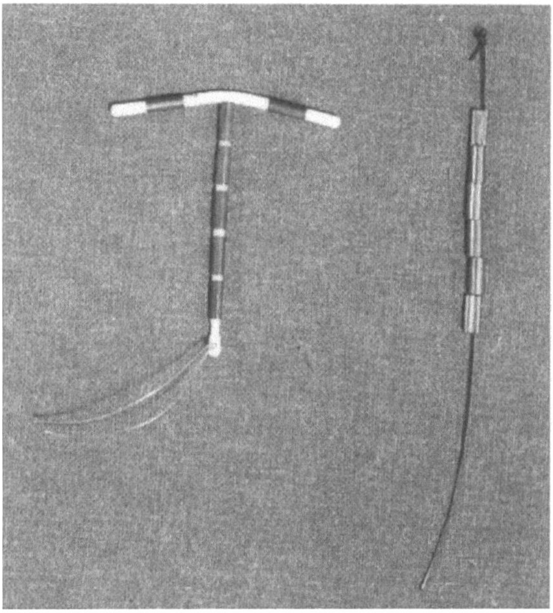

Fig. 14. Left, Cu-T 200 C with five copper sheaths on the vertical member and two on each of the horizontal arms. Next to it, the Gyne-Fix intrauterine implant consisting of six copper sheaths threaded on a monofil plastic string. The Gyne-Fix is fixed to the endomyometrium in the fundus by means of the knot which can be seen at the top end of the string. The device can move freely within the uterine cavity, and it is only the copper that acts as a contraceptive. Because it can move sideways inside the cavity, the spread of the foreign body reaction on the endometrial surface is even wider than with a T with horizontal sheaths. No plastic T carrier is needed in this intrauterine system with copper.

as a medical product will be dealt with (in Germany) under commercial legislation on medical products (Medical Products Law). Its purpose is to enact European Community Directives in national law in order to ensure adequate care for health and the protection of patients, users and third parties in handling, trading and using medical products while at the same time guaranteeing the future of Germany as a business location. The good thing about this law is that it sets Europe-wide quality standards. However, the Directives cover only IUDs and copper-bearing IUDs as yet. Whether or not a gestagen-releasing IUD is a medical product or a medical agent is still an unanswered question. Another undecided issue is whether intrauterine systems like Gyne-Fix are covered by the Law, or whether they will still be handled as medical drugs. The bureaucrats still have a lot of work ahead.

Translator's note. References to German law etc. have been characterised as such in the translation for the benefit of non-German readers.

References

1. Andersson K, Odlind V, Rybo G (1994) Levonorgestrel-releasing and copper releasing (Nova4) IUDs during five years of use: A randomized comparative trial. Contraception 49: 56-72
2. Barash A, Shoham Z, Borenstein R, Nebel L (1990) Development of human embryos in the presence of a copper intrauterine device. Gynefi. Obstet. Invest. 29:203-206
3. Bromham DR (1993) Intrauterine contraceptive devices – A reappraisal. Br Med Bull 49: 100-123
4. Buchan H, Villard-Mackintosh L, Vessey M, Yetes D, Mc Pherson K (1990) Epidemiology of pelvic inflammatory disease in parous women with special reference to intrauterine device users. Br J Obste. Gynecol 97: 780-788

5. Castelisagué X, Douglas TW, Dubrow R (1993) Intrauterine contraception and the risk of endometrial Cancer. Int. J. Cancer 54: 911-916
6. Chi I-C (1993) What we have learned from recent IUD studies: A researcher's perspective. Contraception 48: 81-108
7. Chi I-C (1993) The TCU-A (AG), MLCU 375, and Nova-T IUDs and the IUD daily releasing 20 pg Levonorgestrel - four pillars of IUD contraception for the nineties and beyond? Contraception 47: 325-347
8. Decker K, Reiner R, Hirsch HA (1988) Laparoskopische Befunde bei Verdacht auf Adnexitis. Geburtsh. u. Frauenheilk. 48: 800-803
9. Edelmann DA, Porter CW (1986) The intrauterine device and ectopic pregnancy. Adv. Contracept. 2: 55-63
10. Edelmann DA, van Os WAA (1990) Safety of intrauterine contraception. Adv. Contracept. 6:207-217
11. Edelmann DA, Porter CW (1993) The new intrauterine contraceptive devices: safe and effective. Adv. Contracept. 9: 83-91
12. Farley TMM, Rosenberg MJ, Rowe PJ, Chen JH, Meirik O (1992) Intrauterine devices and pelvic infiammatory disease: an international perspective. The Lancet 339: 785-788
13. Gesenius H (1970) Empfängnisverhütung. Urban und Schwarzenberg, München-Berlin-Wien
14. Hess T, Stepanow B, Knopp MV (1996) Safety of Intrauterine contraceptive devices during MR Imaging. Eur. Radiol. 6. 66-68
15. Hucke J, Campo RL, Kozlowski P, De Bruyne F (1991) Erfahrungen mit der hysteroskopischen oder sonographisch gesteuerten Entfernung einer Intrauterinspirale ohne sichtbaren Faden in der Frühschwangerschaft. Geburtsh. u. Frauenheilk. 51: 31-33
16. Jones HW, Jaffe RB, Cefalo, RC, Bowes WA (1996) IUDs: A state of the art conference. Obstet a. Gynecol. Survey 51: 1-72
17. Koch UJ (1980) Sperm migration in the humen female genital tract with and without intrauterine devices. Acta Europaea Fertilitatis 11: 33-60
18. Koch UJ (1985) Effects of copper IUDs oin cervical cytology and influences on transtubal sperm migration. In: Biomedical Aspects of IUDs. Hasson H, Hafez ESE, van Os WA edts. MTP Press Limited, Lancaster, Boston, The Hague, Dordrecht 2: 25-44
19. Kronmal RA, Whitney CW, Mumford SD (1991) The intrauterine device and pelvic inflammatory disease: The women's health study reanalyzed. J Clin. Epidemiol. 44:109-122
20. Kruczynaki D, Passia D, Berthold D (1991) Lokalisation von Schwermetallen in menschlichen Spermien in Korrelation zu ihrer Motilität. Gyn. Comp. 1: 13
21. Kurz KH (1981) Avoidance of the dimensional incompatibility as the main reason for side effects in intrauterine contraception. Contraceptive Delivery Systems 2: 21-29
22. Lehfeldt H (1975) Efftst GrAfenberq and his Ring. Mount Sinai J. of Med. 4: 345-352
23. Liskin L, Fox G (1982) lUVa: An appropriate contraceptive for many women. Population reports. Baltimore, Maryland 4:101-135
24. Lurie S, Katz Z, Yechezkeli Y, Lifsitz-Mercer B, Shoham Z (1994) Microscopic salpingMe Is not an etiologic factor of tubal pregnancy with intrauterine devices. Int. J. Fertil. 39: 333-336
25. Moyer DL, Shaw ST (1973) Intrauterine devices: biological action. In: Human reproduction: conception and contraception. Hrsg. Hafez ESE, Evans TN. Harper u. Row, Hagerstown, Maryland
26. O'Hanley K, Huber DH (1992) Post parturn IUD's: Keys for success. Contraception 45: 351-361
27. Oppenheimer W (1959) Prevention of pregnancy by the Gräfenberg-Ring-Method. Am J Obstet Gynecol 78:446-451
28. Ortiz ME, Croxatto HB, Bardin CW (1996) Mechanism of action of intrauterine devices. Obstet Gyneco. Surv. 51: 42-51
29. Petta CA, Mc Pheeters M, Chi IC (1996) Intrauterine devices: Learning from the past and looking to the future. J. biosoc. Sci 28: 241-252
30. Richter R (1909) Ein Mittel zur Verhütung der Konzeption. Dtsch. med. Wschr. 35:1525-1528
31. Shannon J, Benrubi GI (1991) Epidemiology of pelvic inflammatory disease. J. Florida M.A. 78:158-161
32. Schwarz H, Mead PB (1991) A new look at IUD-associated infections. Contemporary OB/Gyn 10: 65-92
33. Skouby SO, Molsted-Pedersen L, Kuehl C (1986) Contraception In diabetic women. Acta Endocrinologica 277:125-129
34. Spinnato JA (1997) Mechanism of action of intrauterine contraceptive devices and its relation to informed consent. Am. J. Obstet. Gynecol. 176: 503-506

35. Struthers BJ (1991) Copper IUDs, PID, and fertility in nulliparous women. Advances in contraception 7:211-230
36. Tauber PF, Kloppel LA, Goodpasture JC, Bums J, Ludwig H, Zaneveld LJD (1981) Reduced menstrual blood loss by release of an antifibrlnolytic agent from intrauterine contraceptive devices. Am. J. Obstet. a. Gynecol. 140:322-328
37. Van Kets H, Vrijens M, van Trappen Y, Delbarge W, van der Pas H, Temmermann M, Depypere H, Batar I, Bard P, Martinez F, Iglesias-Cortit L, Shangchun W, Xiaoming C, Chong FZ, Hui WM, Wildemeersch D, Pizarro E, Andrade A, Thiery M (1995) The frameless Gyne Fix Intrauterine Implant. A major improvement in efficacy, expulsion and tolerance. Adv. Contracept. 11: 7-12
38. Wagner H, Predel B, Bröcker W (1975) Biologische Effekte von Intrauterinpessaren. In: Bailer FK, Böttcher, HD: Moderne Kontrazeption. Georg Thieme Verlag Stuttgart
39. Wagner H, Beller FK, Bröcker W (1977) Untersuchungen über die kontrazeptive Wirkung des Gräfenberg-Ringes. Geburtsh. u. Frauenheilk. 37: 124-129
40. Wagner H, Nohlen M (1988) Intrauterine Kontramption bei Jugendlichen? Korasion 4: 37-44
41. Wagner H (1989) Intrauterine Kontrazoption. In: Klinik der Frauenheilkunde und Geburtshilfe Bd. 2: Sexualmedizin - Infertilität - Familienplanung 8: 283-310
42. Xiong X, Suekens P, Wollast E (1995) EUD - use and the risk of ectopic pregnancy: A meta-analysis of case-control studies. Contraception 52: 23-34
43. Zabel M, Lindscheid KR, Mark H (1990) Kupfersulfatallergie unter besonderer Berücksichtigung der internen Exposition. Zeitschr. f. Hautkrankheiten 65: 481-486

8 Intrauterine Hormone-Releasing Systems

Pekka Lähteenmäki

Research and Development

Background

The development of intrauterine contraceptive devices and oral contraceptives has been the major breakthrough in the history of modern contraception. The principle of combining the favourable effects of these two contraceptive methods has been approached by the introduction of intrauterine systems (IUSs) that release steroids. Several steroids have been tested in vitro and in animal models, including clormadinone acetate, medroxyprogesterone acetate, megestrol acetate, norethindrone, levonorgestrel and progesterone [4]. Only the latter two hormones have been utilised in progestogen-releasing IUSs that have reached extensive clinical trials and later been put into use. The first clinical trial of progesterone-releasing IUSs was published in 1970 [28]. Nilsson and co-workers [16] published the first clinical study with levonorgestrel-releasing IUS. These two intrauterine hormone-releasing systems demonstrated that it was possible to combine the favourable effects of oral contraceptives, i.e. good efficacy, decreased menstrual bleeding, decreased menstrual pain and less pelvic inflammatory disease, together with those of intrauterine devices, i.e. good compliance, long-acting method, reversible and no oestrogens.

It is well justified to call these methods IUSs to differentiate them from IUDs. IUSs need to be considered as hormonal contraceptive methods, with the associated benefits and adverse effects. Many of the effects, such as decrease or even cessation of menstrual bleeding that occur during intrauterine administration of progestin, were originally regarded as adverse effects. Once their nature has been more thoroughly characterised, it will be possible to explain to the user that no harm is caused by the changes in the menstrual pattern. Many women appreciate the freedom associated with reduced bleeding or endometrial amenorrhea. Levonorgestrel IUS produces amenorrhea in about 20% of users and can be regarded as a step towards no-bleed contraception.

Systems

There are only two commercially available progestin IUSs. The first intrauterine progesterone-releasing contraceptive system on the market was Progestasert. It was approved in the US in 1976 and has been on the market since then. It is manufactured in the US by Alza Corp. and is currently available in the US, Canada and France. The drug reservoir contains 38 mg of progesterone, with an initial release rate of 65 μg/day. The system is indicated for 1 year of intrauterine contraception in women who are in a stable, mutually monogamous relationship, and who have no history of pelvic inflammatory disease. After 12 months, the women must return to a clinic to have the system removed or replaced.

The intrauterine levonorgestrel-releasing system, Mirena, consists of a levonorgestrel-polydimethylsiloxane elastomer sleeve, consisting of 1:1 mixture of polymer and 52 mg of steroid, mounted on a supporting T-body (32x32 mm) made of polyethylene. The body is the same as used in the Nova T copper IUD. The sleeve is covered with a drug-release-controlling membrane of medical grade polydimethylsiloxane. The system releases the active ingredient, levonorgestrel, over a period of up to 5 years, at a practically constant rate. The initial release rate of Mirena is 20 μg/day, and at the end of 5 years, the release is still above 10 μg/day. It is manufactured by Leiras Oy, Turku, Finland, the subsidiary of Schering AG, Berlin, Germany. Mirena was first introduced in Finland in 1990 and is currently marketed by Schering in more than 20 countries.

Local Suppression of Endometrium by Progestins

Since progestin-releasing IUSs are in intimate contact with endometrium, the greatest changes during exposure are to endometrial morphology. Intrauterine administration of 20 μg levonorgestrel daily leads to strong suppression of the endometrium. Its glands become atrophic and its stoma decidualized [18, 30]. The mucosa is thin and the stoma swollen. The epithelium is inactive. These histological changes are uniform within a month of levonorgestrel IUS use, and the picture does not change according to the phase of the menstrual cycle [30]. Additional microscopic changes, such as stromal leucocyte infiltrations, sometimes containing plasma cells and usually accompanied by small necroses and scarring, are present in samples taken during the levonorgestrel IUS, and are similar to those observed with copper IUDs [30].

The local release of progestin also has important effects on the biochemistry of the endometrium. The synthesis of estradiol receptors is downregulated during progesterone administration [11], making endometrium insensitive to oestrogen stimulus. This would explain why the endometrium does not show normal growth in response to the circulating oestrogen levels. Although this has not been shown with local administration of levonorgestrel, there is little reason to believe the situation to be different. Furthermore, local levonorgestrel increases the synthesis of insulin-like growth factor-binding proteinin-1 in the decidualized cells of the endometrium [23]. A recent report describes an "inappropriate" expression of glycodelin A in endometrium between cycle days 7 and 16 in women who have Mirena inserted [15]. Both of the latter two proteins may have a role in the clinical contraceptive efficacy of Mirena. IGF-binding protein-1 has been shown to regulate the effect of estradiol on endometrium, mediated by IGF [23]. Glycodelin A has been shown to have contraceptive properties in vitro [15]. It inhibits potently and dose dependently the binding of sperm to the zona pellucida [20].

Minimal Effects on the Ovary and Pituitary

Mirena releases levonorgestrel into the uterine cavity, where it is quickly absorbed via the capillary network into the systemic circulation (Fig. 1). Maximum plasma levels are reached within a few hours. Plasma levonorgestrel concentrations reach a plateau of 100-200 pg/ml after the first few weeks [19] (Fig. 2). Plasma concentrations achieved by Mirena are lower than those seen with Norplant, the combines oral contraceptives and the minipill. Although levonorgestrel concentrations are fairly stable, there is significant interindividual variation [19].

Plasma levonorgestrel is mainly bound to sex-hormone-binding-globulin (SHBG). This affinity for levonorgestrel may inhibit the metabolic degradation of levonorgestrel [10].

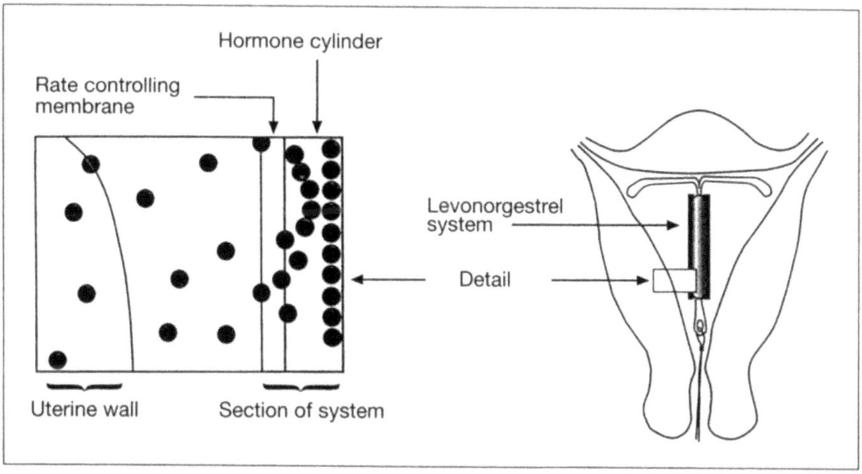

Fig. 1. Mirena in the uterine cavity. Sustained release of levonorgestrel from the system gives a high local concentration in the endometrium, but lowest systemic blood concentration of any levonorgestrel hormonal contraceptive

Fig. 2. Plasma levonorgestrel concentrations in Mirena users over 5 years. Individual concentrations remain relatively constant throughout the use, but the interindividual variation may be wide [19].

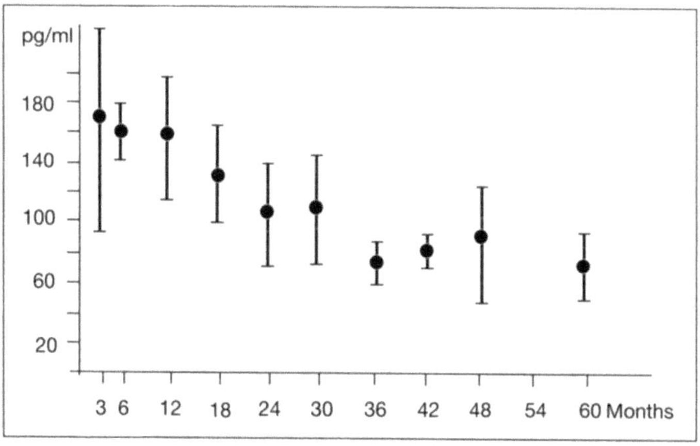

Table 1. Plasma estradiol (mean±SE) concentrations (pg/ml) in women using Mirena

	3 months	1 year	2 years	5 years	7 years
Estradiol	168	105	128	110	112
SE	29	10	10	14	17
N	33	53	42	32	34

In the majority of women, serum levonorgestrel concentration is not high enough to inhibit ovulation. Up to 85% of women using Mirena are ovulatory [26]. However, the midcycle peaks of luteinizing hormone (LH) and follicle-stimulating hormone (FSH) are often blunted [7]. For complete inhibition of ovulation, a daily intrauterine release of 50 μg/day is needed [14]. With 20 μg/day, release of levonorgestrel ovarian estradiol production is not disturbed. The individual estradiol concentrations fall into the range typical of normal menstrual cycles (Table 1) and usually no menopausal values are found. There is no difference between menstruating and amenorrheic women [14]. This is important as a guarantee that women using Mirena are not exposed to hypo-oestrogenism, leading to osteoporosis.

Mirena Prevents Fertilisation

So far, it has been impossible to conclusively demonstrate a single mode of action for contraceptive efficacy of Mirena (Table 2). The classical progestin effect causes thickening of the cervical mucus. The local progestin effect prevents endometrial growth [30]. The local progestin seems to create a hostile environment for fertilisation, while inhibiting sperm mobility and function inside the uterus and ovarian tubes [37]. Similar to copper IUD users, recovery studies have been unable to find normally fertilised eggs in Mirena users [21]. As described earlier, some specific changes in the function of endometrium also contribute or may even play a key role in the contraceptive efficacy of Mirena. Glycodelin A has been shown to be expressed in endometrium during Mirena use [15].

High Contraceptive Efficacy with Full Reversibility

The efficacy of Mirena for contraceptive use has been established in a number of studies. The four main studies (Table 3) demonstrate that the 5-year Pearl index for Mirena is 0.1. The clinical comparative studies gather data from more than 12,000 woman-years of Mirena use. Some of these clinical studies have covered up to 7 years of use.

Table 2. The proposed mechanisms of action contributing to contraceptive efficacy of Mirena

Thickening of cervical mucus
Suppression of endometrial development
Hostile environment in the uterus and Fallopian tubes preventing fertilisation
Disturbance in normal ovulation
Stimulation of endometrial proteins leading to inhibition of fertilisation (glycodelin A)

Table 3. Main studies documenting the clinical efficacy of Mirena. Overall experience in clinical studies covers more than 12 000 woman years

Study	Duration	Woman years	Mirena users	Control	Pearl Index
Pilot	5	884	281	Nova T	0.1
Population Council	7	2831	1124	Copper T	0.2
Multicenter in Europe	5	5615	1821	Nova T	0.1
Indian Medical Council	3	882	475	Several	0.0

Table 4. Pregnancy rates for different age groups in European multicenter study comparing Mirena and Nova T copper IUD. There is an age-dependent difference in contraceptive efficacy for copper IUD users but, for Mirena users, the efficacy is independent of the user's age [4].

Age (years)	Mirena	Nova T
<25	0.0	2.9
25-30	0.1	1.5
31-35	0.1	0.8
>35	0.2	0.6

The clinical efficacy of Mirena in contraception is not age dependent. The European multicentre study [4, 13, 35] clearly demonstrated that, unlike copper IUDs, Mirena is as effective in young fertile women as in women in their later reproductive years (Table 4).

It is important to know that all endometrial changes occurring during the use of intrauterine progestin-releasing systems are completely reversible. The normal endometrial morphology and function resumes as soon as the device has been removed [30]. The fertilisation rates after removal of Mirena are similar to those seen after removal of copper IUDs [17]. The cross-cumulative conception rate is 79.1 at 1 year after removal [2], which is comparable to the normal conception rate.

A matter of concern has been the fact that both Progestasert and a low-dose (2 µg/day) levonorgestrel IUS developed by the World Health Organization (WHO) have resulted in increased risk of ectopic pregnancy. With Progestasert, the relative risk is increased several fold compared with copper IUDs [31]. A clinical trial of WHO with the levonorgestrel IUD releasing 2 µg daily was discontinued because of the increase in ectopic pregnancies [36]. In contrast, Mirena releasing 20 µg daily decreases the ectopic pregnancy risk relative to most copper IUDs [31]. From the studies published, the estimated risk of ectopic pregnancy with Mirena is about 1 in 5000 woman-years.

Menstrual Changes for Everyone

The use of Mirena is characterised by bleeding-pattern changes in all women. The major change is an overall reduction in the menstrual volume, which becomes even more prominent after long-term use. Also, most women experience additional bleeding and spotting during the first 1-6 months after insertion of Mirena. The reason for the change in bleeding pattern is the endometrial atrophy caused by local progestin. These changes are reversible, returning to the original state immediately after removal of the IUS.

Not only does the volume of menstrual bleeding decrease [16, 27], but also the number of bleeding days decreases during Mirena use [33]. Compared with copper IUD users, the median number of bleeding days decreases quickly in Mirena users. They also have significantly fewer days of menstrual bleeding than copper IUD users from the second month on. After 8 months, half of the Mirena users experience no menstrual bleeding (Fig. 3). Although the interindividual variation in the total num-

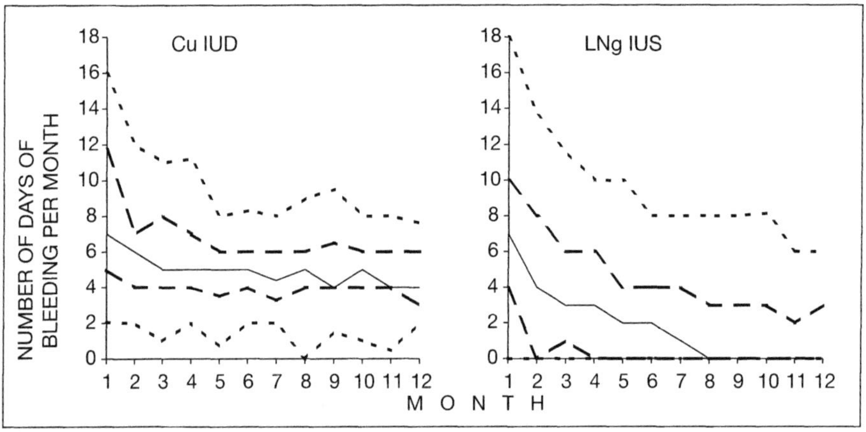

Fig. 3. Number of days of menstrual bleeding per month during the first year of use of copper IUD *(left)* or Mirena *(right)*. *Solid line* depicts the median, *dotted lines* the 10th, 25th, 75th and 90th percentiles. From the second month onwards Mirena users experience significantly fewer days of bleeding compared with copper IUD users. From 8 months onwards, more than 50% of Mirena users experience no bleeding, but can have light spotting

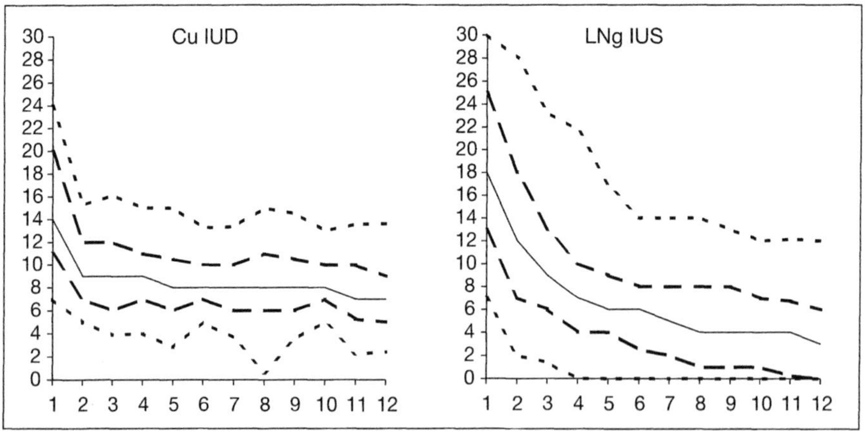

Fig. 4. The sum of the menstrual bleeding and spotting days per month during the first year after insertion of Nova T *(left panel)* or Mirena *(right panel)*. Median *(solid line)* and 10th, 25th, 75th and 90th percentiles *(dotted lines)* are depicted. Although the interidividual variation of the sum of bleeding and spotting days is initially higher in Mirena users, the spotting is decreased to the same level as in copper IUD users from 6 months onwards

ber of bleeding and spotting days is greater in Mirena users initially (Fig. 4), after 6 months, the variation is the same as in copper IUD users. This means that in Mirena users, menstruation is mainly scanty spotting. It is impossible to predict the individual behaviour of menstruation in the new user. The key message for counselling is to expect, at 3-6 months, significant improvement for those users who had excessive spotting at the beginning. When both menstrual bleeding and spotting are analysed (Fig. 4), 5% of women have no bleeding after 4 months of Mirena use and 20-25% of women experience no bleeding at all after 12 months of use [33].

Other subjective side effects are common during the first month after insertion and subside during the prolonged use. Table 5 gives the incidence of adverse effects reported at 3 months and 5 years by more than 1% of 821 women who were questioned non-specifically about the systems in use (Leiras data on file).

Table 5. Percentage of women reporting side effects after the non-leading question during the first 3 months and fifth year of use of Mirena in the European multicenter study [4].

Side effects	3 months	5 years
Lower abdominal pain	10.5	2.1
Acne or other skin problems	3.5	1.2
Back pain	3.1	1.0
Mastalgia	3.1	1.0
Headache	2.8	1.6
Vaginal discharge	2.7	<1
Mood changes	2.5	<1
Nausea	2.4	<1
Edema	1.1	<1

Choice of Users

The ideal user of a progestin IUS (as well as of a copper IUD) is a parous woman over 25 years of age that is living in a mutually monogamous relationship. Women under 25 years of age seem to be at a higher risk of contracting sexually transmitted diseases. There is no upper age limit for use of progestin IUS; in fact, it seems to be an ideal method of contraception in the transition from late reproductive years to menopause. Intrauterine contraception may not be the first choice for young women. If this is the eventual choice, a progestin IUS should be preferred to copper IUD because of its reported protective effect against pelvic inflammatory disease [4, 35].

Progestin IUSs should always been considered as an option before recommending that a woman undergo sterilisation. An IUS is a reversible method and, therefore, especially worthy of consideration for younger women, e.g. in their 30s, who may later want more babies. Insertion of an IUS is a simple procedure compared with sterilisation.

Both Postmenstrual and Postabortal Insertions Are Suitable

The progestin IUS should be inserted within 7 days from the onset of menstrual bleeding to guarantee effectiveness from the very beginning. The local signs and symptoms of genital infection must be noted and, if present, appropriate diagnostic and therapeutic measures should be taken before insertion. It is mandatory to review carefully the insertion technique of the systen. Inappropriate insertion technique may result in poor performance of the method, resulting in expulsions and pregnancies. Although perforations are not a common problem, partial penetration of an IUS into myometrium increases bleeding and pain. If the pain beyond normal postinsertional cramps occurs or if excessive bleeding continues, the proper location of the IUS can be verified by ultrasonography. Routine ultrasonography is not necessary if an experienced provider does the insertion.

Mirena has been successfully inserted in women immediately after a first trimester abortion [4, 9]. In fact, the analysis of menstrual bleeding after postmenstrual and postabortal insertion of Mirena and copper IUD suggests even better menstrual performance of Mirena in postabortal insertions [33].

Intrauterine Progestin Administration Gives Health Benefits

Mirena has proven to be a contraceptive method that brings about both contraceptive (Table 6) and non-contraceptive health benefits (Table 7). Intrauterine administration of levonorgestrel reduces the amount of menstrual bleeding. Local administration inactivates the growth of endometrium, which can be documented both histologically

Table 6. Contraceptive benefits of Mirena

Contraceptive benefit
High efficacy with Pearl rate 0.1
Active for 5 years
Decreases the need for abortions
Efficacy is not age dependent
Decreases the number of ectopic pregnancies
Hormonal side effects are not common
Reversible
Also appropriate for men who cannot tolerate oestrogens
Average annual continuation rate is 80%
Insertion can occur immediately after first trimester abortion

Table 7. Non-contraceptive benefits of Mirena

Non-contraceptive benefit
Reduction of menstrual blood loss
Effective treatment of menorrhagia
Reduces the cost of menstrual hygiene
Reduces the number of bleeding days
Improves haemoglobin and body iron stores
Decreases dysmenorrhea
Decreases the incidence of pelvic inflammatory disease
Decreases the development of fibroids
Effective treatment of endometrial hyperplasia
Easy removal

[30] and ultrasonographically [22]. Clinically, this is seen as a reduction in menstrual bleeding. Objective measurements in normally menstruating women have shown a reduction of menstrual blood loss by 30-40 ml/cycle (Fig. 5) [16, 27]. Most women regard the reduction in menstrual bleeding as an improvement of the quality of life. This also reduces the cost of menstrual hygiene. However, it is very important to counsel women about the expected changes in their menstrual pattern before the insertion of Mirena.

The ability of Mirena to decrease menstrual blood loss can be utilised therapeutically to treat menorrhagic women. Menstrual blood loss diminished from 176 ml to 24 ml (86%) after 3 months of use and to 5 ml (97%) after 12 months of Mirena use [5]. In a comparison with medical treatments of menorrhagia, Mirena was superior to oral contraceptives, non-steroidal anti-inflammatory drugs and fibrinolysis inhibitors (Fig. 6) [1]. The reduction in menstrual blood loss is reflected in increased blood haemoglobin and body iron store [8].

While decreasing the menstrual flow, Mirena also decreases dysmenorrhea [4]. In Finland and other Nordic countries, dysmenorrhea is a treatment indication for Mirena. It also has positive preventative effects on sexual health. One study demonstrated the protective effect of Mirena on pelvic infections [6, 35]. Another study demonstrated decreased development of uterine enlargements, i.e. fibroids in Mirena users compared with copper IUD users [32]. Mirena has also been used for the successful treatment of endometrial hypoplasia [24, 25]. Therefore, it is easy to hypothesise, based on the theoretical background and clinical evidence, that the use of Mirena would prevent the development of endometrial hypoplasia. Mirena has been used successfully in hormonal replacement therapy as a progestin component for women who have their uterus intact [3].

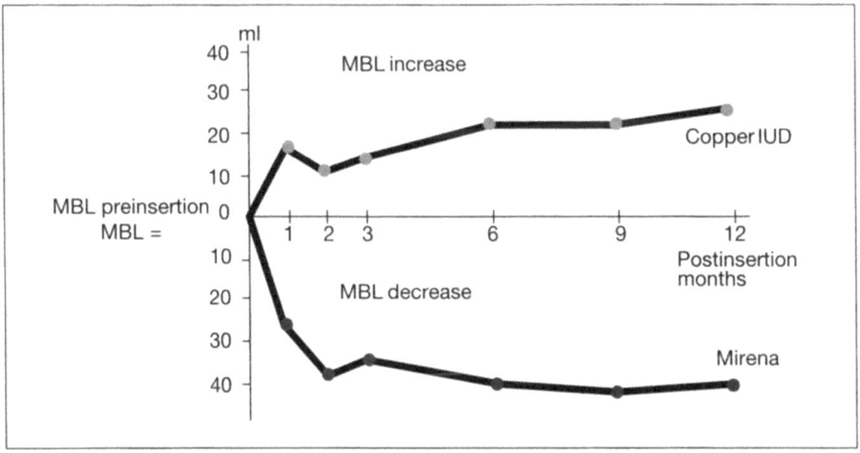

Fig. 5. Change of measured menstrual blood loss per month compared with preinsertion volume in women having either a copper IUD or Mirena. The menstrual blood loss increased in copper IUD users about 20 ml per month during the first year of use, whereas it decreased about 40 ml in women using Mirena [27].

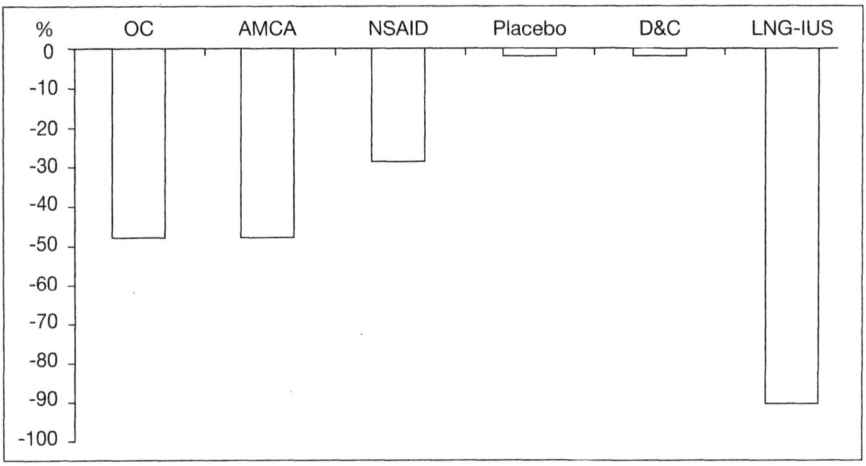

Fig. 6. Percentage reduction of menstrual blood loss in women suffering from menorrhagia (blood loss more than 80 ml per month). Mirena users had a reduction of more than 90% at 12 months. The treatment with oral contraceptives (OC), fibrinolysis inhibitors (AMCA), prostaglandin synthesis inhibitors (NSAID), placebo or dilatation and curettage (D&C) were less effective [1].

Counselling of Clients Is Essential for Successful Use

Mirena is a new method of contraception with some special features. Therefore, extensive counselling of both users and providers is essential for its successful application. Women should be advised that, during the first 2 months of use, harmless irregular and scanty spotting may occur. Menstruation will be shorter and of a lesser volume. In many women, bleeding may not occur at all. Oligoamenorrhea is not a sign of pregnancy or menopause. The women can be reassured that their ovarian function is continuing even in the absence of menstruation. When adequately advised beforehand, most women learn to like the change. Advice on the high level of effectiveness

Fig. 7. User satisfaction of women who have previously used copper IUD, after 12 months of Mirena use. More than 70% were much more or a little more satisfied with Mirena use than copper IUD use [29].

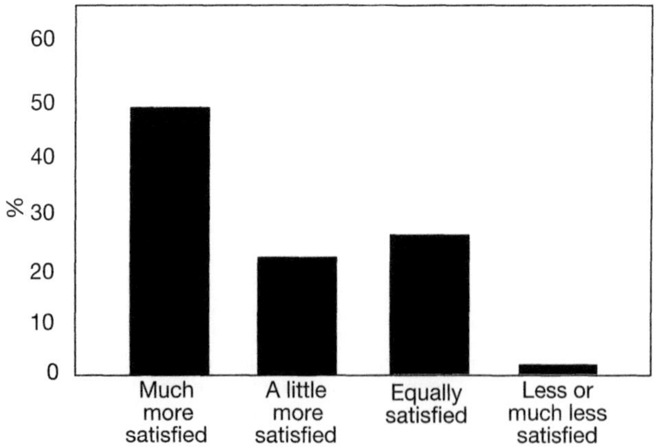

of the method is important to motivate women using this method. She should also be told that the benefits, such as increased haemoglobin, better iron stores, general well being and relief from menstrual dysmenorrhea, are a consequence of Mirena use.

During the first months after insertion, the user may suffer episodic headaches, swelling, breast tenderness and skin problems, but these hormonal side effects usually disappear. Mirena may be expelled like other IUDs. If normal menstruation returns, it is most probably an indication of expulsion and the user should contact the clinic. Furthermore, if the woman has episodes of heavy bleeding, it may be a sign of penetration of the device into myometrium; such bleeding should not occur during the normal use of Mirena.

Mirena can also be used by women who have problems with other contraceptive methods. Women who have previously had a copper IUD were asked to compare their experience with Mirena [29]. The majority of women reported much more or a little more satisfaction with Mirena than with a copper IUD (Fig. 7). Some users may have experienced accidental pregnancy, increased or heavy bleeding or increased dysmenorrhea; Mirena has been effective in these women and it is a good alternative for women who have a contraindication for methods that involve oestrogen.

References

1. Andersson K (1993) Intrauterine release of levonorgestrel. A contraceptive and therapeutic system. The department of obstetrics and gynecology, University of Gothenburg
2. Andersson K, Batar I, Rybo G (1992) Return to fertility after removal of a levonorgestrel releasing intrauterine device and Nova-T. Contraception 46:575-584
3. Andersson K, Mattson L-Å, Rybo G, Stadberg E (1992) Intrauterine release of levonorgestrel - a new way of adding progestogen in hormonal replacement therapy. Obstet Gynecol 79:963-967
4. Andersson K, Odlind V, Rybo G (1994) Levonorgestrel-releasing and copper-releasing (Nova T) IUDs during five years of use: a randomized comparative trial. Contraception 49:56-72
5. Andersson K, Rybo G (1990) Levonorgestrel-releasing intrauterine device in the treatment of menorrhagia. Br J Obstet Gynaecol 97:690-694
6. Andersson K, Rybo G (1994) Levonova. Intrauterine release of 20 micrograms of levonorgestrel/24 hours. Workshop Contraceptive Methods, Läkemedelsverket, Uppsala, Sweden, 2:59-71
7. Barbosa I, Olsson S, Odlind V (1988) Ovarian function during use of a levonorgestrel releasing IUD. Contraception 1990; 42: 51
8. Faundes A, Alvarez F, Brache V, Tejada AS (1988) The role of the levonorgestrel IUD in the prevention and treatment of iron deficiency anemia during fertility regulation. Int J Gynecol Obstet 26:429-433
9. Heikkilä M, Lähteenmäki P, Luukkainen T (1982) Immediate postabortal insertion of a levonorgestrel-releasing IUD. Contraception 26:245-259
10. Jia MC, Zhou LY, Ren S, Dong L, Xiao B (1992) Serum levels during normal menstrual cycle and after insertion of levonorgestrel-releasing IUD. Adv Contracept 8:33-40
11. Jänne O, Ylöstalo P (1980) Endometrial estrogen and progestin receptors in women bearing a progesterone-releasing intrauterine device. Contraception 22:19-23
12. Kulkarni BD, Avila TD, Pharriss BB, Scommegna A (1973) Contraception 8:299-314
13. Luukkainen T, Allonen H, Haukkamaa M, et al. (1987) Effective contraception with the levonorgestrel-releasing intrauterine device. 12-month report of a European multicenter study. Contraception 36:169-179
14. Luukkainen T, Lähteenmäki P, Toivonen J (1990) Levonorgestrel-releasing intrauterine device. Ann Med 22:85-90
15. Mandelin E, Koistinen H, Koistinen R, Affandi B, Seppälä M (1997) Levonorgestrel-releasing intrauterine device-wearing women express contraceptive glycodelin A in endometrium during midcycle: another contraceptive mechanism? Hum Reprod 12:2671-2675

16. Nilsson CG (1977) Comparative quantitation of menstrual blood loss with a D-norgestrel-releasing IUD and a Nova-T-copper device. Contraception 15:379-387
17. Nilsson CG (1982) Fertility after discontinuation of levonorgestrel-releasing intrauterine devices. Contraception 25:273-278
18. Nilsson CG, Luukkainen T, Arko H (1978) Endometrial morphology of women using a D-norgestrel-releasing intrauterine device. Fertil Steril 29:397-401
19. Nilsson CG, Lähteenmäki P, Luukkainen T, Robertson DN (1986) Sustained intrauterine release of levonorgestrel over five years. Fertil Steril 45:805-807
20. Oehninger S, Coddington CC, Dodgen GD, Seppälä M (1995) Factors affecting fertilization: endometrial placental protein 14 reduces the capacity of human spermatozoa to bind to the human zona pellucida. Fertil Steril 63:377-383
21. Ortiz ME, Croxatto HB (1987) The mode of action of IUDs. Contraception 36:37-53
22. Pakarinen P, Luukkainen T, Laine H, Lähteenmäki P (1995) The effect of local intrauterine levonorgestrel administration on endometrial thickness and uterine blood circulation. Hum Reprod 10:2390-2394
23. Pekonen F, Nyman T, Lähteenmäki P, Haukkamaa M, Rutanen E M (1992) Intrauterine progestin induces continuous insulin-like growth factor-binding protein-1 production in the human endometrium. J Clin Endocrinol Metab 75:660-664
24. Perino A, Quartararo P, Catinella E, Genova G, Cittadini E (1987) Treatment of endometrial hyperplasia with levonorgestrel releasing intrauterine devices. Acta Eur Fertil 18:137-140
25. Scarselli G, Tantini C, Colafranceschi M et al. (1988) Levo-norgestrel-Nova-T and precancerous lesions of the endometrium. Eur J Gynaecol Oncol 9:284-286
26. Scholten PC, Christaens GC, Haspels AA (1987) Intrauterine steroid contraceptives. Wien Med Wochenschr 137:479-483
27. Scholten PC, Christiaens GCML (1985) Menstrual blood loss with levonorgestrel Nova T and multiload Cu 250 IUDs. Third SAC Annual Meeting, Bordeaux, France
28. Scommegna A, Pandya GN, Christ M, Lee AW, Cohen MR (1970) Fertil Steril 21:201-210
29. Shain RN, Ratsula K, Toivonen J, et al. (1989) Acceptability of an experimental intracervical device: results of a study controlling for selection bias. Contraception 39:73-84
30. Silverberg SG, Haukkamaa M, Arko H, Nilsson CG, Luukkainen T (1986) Endometrial morphology during long-term use of levonorgestrel-releasing intrauterine devices. Int J Gynecol Pathol 5:235-241
31. Sivin I (1995) IUDs and ectopic pregnancy. Contraception 52:321-322
32. Sivin I, Stern J (1994) Health during prolonged use of levonorgestrel 20 µg/D and the copper TCU 380AG intrauterine contraceptive devices. Fertil Steril 61:70-77
33. Suvisaari J, Lähteenmäki P (1996) Detailed analysis of menstrual bleeding patterns after postmenopausal and postabortal insertion of a copper IUD or a levonorgestrel-releasing intrauterine system. Contraception 54:201-208
34. Tietze C, Lewit S (1973) Recommended procedures for the statistical evaluation of intrauterine contraception. Stud Fam Plann 4:35-42
35. Toivonen J, Luukkainen T, Allonen H (1991) Protective effect of intrauterine release of levonorgestrel on pelvic infection. Three years comparative experience of levonorgestrel- and copper-releasing intrauterine devices. Obstet Gynecol 77:261-264
36. WHO (1995) A randomized double-blind study of the effects of two low-dose combined oral contraceptives on biochemical aspects. Report from a seven-centred study. WHO special programme of research, development and research training in human reproduction. Task force on oral contraceptives. Contraception 32:223-236
37. Videla Rivero L, Etchepareborda JJ, Kesseru E (1987) Early chorionic activity in women bearing inert IUD, copper IUD and levonorgestrel-releasing IUD. Contraception 36:217-226

9 Vaginal Rings for Contraceptive Use

John R. Newton

Introduction

Steroids released from vaginal rings avoid first pass hepatic metabolism, producing high bio-availability. It has long been recognised that drug absorption occurs across the vaginal mucosa (Macht, 1918). The first vaginal ring study was that described by Mishell et al, 1970. Using a progestogen medroxyprogesterone acetate, sufficiently high serum progestogen levels were produced to induce anovulation. Further studies with this ring were hindered by the discovery of the possible potential carcinogenic effect of MPA on beagle bitches. Research and development then concentrated on vaginal rings, incorporating lower doses of progestogens, or combined rings with an oestrogen and a progestogen.

From the first design, vaginal rings have undergone considerable modification. Initially the progestogen was mixed with a silastic polymer into a toroidal shaped ring of 70-80 mm in diameter.

These rings unfortunately had a burt effect following initial placement in the vagina, then declined to a steady level. Further design then incorporated a core (active) type ring with the steroid contained in a polymer core surrounded by an outer polymer membrane (Akinla et al, 1976). Various other methods of steroid incorporation were then investigated, with further development of an active core ring surrounded by an active silastic membrane, leading to the multi-compartment rings used in clinical studies. These included both progestogen-only and combined oestrogen and progestogen rings. The release rates were altered by varying either the thickness of the wall, or by altering the relative length of the chamber containing the active steroid in either the progestogen-only, or combined rings.

Further development by the World Health Organisation resulted in a series of studies leading to a clinically effective levonorgestrel releasing progestogen-only vaginal ring (WHO 1990, Papers a, b, c and d). These rings could be used for a period of 12 weeks and were then replaced with a new ring. During this time their contraceptive efficacy was maintained by the effect on the cervical mucus (blockade) and effects on the endometrium and interruption of ovulation in a significant number of cycles.

The use of vaginal rings in the puerperium was also investigated as there was a need to demonstrate a use effectiveness of a progesterone releasing ring in those nursing mothers who required additional contraception. This core design releasing 10 mg of progesterone a day, was investigated in a comparative study with a group of nursing mothers using the Copper T 200 IUCD (Diaz et al, 1985). The ring was found to be effective despite up to 28% of women having bleeding episodes of greater than, 6 days in every 30 days.

A further approach to a progestogen-only ring was that using 3-keto-desogestrel (Hammond et al, 1984, Bergink et al, 1983). These dose-finding studies indicated that a progestogen release of 3-keto-desogestrel at 75 pg per day, would inhibit ovulation completely. We then embarked on a series of studies looking at progestogen-only rings releasing 3-keto-desogestrel (Jackson and Newton, 1989) and combined rings releasing a low dose oestrogen and 3-keto-desogrestrel (Davies et al, 1995) – see later section on desogestrel combined rings.

The Population Council continued to investigate this method of contraception, using doses of oestrogen and progestogen aimed at ovulation inhibition and minimising menstrual irregularity. A shell design was used for this type of ring, which released levonorgestrel and oestradiol from a 50 mm ring, or in a slightly larger ring, 290 mg of levonorgestrel and 180 µg of oestradiol. With both these rings, a failure of 3 per 100 women years was found (Sivin, 1981). Other progestogen combinations have been tried including the novel progestogen ST1435. Ovulation was suppressed and cycle control was satisfactory (Laurikka et al, 1990). Preliminary work with the combination of ethinyl oestradiol 50 µg and 120 µg of 3-keto-desogestrel per day, used for 12 weeks, were then investigated (Olsson et al, 1990 and Davies et al, 1994).

Progestogen-only Vaginal Rings

The main clinical data on progestogen-only rings, comes from the WHO Studies of the 20 µg release rate vaginal ring used continuously for a period of 12 weeks.

Levonorgestrel 20 µg/Day Release Vaginal Ring

From the early 1980's WHO conducted a series of research trials to investigate a progestogen-only vaginal ring releasing 20 µg/day of levonorgestrel. This toroidal ring of 55.6 mm by 9.5 mm was made of polysiloxane elastomer, and contained an active drug core of 5 mg of levonorgestrel. The release rate was 20 µg/day. Studies between 1980 and 1986 in 19 centres world-wide investigated efficacy, expulsion, body weight and bleeding patterns.

The efficacy study WHO (1990a) looked at 1,005 women with 8176.74 women months of use. The intrauterine pregnancy rate at one year of use was 3.6/100 women, while the principle reasons for discontinuation were menstrual disturbance (17.2% at one year), repeated expulsion of the ring (7.1%) and vaginal symptoms (6.0%). This failure rate compared favourably with a low oestrogen combined contraceptive pill and was less than half that seen with progestogen-only oral contraception in WHO randomised studies (WHO 1982, a and b). Table 1 gives the discontinuation rates for menstrual problems, while Table 2 gives similar results for vaginal related reasons.

WHO (1990b) looked specifically at the expulsion rates and removals in this same cohort of women. The overall life table discontinuation rate due to expulsion was 7.1% at one year, being highest in Asian and lowest in European women from the 19 centres. Following a first expulsion, the second expulsion rate was found to be 45% within the next 6 months. The majority of expulsions were associated with defaecation, 57% of the total, urination (12%) and menstruation (17%). The rings

Table 1. Cumulative discontinuation rates (95% Confidence Interval, CI) for menstrual problems

Discontinuation reason	Months			
	3	6	9	12
Prolonged bleeding				
rate	2.2	3.9	4.2	4.6
Cl	(1.3-3.2)	(2.6-5.3)	(2.8-5.6)	(3.2-6.1)
n	19	29	34	36
Heavy bleeding				
rate	1.2	2.6	3.3	3.7
Cl	(0.3-1.5)	(1.5-3.7)	(2.0-4.6)	(2.3-5.0)
n	9	19	23	26
Intermenstrual bleeding				
rate	2.2	4.6	5.9	6.2
Cl	(1.3-3.2)	(3.2-6.1)	(4.2-7.5)	(4.5-8.0)
n	20	37	46	48
Other menstrual*				
rate	1.0	1.4	1.5	1.7
Cl	(0.3-1.6)	(0.6-2.1)	(0.7-2.4)	(0.8-2.6)
n	8	11	12	13
Amenorrhoea**				
rate	0.4	1.4	2.0	2.2
Cl	(0-0.8)	(0.5-2.2)	(1.0-3.1)	(1.1-3.3)
n	3	10	14	15
All menstrual problems				
rate	6.8	13.2	15.9	17.2
Cl	(5.1-8.4)	(10.9-15.5)	(13.8-18.4)	(14.5-19.8)
n	59	106	129	138

* More frequent or shorter periods, oligomenorrhoea, hypermenorrhoea

** Amenorrhoea was defined as a period not having started more than 42 days since the onset of the previous one and a negative pregnancy test. The range was 48-184 days

Table 2. Cumulative discontinuation rates (95% Confidence Interval, CI) for vaginal-related reasons

Discontinuation reason	Months			
	3	6	9	12
Discharge				
rate	1.0	2.0	3.0	3.5
Cl	(0.4-1.7)	(1.0-3.0)	(1.7-4.2)	(2.1-4.9)
n	9	16	22	25
Irritation				
rate	0.9	1.0	1.2	1.2
Cl	(0.3-1.5)	(0.4-1.7)	(0.5-1.9)	(0.5-1.9)
n	8	9	10	10
Infection				
rate	0.3	0.7	1.2	1.4
Cl	(0-0.7)	(0.1-1.3)	(0.4-2.0)	(0.5-2.3)
n	3	6	9	10
Total				
rate	2.3	3.8	5.3	6.0
Cl	(1.3-3.2)	(2.4-5.1)	(3.7-6.9)	(4.3-7.8)
n	20	31	41	45

were removed by 12% of women for a variety of reasons. The main reasons were vaginal discharge and irritation, bleeding, pain and dyspareunia, whilst others removed the ring prior to defaecation or urination and then replaced it. Nevertheless the availability of the ring allowed women to control its use and was not necessarily related to method use.

A further paper (WHO 1990c) investigated the possible relationship between body weight and pregnancy. This study confirmed an increased risk of pregnancy with increased body weight. Those of 40 kg had a rate of 1.7%, whilst those of 80 kg had an increased chance of pregnancy of 9.8% at 1 year of use.

As with all progestogen-only methods, menstrual disturbance was the most common side-effect. The bleeding pattern, using the standard WHO 90 day reference period analysis, was investigated by WHO (1990d). Half the users had patterns similar to normal untreated patterns, whilst a quarter experienced irregular bleeding. A further 10% had shortened cycles and 10% prolonged cycles, thus emphasising the need for effective pre-use counselling. Those with the worst bleeding patterns tended to discontinue early, and were influenced by their more recent menstrual irregularity.

Progestogen-only Studies of 3-Keto-Desogestrel Progestogen-only Rings

We investigated the pharmacokinetic and pharmacodynamic effects of a progestogen-only ring releasing 30 μg of 3-keto-desogestrel (Jackson and Newton, 1989a and b). In this study we compared a similar ring with levonorgestrel 20 μg release rate per day and all formulations containing either 30 μg of levonorgestrel or 60 μg of desogestrel. This study examined the respective plasma levels of the progestogens resulting from the 2 methods of administration and their effects on ovulation. The steady state plasma levels with the 3-keto-desogestrel ring did not differ from those seen with the 16 μg desogestrel tablets. The release rate from the levonorgestrel containing ring was in a similar relationship to the release rate from the levonorgestrel tablet. Ovulation was inhibited in 4 of the 10 subjects in the levonorgestrel ring group, 8 out of the 10 with the levonorgestrel tablet group, while no ovulation was seen with the keto-desogestrel tablet or the desogestrel vaginal ring.

All treatments were associated with persistent follicle formation, but there was no significant difference between groups. Using ultrasound scanning and standardised investigation of cervical mucus, the classification of the ovarian reaction, follicular development without ovulation and persistent follicles, was investigated.

The two progestogen-only vaginal rings were found to offer lower dose steady state release characteristics of significant advantage over the oral formulations, preventing the peaks and troughs often seen with the oral formulation.

In the recovery cycle, following treatment, 9 out of the 10 in the levonorgestrel ring group, 6 out of the 10 in the levonorgestrel tablet group and 7 out of the 10 in the desogestrel tablet group and 5 out of the 10 in the 3-keto-desogestrel ring group achieved ovulation within 30 days.

There was no evidence of persistent follicular suppression. This detailed pharmacodynamic study prompted us to investigate further the suitability of the progestogen-only vaginal ring (Jackson et al, 1994).

Effect on Vaginal Flora

Given the incidence of discontinuation, due to vaginal symptoms, as seen in the WHO 1990 studies. We further investigated the effect of a combined contraceptive ring releasing ethinyl oestradiol and 3-keto-desogestrel on the vaginal flora (Davies et al, 1992). During this period of study, when all relevant vaginal commensuals and pathogens were screened for, no serious abnormality or incidence of increase in abnormal vaginal flora was seen during the study period.

Extended Use of Vaginal Rings and Their Effect on Vaginal Bleeding Patterns

Given the regime of the combined ring, used for 21 days and then removed for 7 days, we further investigated the effect of extended use on ovarian activity and bleeding patterns (Davies et al, 1992b) with the combined ethinyl oestradiol 3-keto-desogestrel ring. As increase in use beyond 21 days occurred, so the increase in irregular bleeding and spotting occurred, with the majority of subjects seeing irregular vaginal bleeding patterns with extended use. Despite this irregularity, continued cervical mucus blockade and endometrial suppression was seen with no evidence of ovulation. However, extended use beyond 3-4 weeks may limit the acceptability of vaginal rings with this formulation. The increased percentage of subjects with bleeding and spotting during extended use rose from less than 20% at 21 days to more than 80% at 56 days of continuous use. These studies have been reviewed and summarised in Newton, 1996.

The effect of different insertion regimes on side-effects with a different combined vaginal ring has been investigated by Weisberg et al, 1997. Here the vaginal ring released 20 µg ethinyl oestradiol and 1 mg norethindrome acetate daily over 2 successive cycles, with a new ring in each of 3 different insertion regimes. A total of 129 women completed the study, with 831 women months of experience. The overall incidence of side-effects was similar in the 2 centres studying this ring and there were no significant differences between the insertion regimes. The study by Weisberg et al, 1997, was to determine whether night-time insertion, rather than morning insertion of the ring, or a timed insertion/removal regime would reduce the incidence of transient nausea and other side-effects. Data on efficacy and acceptability were also collected.

The most prominent effect was transient nausea following the insertion of a new ring, lasting from 0.5 to 48 hours, but there was no difference between the 2 insertion regimes, although the incidence tended to be higher with a night-time insertion (34%) and lowest with an early evening insertion and temporary removal during the first night (27%). Transient vomiting occurred in about 10% of the women in the first 24 hours after the first insertion. This study demonstrated that the CVR, known to be effective and generally well tolerated, caused a higher incidence of transient nausea after insertion of a new ring, possibly due to the accumulation of ethinyl oestradiol on the ring surface during storage. However, acceptability was still high and the authors recommend that this combined ring merits further observation and development.

Other Combined Rings

Many groups have attempted combined vaginal ring formulation, using a variety of different progestogens and oestrogens.

The Population Council developed a vaginal ring releasing 280 µg to 300 µg of levonorgestrel and 100 µg of oestradiol a day, using the standard insertion regime of 3 weeks in and 7 days out. The serum levels of levonorgestrel range from 1 to 3 nanomol/ml and was relatively constant with each treatment cycle of the ring in situ. This level was sufficient to produce anovular cycles and the endogenous plasma progesterone levels remained low.

There were no significant changes in glucose metabolism and liver function during vaginal ring use. The levels of levonorgestrel were similar to those following oral ingestion of a combined COC containing a much higher dose of levonorgestrel at 0.3 mg. Withdrawal bleeding occurred after removal of the ring, usually within 1 to 5 days, with a mean of 2.6 days, and a mean of 4.5 days bleeding. Interestingly only 7% of cycles recorded break through bleeding or spotting.

The Population Council continued to study this combined ring and looked at different sizes of the shell ring of 50 mm and 58 mm. These were compared with a combined oral contraceptive pill containing 150 µg of levonorgestrel and 30 µg of ethinyl oestradiol in a large multi-centre study (Sivin et al, 1981). The net one year pregnancy rates were 1.8 and 1.0 per 100 women for the two sizes of vaginal ring, which was not significantly different from the pregnancy rate of the combined oral contraceptive pill at 2.0 per 100 women.

The continuation rates at one year for the vaginal rings, were about 50% and significantly better than that seen with COC users. The major advantage of this combined ring was its contraceptive efficacy and minimal side-effects. The major disadvantage was the progesterone dominance, due to the use of levonorgestrel with an oestrogen of low potency. There was a significant decrease in high density lypoprotein cholesterol and a small increase in low density lypoprotein cholesterol, resulting in changes in the LDL/HDL ratio.

Other rings that were investigated were a combination of norethindrone (NET), plus oestradiol 850 µg plus 200 µg of oestrogen, - which inhibited ovulation. However, bleeding control was poor and there was significant break through bleedings.

ST 1435, the synthetic steroid which is inactive orally, but active when administered in a vaginal ring, was used with ethinyl oestradiol 60 mg (ST 1435 plus 122 mg ethinyl oestradiol). This was effective in a pilot study and serum levels suppressed ovulation. This ring was thought to be worthy of further development.

Oestradiol Vaginal Rings for Specific HRT Symptoms

Most of the development work has been with rings for contraceptive purposes. However, recent developments and studies have indicated a useful development of a vaginal ring releasing a low dose of oestrogen in order to alleviate the tiresome urogenital symptoms associated with the menopause. This ring system releases low levels of oestradiol (Barentsen, 1997). In a cross-over study the authors looked at a silicone vaginal ring of core design with an oestradiol loaded core containing 2 mg Micronized 17 beta oestradiol, release rate 7.51/4 g per 24 hours for 90 days.

This study, which looked at 168 women in a cross-over design showed significant alleviation of symptoms within the 12 week period of study, when compared with a vaginal oestrogen cream.

Further studies by Ayton et al, 1996, showed that a similar oestrogen vaginal ring alleviated the symptoms of vaginal dryness and dyspareunia and resolution of atrophic signs, with superior acceptability to vaginal cream.

Other studies – Henriksson et al, 1996, and Kalogirou, 1996, also confirm the superior effect of vaginal ring release of oestrogen compared with oral or other routes of delivery of oestrogen. It was found to be highly effective, well accepted and a useful long-term treatment of urogenital disorders caused by oestrogen deficiency in post-menopausal women.

Progesterone Rings for Use in the Puerperium

Following the in vitro release rate studies of a progesterone core-loaded ring by Matlin et al, 1992, progesterone releasing rings of different release rate characteristics were investigated in a pilot study. This pilot study compared three different initial rates of 5 mg, 8 mg and 20 mg per day (Landgren et al, 1991). The 5 mg and 8 mg per day rings were a core-loaded progesterone shell ring. The 20 mg a day ring was homogenously distributed progesterone throughout the mass of the ring.

The total progesterone levels (area under the curve) were directly related to the release rates. The decrease in progesterone levels were 25%, 31% and 47% for the rings of the three release rates at 90 days after insertion.

There was therefore good correlation between the in vitro and in vivo data, which indicated that progesterone released from a ring would be a suitable puerperal contraceptive for those who might not be fully breast feeding. This was therefore investigated in a comparative study (Sivin et al, 1997). This study compared the Copper T 380 A IUD in 734 women with 802 vaginal ring users, who used a progesterone releasing ring with an average release rate of 10 mg per day for a 3 month period. Evaluation included measures of lactational performance as well as contraceptive efficacy and safety to mother and child. The study was in nine clinics.

The one year pregnancy rate of 1.5 per 100 for the vaginal ring did not differ significantly from the Copper T 380 A IUD. More than half the ring subjects were continuing six months post-administration and a quarter were still using the ring and breast feeding one year after admission. Women with the IUD, however, had higher continuation rates at both time points. Vaginal ring users had more complaints of vaginal problems, but had fewer vaginal disorders on examination. Lactational performance, health and weight gain of the infants were similar among both vaginal ring users and IUD users. The use of progesterone releasing vaginal rings may be of use in countries where lactational contraception is necessary.

Vaginal Lesions and Vaginal Rings

Following a report in 1994 by Bounds et al of vaginal lesions related to the use of a levonorgestrel releasing vaginal ring, a series of studies were initiated by the Population Council and WHO to investigate whether there was any relationship between contraceptive use and vaginal lesions. In 1996 WHO confirmed the results of a multi-centre study that was set up to examine if pressure effects caused any vaginal or cervical lesions. In this study serial colposcopy was carried out on 166 volunteers, who used a placebo ring of new 'flexibility' compared with the control group using a non-vaginal non-hormonal method of contraception. Only in one centre were lesions seen in 12 of the 50 volunteers, who developed new vaginal or cervical lesions (16) during follow up. Of these lesions 81% were on the cervix and many were associated with trauma or infection. There was no difference between control and placebo ring group, suggesting that the new ring design can be considered suitable for further development.

This is supported by the recent Population Council multi-centre study (1998) and I am grateful to Dr. Harold Nash and to Dr. Elof Johansson of the Population Council for permission to report the preliminary results of the study, which indicate no significant difference between vaginal ring users and other methods of contraception. In this study micro-lesions were seen in some cases in this multi-centre international study on the vagina or cervix but were more related to the recent act of intercourse or to tampon use, rather than to the contraceptive method.

Conclusions

For many years the vaginal ring delivery system for either progestogen-only or combined progestogen and oestrogen use, as a method of contraception, has been extensively investigated. It is now clear that modern flexible shell-type rings with an active core, containing either a progestogen or a combined oestrogen and progestogen, may offer significant advantages to a certain group of women who prefer total control of their own contraceptive method. Regimes indicate that a progestogen-only vaginal release ring will require replacement every 12 weeks, whilst with a combined ring the standard oral contraceptive cycle of "21 days in and 7 days out" may be the best way forward. Extended use of combined vaginal rings leads to an increase in intermenstrual bleeding and break-through bleeding, which does not increase acceptability.

Significant studies have indicated the lack of change in vaginal flora and the lack of effect on ovarian morphology. The multi-factorial effect of this vaginal ring as a contraceptive cervical mucus and the endometrium, with in some cases an effect on ovulation due to the dose used in the vaginal ring.

Further design work has improved retention and flexibility of the shape of the toroidal ring, which leads to high acceptability and warrants further investigation. Studies clearly indicate the need for effective counselling and careful case selection with a need to make certain that lifestyle matches the designed ring use schedule, particularly with respect to removing the ring before defaecation and urination, replacing the ring thereafter, and monitoring carefully the time that the ring is left in place.

Initial worries about vaginal lesions appear to have been resolved with recent studies from the Population Council and WHO.

This method should prove to be an acceptable form of contraception and one worth pursuing.

As far as the ring system for delivery of oestrogen to alleviate some menopausal symptoms is concerned, studies indicate the quite significant advantage offered by low release oestrogen containing soft vaginal rings for the treatment of menopausal urogenital symptoms.

References

Akinla O et al. (1976) Intravaginal contraception with the synthetic progestin R2323, Contraception, 14: 671-678

Alvarez-Sanchez F et al. (1992) Evaluation of four different contraceptive vaginal rings: steroid serum levels, luteal activity, bleeding control and lipid profiles, Contraception, 46: 387-398

Ayton RA et al. (1996) A comparative study of safety and efficacy of continuous low dose oestradiol released from a vaginal ring compared with conjugated equine oestrogen vaginal cream in the treatment of postmenopausal urogenital atrophy, Brit. J. of Obs. & Gynae., April 1996, Vol. 103: 351-358

Barentsen R et al. (1997) Continuous low dose estradiol released from a vaginal ring versus estriol vaginal cream for urogenital atrophy, Eur. J. of Obs. & Gynae. and Rep. Biology, 71, 73-80

Berjink EW et al. (1983) Binding of progestogens to receptor proteins in MCF-7 cells, J. Steroid Biochem. 19: 1563-1570

Bounds W et al. (1993) A preliminary report of unexpected reactions to a progestogen releasing contraceptive ring, European Journal of Reproductive Biology, 48(2), 123-125

Davies GC (1992)et al. The effects of a combined contraceptive ring releasing ethinylestradiol and 3-ketodesogestrel on vaginal flora, Contraception; 45:511-8

Diaz S et al. (1985)Fertility regulation in nursing woman: Progesterone plasma levels and contraceptive efficacy of a progesterone releasing vaginal ring, Contraception, 32: 603-622

Gabrielsson J et al. (1996) Pharmacokinetic data on estradiol in light of the estring® concept, Acta Obstetricia et Gynaecologica Scandinavica 75: 26-31

Hammond GL et al. (1984) Serum steroid binding protein concentrations and distributions of progestogens and bioavailability of testosterone during treatment with contraceptives containing desogestrel or levonorgestrel, Fertil. Steril., 42: 44-51

Henriksson L et al. (1996) A one-year multicenter study of efficacy and safety of a continuous, low-dose, estradiol-releasing vaginal ring (Estring) in postmenopausal women with symptoms and signs of urogenital ageing, Am.J. Obstet Gynecol, January 1996: 85-92

Henriksson L et al. (1995) Randomized comparison of a new estradiol-releasing vaginal ring versus estriol vaginal pessaries. Letter to Editor, Am. J. Obstet. Gynecol, August 1995: 670-1

Jackson R and Newton J (1989) Pharmacodynamics of a contraceptive vaginal ring releasing 3-keto-desogestrel, Contraception, 39: 655-664

Jackson X, Li F and Newton JR (1994) A study comparing the ovarian effects of levonorgestrel and desogestrel given orally and by vaginal ring, J. of Obs. & Gynae. (1994) 14: 277-284

Kalogirou D et al. (1996) A comparative study of the effects of an estradiol-releasing vaginal ring combined with an oral gestagen versus transdermal estrogen combined with a levonorgestrel-releasing IUD - Clinical Findings and Endometrial Response, Int. J. Fetil. 41(6): 522-527

Landgren B-M et al. Progesterone-releasing vaginal rings for use in postpartum contraception. II. Pharmacokinetic profiles in women

Laurikka-Routti M et al. (1990) A contraceptive vaginal ring releasing ethinyl estradiol and the progestin ST-1435: Bleeding control, serum steroid concentration, serum lipids and steroid chemistry. Contraception, 42: 111-120

Macht DI (1918) The absorption of drugs and points through the vagina, J. Pharmacol Pathol., 10: 509-513

Matlin SA et al. (1992) Progesterone-releasing vaginal rings for use in postpartum contraception. I. In vitro release rates of progesterone from core-loaded rings, Contraception, 45: 329-341

Mishell DR et al. (1970) Contraceptive effect of varying doses of progestogen in silastic vaginal rings, Fertil. Steril., 21: 99-103

Mishell DR (1970) et al. Contraception by means of a silastic vaginal ring impregnated with medrosy-progesterone acetate, A. J. Obstet. Gynecol., 107: 100-107
Mishell DR et al. (1972) Inhibition of ovulation with cyclic use of progestogen impregnated intravaginal devices, A. J. Obstet. Gynecol., 113: 927-932
Mishell DR Jr. Vaginal Contraceptive Rings, Ann. Med. 25, 191-197
Newton JR (1996) New hormonal methods of contraception, Bailliere's Clinical Obstetrics and Gynaecology, Vol. 10/No. 1, April 1996; 94-5
Newton JR, Davies GC A study to evaluate ovarian function, acceptability and side effects during extended continuous use of a contraceptive vaginal ring releasing 0.120 mg Org 3236 and 0.015 mg ethinylestradiol per day in healthy female volunteers
Newton JR (1996) New hormonal methods of contraception, Bailliere's Clinical Obstetrics and Gynaecology, Vol. 10/No. 1, April 1996; 94-5
Olsson SE et al. (1990) Contraception with a vaginal ring releasing 3-ketodesogestrel and ethinylestradiol, Contraception, 42: 563-572
Roumen FJME et al. (1996) The cervico-vaginal epithelium during 20 cycles' use of a combined contraceptive vaginal ring, Human Reproduction, Vol. 11, No. 11: 2443-2448
Sivin I (1981) A multicenter study of levonorgestrel-estradiol contraceptive vaginal rings. An international comparative trial, Contraception, 24: 341-392
Sivin I et al. (1997) Contraceptives for Lactating Women: A Comparative Trial of a Progesterone-Releasing Vaginal Ring and the Copper T 380 A IUD, Contraception; 55: 225-232
Weisberg E et al. (1997) Effect of Different Insertion Regimens on Side Effects with a Combination Contraceptive Vaginal Ring, Contraception; 56:233-239
WHO (1996) Annual Report on the special programme on human reproduction – section on long-acting methods of contraception, Published by WHO, Geneva
WHO 1996 Annual Technical Report, P. 9, published WHO Geneva 1997, Ed. Van Look, PFA
WHO task force on long-acting methods of contraception: Microdose intravaginal levonorgestrel contraception. A multi-centre clinical trial
WHO (1990a) task force on long-acting methods of contraception: Contraceptive efficacy and side-effects: Contraception, 41(2), 105-123
WHO (1990b) task force on long-acting methods of contraception: Expulsions and removals: Contraception, Vol. 41(2), 125-141
WHO (1990c) task force on long-acting methods of contraception: The relationship between pregnancy rate and body weight: Contraception, Vol. 41(2), 143-149
WHO (1990d) task force on long-acting methods of contraception: Bleeding patterns: Contraception, 41(2), 151-168
WHO (1982) Task Force on Oral Contraceptives. A randomised double-blind study of six combinated oral contraceptives. Contraception 25: 231-241
WHO (1982) Task Force on Oral Contraceptives. A randomised double-blind study of two combined and two progestogen-only contraceptives. Contraception 25: 243-252

10 Use of Anti-progestins in Female Contraception

E. E. Baulieu

The only antiprogestin active, safe and ready for clinical use in contraception studies is the synthetic steroid mifepristone (RU486). Other antiprogestins do have similar activities to mifepristone, but have not been tested in human.

Mifepristone is essentially known for its anti-progesterone activity and its application to early pregnancy termination. The compound has been registered for this indication and used in 500,000 women in France, Great Britain and Sweden, and more than 3 million women/year recently, in China. Its efficiency in pregnancies up to 50 days of amenorrhea is ≥95% when a dose of 200 mg is orally administered once, followed about 48 h later by intake of a small amount of an orally active prostaglandin (400-600 μg of misoprostol) or a vaginal suppository (0.5-1mg of gemeprost).

The mechanism of action of RU486 involves the intracellular receptors of the antagonized hormones (progesterone and glucocorticosteroids), but only the antiprogesterone effect is involved in pregnancy termination. At the molecular level, the most important features are high binding affinity to the receptor ($K_D \leq 1$ nM), interaction of the phenyl-aminodimethyl group in the 11β-position with a specific region of the receptor binding pocket, and RU486-induced transconformation differences in the ligand-binding domain. These particularities have consequences at different steps of the receptor function compared with agonists. However, the reasoning cannot be limited to the RU486-receptor interaction and, for instance, there is the possibility of a switch from antagonistic property to agonist activity, depending on the intervention of other signaling pathways (i.e., the cAMP system). For the use of mifepristone in contraception, one has to take into account the period of the cycle for which the compound is administered. The number of days of administration and the amount of each intake will vary accordingly.

Occasional Late Luteal-Phase Administration

In two studies [1, 2], it has been demonstrated that RU486 could be used as a luteal phase occasional contraceptive, when 400 mg or 600 mg are given once or twice on the day of (or the day before) expected menses in women at risk of pregnancy. The efficacy of RU486 (given alone, without phostaglandin) was the same as in early pregnancy termination (approximately 80% in women with elevated beta-hCG). Therefore, since the risk of pregnancy is about 20% in normal young couples, the global efficiency if a woman is at risk to be pregnant is therefore -96%. Such an occasional late luteal-phase administration is also described as "contragestive" [3].

Monthly Premenstrual (Late Luteal Phase) Administration (Monthly Mense Inducer)

The administration of mifepristone late in the cycle may modify the timing of ovulation during the next cycle, leading to some irregularity in the ovulation schedule, and this effect as well as a small risk of pregnancy (as discussed in the preceding paragraph) explains why the administration on a regular monthly basis has not yet been successful. Giving RU486 approximately 2 days before the expected day of menses over several months proved unsuccessful [4], since the failure rate (20%) renders the administration of RU486 alone impracticable on a regular monthly basis, and also because, at the doses used (200-100 mg), RU486 induced cycle irregularities with retardation of the next ovulation. The possibility that lower doses of RU486 combined with prostaglandin may circumvent these difficulties is currently under evaluation.

Early Luteal-Phase Administration: Anti-Implantation

Progesterone acts on the endometrium to prepare for implantation, and experiments in animals have shown that endometrial receptivity and embryo implantation can be modified by anti-progestins [5-9]. RU486 has been shown to induce epithelium cell apoptosis.

Treatment with two doses of 200 mg RU486 was performed in women on day 2 and day 3 post-LH surge, who had had unprotected intercourse at least once during the previous three days – 1 day after ovulation [10]. Of over 157 cycles, only one pregnancy occurred. The main drawback of such an anti-implantation method is its impracticability, necessitating the detection of ovulation. In any case, larger samples are necessary in order to have a precise quantitation of the efficacy of the method.

Emergency Post-coital Contraception

Two studies [11, 12] have suggested that mifepristone, given as a single 600 mg dose within 72 h of unprotected intercourse, is at least as efficient as a high dose of estrogen or estro-progestative preparation, and better tolerated. Larger trials are under way to confirm these results, to define the optimal dose of RU486, and to evaluate its consequences on menstrual cyclicity.

Ovulation Suppression

A number of observations demonstrate that progesterone contributes to ovulation. The administration of RU486 (1-5 mg/day) during the follicular phase delays or suppresses ovulation, an effect that may be due to antiprogesterone action in ovaries, and to a suppressive effect of RU486 on gonadotropins [13-24]. This may be obtained even with very low doses of RU486 [25]. Thus, a new method of estrogen-free contraception could be proposed. However, such a method raises the question of a prolonged estrogen activity, since, contrarily to what has been reported for monkeys, daily administration of RU486 (200 mg) for several months in women may be associated with endometrial hyperplasia [26]. It has been suggested that this problem can be avoided by using an antiprogestin and a progestin sequentially [27], but the contraceptive activity of such a scheme remains to be evaluated.

Endometrial Contraception With Daily Delivery of Very Low Dose of RU486

Continuous exposure to a very low dose of RU486 (i.e., equivalent of 0.5 mg/day in women) may prevent implantation and possibly even fertilization without any change in ovulation and in estrogen and progesterone secretion pattern, as observed in the guinea pig and in baboons [28]. Studies in monkeys performed at the Jones Foundation (Virginia, USA) have indicated the remarkable efficacy of this very low dose administration (G. Hodgen, personal communication). In women, it is necessary to determine the maximal dose that does not suppress or delay ovulation, but that can effect the endometrium. Such a dose should certainly be well below 1 mg/day, because this dose has been shown to suppress ovulation in some women (~20%). If such a dose can be found, as preliminary data indicate [29, M. Bygdeman, personal communication], and if the contraceptive effect is proved, such administration could become a very promising estrogen-free method. The action of RU486 in interfering with sperm may be space involved in this effect on fertilization [30, 31].

As bold face, these studies indicate the potential of mifepristone for contraception, and both clinical studies and laboratory experiments suggest that the prolonged administration of the compound in small dose is basically safe. Besides the antiprogesterone effect, it should be noticed that mifepristone respects the endogenous estrogen levels in women (contrary to the administration of GnRH agonists) and that the anticortisol activity of mifepristone does not create side-effects at the envisaged doses.

However, the fact that contraception is associated with the concept of "preventive" medicine as well as that the very mandatory medical attitude "primum non nocere", imposes long-term toxicity studies that will not make mifepristone ready for contraceptive purpose before several years.

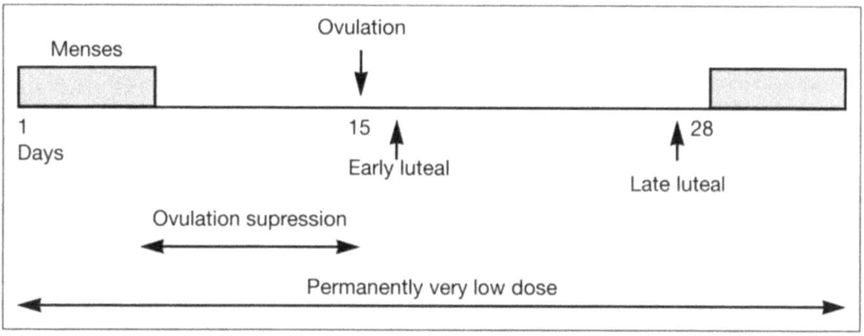

Fig. 1. Scheme of the menstrual cycle in women and timing of mifepristone administration for different methods of contraception. Late luteal administration may be occasional or monthly (see text). Administration of mifepristone for emergency post-coital contraception is not represented in this figure

References

1. Dubois C, Ulmann A, Baulieu EE (1988) Contragestion with late luteal administration of RU486 (mifepristone). Fertil Steril 50:593
2. Bosc MJ, Germain G, Nicolle A, et al. (1985) The use of antiprogesterone compound RU486 to control timing of parturition in rats. In: E.E. Baulieu, SJ. Segal (eds) The antiprogestin steroid RU486 and human fertility control. Plenum Press, New York, pp 69-70
3. Baulieu EE (1989) Contragestion and other clinical applications of RU486, an antiprogesterone at the receptor. Science 245:1351-1357
4. Van Santen M, Haspels AA (1987) Failure of mifepristone (RU486) as a monthly contragestive, «lunarette». Contraception 35:433
5. Batista MC, Bristow TL, Mathews J, et al. (1991) Daily administration of the progesterone antagonist RU486 prevents implantation in the cycling guinea pig. Am J Obstet Gynecol 165:82
6. Gravanis A, Zorn JR, Tanguy G, et al. (1984) The "disharmonic luteal phase" syndrome: endometrialprogesterone receptor and estradiol dehydrogenase. Fertil Steril 42:730
7. Herrmann WL, Schindler AM, Wyss R (1985) Effects of the antiprogesterone RU486 in early pregnancy and during the menstrual cycle. In: EE Baulieu, SJ Segal (eds) The antiprogestin steroid RU486 and human fertility control. Plenum Press, New York, pp 179-198
8. Schaison G, George M, LeStrat N, et al. (1985) Effects of an antiprogesterone steroid RU486 during midluteal phase in normal women. J Clin Endocrinol Metab 61:484
9. Swahn ML, Johannisson E, Daniore V, et al. (1988) The effect of RU486 administered during the proliferative and secretory phase of the cycle on the bleeding pattern, hormonal parameters and the endometrium. Hum Reprod 3:915
10. Gemzell-Danielsson K, Svalander P, Swahn, ML, et al. (1994) Effects of a single postovulatory dose of RU486 on endometrial maturation in the implantation phase. Human Reprod 9:2398
11. Glasier AK, Thong J, Dewar M, et al. (1992) Mifepristone (RU486) compared with high-dose estrogen and progestogen for emergency postcoital contraception. New Engl J Med 327:1041
12. Webb AMC, Russel J, Elstein M (1992) Comparison of Yuzpe regimen, danazol, and mifepristone (RU486) in oral postcoital contraception. BMJ 305:927
13. Batista MC, Cartledgde TP, Zellmer AW, et al. (1992) Evidence for a critical role of progesterone in the regulation of the midcycle gonadotropin surge and ovulation. J Clin Endocrinol Metab 74:565
14. Baulieu EE (1975) Antiprogesterone effect and midcycle (periovulatory) contraception. Eur J Obstet Gynecol Reprod Biol 4:161
15. Cohn M, Stewart P (1991) Pretreatment of the primigravid uterine cervix with mifepristone 30 h prior to termination of pregnancy: a double blind study. Br J Obstet Gynaecol 98:778
16. Collins RL, Hodgen GD (1986) Blockade of the spontaneous midcycle gonadotropin surge in monkeys by RU486. A progesterone antagonist? J Clin Endocrinol Metab 63:1270
17. Garzo VG, Liu J, Ulmann A, et al. (1988) Effects of an antiprogesterone (RU486) on the hypothalamic-hypophyseal-ovarian-endometrial axis during the luteal phase of the menstrual cycle. J Clin Endocrinol Metab 66:508
18. Ledger WL, Sweeting VM, Hillier H, et al. (1992) Inhibition of ovulation by low-dose mifepristone (RU486). Human Reprod 7:945
19. Liu JH, Garzo G, Morris S, et al. (1987) Disruption of follicular maturation and delay of ovulation after administration of the antiprogesterone RU486. J Clin Endocrinol Metab 65:1135
20. Luukkainen T, Heikinheimo O, Haukkamaa M, et al. (1988) Inhibition of folliculogenesis and ovulation by the antiprogesterone RU486. Fertil Steril 49:961
21. Shoupe D, Mishell DR, Page MA, et al. (1987) Effects of an antiprogesterone RU486 in normal women. II. Administration in the late follicular phase. Am J Obstet Gynecol 157:1421
22. Croxatto HB, Salvatierra AM, Croxatto HD, et al. (1993) Effects of continuous treatment with low dose mifepristone throughout one menstrual cycle. Human Reprod 8:201
23. Permezel JM, Lenton EA, Roberts I, et al. (1989) Acute effects of progesterone and the antiprogestin RU486 on gonadotropin secretion of the follicular phase of the menstrual cycle. J Clin Endocrinol Metab 68:960
24. Gravanis A, Schaison G, George M, et al. (1985) Endometrial and pituitary responses to the steroidal antiprogestin RU486 in postmenopausal women. J Clin Endocrinol Metab 60:156
25. Croxatto BB, Salvatierra AM, Fuentealba B, et al. (1995) Follicle stimulating hormonegranulosa cell axis involvement in the antifolliculotrophic effect of low dose mifepristone (RU486). Human Reprod 10:1987

26. Murphy AA, Kettel LM, Morales AJ, et al. (1995) Endometrial effects of long-term, low-dose administration of RU486. Fertil Steril 63:761
27. Croxatto HB, Salvatierra AM, Fuentealba B, et al. (1994) Effect of the antiprogestin onapristone on follicular growth in women. Human Reprod 9:1442
28. Greene KE, Kettel LM, Yen SSC (1992) Interruption of endometrial maturation without hormonal changes by an antiprogesterone during the first half of luteal phase of the menstrual cycle: a contraceptive potential. Fertil Steril 58:338
29. Germzell-Danielsson K, Westlund P, Johannisson E, et al. (1996) Effect of low weekly doses of mifepristone on ovarian function and endometrial development. Human Reprod 11:256
30. Baldi E, Casano P, Falsetti C, et al. (1994) Intracellular calcium accumulation and responsiveness to progesterone in capacitating human spermatozoa. J Androl 12:323
31. Yang J, Serres C, Philibert D, et al. (1994) Progesterone and RU486: opposing effects on human sperm. Proc Natl Acad Sci U S A 91:529

11 Antiprogestins – A New Challenge for Female Contraception

Marc Bygdeman, Kristina Gemzell Danielsson, Lena Marions, Marja-Liisa Swahn

Introduction

Mifepristone (Roussel Uclaf, Paris, France) is an antiprogestin which binds to the progesterone receptor, thereby preventing progesterone from expressing its biological effect. Mifepristone, in combination with a prostaglandin analogue, is used for termination of early pregnancy in several countries, including Sweden [3, 17]. The use of antiprogestins for contraceptive purposes is currently being evaluated and recent results indicate that this may very well be possible.

Effect of Antiprogestin During the Menstrual Cycle

High Doses

Administration of antiprogestins during the follicular phase of the menstrual cycle delays the oestrogen rise and the luteal-hormone (LH) surge. Follicular development is delayed or arrested and ovulation is inhibited as long as treatment is continued [12]. Even if ovulation is inhibited, some follicular development occurs and sufficient amounts of estradiol are produced to result in withdrawal bleeding if a short period of gestagen therapy is given [10]. After cessation of treatment, there is a resumption of follicular growth or a recruitment of new follicles and the following luteal phase is usually normal [16]. The effect of antiprogestin on follicular development and ovulation could stem from direct influences on the ovary, indirect influences via the hypothalamic pituitary axis, or both. The results of several studies indicate that the preovulatory increase in progesterone (of ovarian origin) reinforces positive feedback of oestrogen in triggering the midcyle LH surge, and that the inhibitory effect of antiprogestin on ovulation is mediated by a blocking effect of progesterone at the pituitary [1, 2].

The effect of mifepristone on the endometrium during the follicular phase is related to inhibition of ovarian function. In contrast, during the luteal phase, it seems to be due to withdrawal of the effects of progesterone on the endometrium. If a high dose of mifepristone (200 mg) is given immediately after ovulation, on day LH+2, plasma levels of ovarian steroids and the menstrual cycle are not influenced, although occasional spotting may occur [5]. However, at the time of implantation, LH+2 to LH+8, a marked effect on endometrial development and function have been demonstrated [5]. The secretory changes of the endometrium were significantly inhibited, as was the normal downregulation of the progesterone receptor concentration. The reduction in the amount of uterine fluid at midluteal phase compared with that at ovulation was

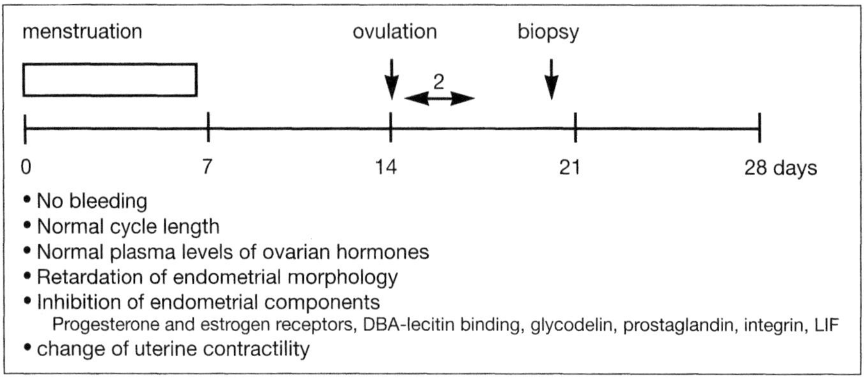

Fig. 1. The effect of 200 mg mifepristone administered on day LH+2 on the menstrual cycle and the endometrium. A biopsy was taken on cycle day LH+6 to LH+8

less pronounced and the concentration of $PGF_{2\alpha}$ in uterine fluid was significantly reduced. The same was true for 17β-hydroxysteroid dehydrogenase, glycodelin and the secretory activity measured by DBAlectin staining [4, 5, 11, 14, 15]. Also, the expression of leukaemia inhibitory factor (LIF) and integrin subunits β3 and α4 in glandular cells were significantly reduced at implantation time [6, 13] (Fig. 1).

Treatment in the mid- or late luteal phase will result in bleeding a few days after initiation of therapy and in shedding of the endometrium. In some women, the bleeding will occur in spite of normal progesterone levels and, in these cases, will be followed by a second bleeding at approximately the expected time of menstruation [11, 15, 16].

Low Doses

The endometrium seems more sensitive to antiprogestin treatment than to the ovulation process. Weekly administration of 2.5 mg or 5 mg mifepristone for 2 months, starting on day 2 of the first cycle, did not stop ovulation but did cause some inhibiti-

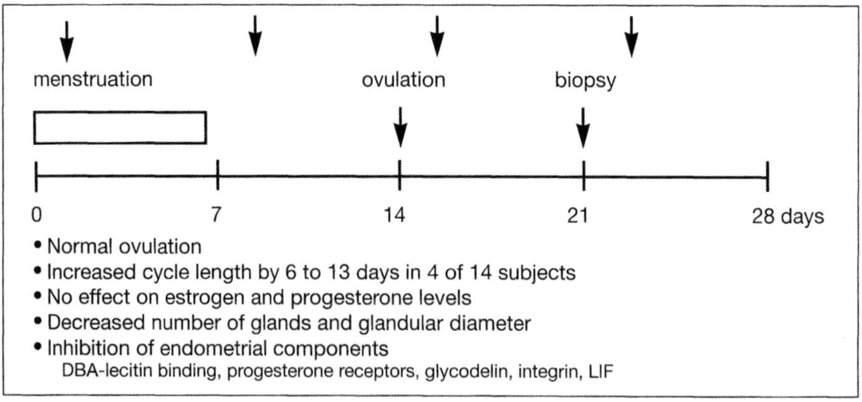

Fig. 2. The effect of 5 mg mifepristone, administered once weekly, on the menstrual cycle and endometrium. A biopsy was taken on cycle day LH+6 to LH+8

on of endometrial development (measured in the midluteal phase) relative to a control cycle. Inhibition of the normal downregulation of progesterone receptor concentration and a significant reduction in DBA-lectin binding and in glycodelin serum concentrations were also found [8] (Fig. 2). Daily doses of 0.5 mg mifepristone for 3 months did not have any inhibitory effects on ovulation and did not disturb the menstrual pattern. Nevertheless, endometrial development appeared to be slightly retarded and glandular diameter was significantly reduced. Furthermore, significant decreases in DBA-lectin binding and endometrial expression of glycodelin were observed at the time of implantation [8]. Both with low weekly and low daily doses of mifepristone, the endometrial glandular LIF and integrin expression were inhibited at the expected time of implantation [2, 6].

Contraceptive Use of Antiprogestins

The anti-ovulatory effect and the effect of mifepristone on the endometrium might be used for contraceptive purposes. This possibility has been evaluated in a few pilot studies. Whether the effect on the endometrium was sufficient to prevent implantation was tested in a clinical study, in which 200 mg mifepristone was administered once monthly (on day LH+2) for up to 12 months to 21 sexually active women; this was their only contraceptive method. The day of the LH peak was measured by the women. Over 121 cycles, the women had had intercourse during the fertile period (3 days before and 1 day after ovulation). Only one pregnancy occurred [7] (Table 1).

Treatment with antiprogestin is also a highly effective method for emergency contraception. In two studies, 600 mg mifepristone was administered within 72 h, following a single episode of unprotected intercourse. The treatment was compared with the Yuzpe regimen (ethinyl estradiol and levonorgestrel). The outcome indicated that mifepristone was at least as effective as the Yuzpe regimen and that it was associated with a significantly lower frequency of gastrointestinal side effects. A drawback of the mifepristone treatment is that, in up to 25% of the women, menstruation was delayed 7-10 days [9, 19]. In a recent multicentre study conducted by the World Health Organization (WHO), it was shown that the dose of antiprogestin could be reduced to 10 mg without a decrease in efficacy [WHO, unpublished observations]. The high efficacy of mifepristone is most likely due to the fact that if treatment is given just prior to ovulation, ovulation is delayed, and if given following coitus that takes place at the time of ovulation, its effects on the endometrium inhibit implantation.

Table 1. Contraceptive effect of mifepristone: number of cycles with one intercourse from 3 days before to 1 day after ovulation

Treatment (mg)	Subjects (*n*)	Cycles (*n*)	Number of pregnancies (n)	Total Intercourse (n)	Pregnancy rate at ovulation	Time
200	21	161	121	1	0.008	Day LH+2
5.0	18	60	45	3	0.067	Once weekly
WHO trial*	72	35			0.486	

* Fertile women having unprotected intercourse during the time period 3 days before to 1 day after the peak mucous day [18]

As described previously, even low doses of mifepristone that do not inhibit ovulation have an effect on endometrial development and function. In a recent study, the contraceptive effect of 5 mg mifepristone administered once weekly starting on day 2 of the menstrual cycle was evaluated [20]. The study was aimed at 20 women who were treated for 6 months. For ethical reasons, it was decided prior to the start that the study would be terminated if more than two pregnancies occurred. Since this was the case, only 18 women were treated (during the first 6 months or during 63 cycles). Based on those cycles in which the woman had intercourse 3 days before to 1 day after ovulation, the probability of pregnancy was 0.067; this value seems lower than that reported in the WHO study [18] for which no contraceptive method was used. According to Wilcox et al. [21], it is also significantly lower than the expected number of pregnancies. The contraceptive effect is, however, not sufficient for routine clinical use.

Conclusions

Antiprogestin has a number of effects during the menstrual cycle. These include inhibition of ovulation and influences on the development and function of the endometrium during the luteal phase of the cycle – effects which may be used for contraceptive purposes. So far, once-monthly administration of mifepristone immediately after ovulation, and treatment following a single episode of unprotected intercourse (emergency contraception) have been shown in clinical studies to be highly effective in preventing pregnancy.

Acknowledgements. Most of the studies summarised here have been supported by the WHO, Geneva, Switzerland, by the Knut and Alice Wallenberg Foundation and by the Swedish Medical Research Council (05696).

References

1. Batista MC, Cartledge TP, Zellmer AW, Nieman LK, Loriaux DL, Merriam GR (1994) The antiprogesterone RU 486 delays the midcycle gonadotrophin surge and ovulation in gonadotrophin-releasing hormone induced cycles. Fertil Steril 62:28-34
2. Batista MC, Cartledge TP, Zellmer AW, Nieman LK, Merriam GR, Loriaux DL (1992) Evidence for a critical role of progesterone in the regulation of the midcycle gonadotropin surge and ovulation. J Clin Endocrinol Metab 74:565-570
3. Bygdeman M, Swahn ML (1985) Progesterone receptor blockage. Effect on uterine contractility and early pregnancy. Contraception 32:45-51
4. Gemzell Danielsson K, Hamberg M (1994) The effect of antiprogestin (RU 486) and prostaglandin biosynthesis inhibitor (Naproxen) on uterine fluid PGF2a concentrations. Hum Reprod 9:1626-1630
5. Gemzell Danielsson K, Svalander P, Swahn ML, Johannisson E, Bygdeman M (1994) Effect of a single postovulatory dose of RU 486 on the endometrial maturation in the implantation phase. Hum Reprod 9:2398-2404
6. Gemzell Danielsson K, Swahn ML, Bygdeman M (1997) The effect of various doses of mifepristone on leukaemia inhibitory factor expression in the midluteal phase – an immunohistoctemical study. Hum Reprod 12:1293-1297

7. Gemzell Danielsson K, Swahn ML, Svalander P, Bygdeman M (1993) Early luteal phase treatment with RU 486 for fertility regulation. Hum Reprod 8:870-873
8. Gemzell Danielsson K, Westlund P, Johannisson E, Swahn ML, Seppais M, Bygdeman M (1997) Effect of low weekly doses of mifepristone on ovarian function and endometrial development. Hum Reprod 12:124-131
9. Glasier AF, Thong Kj, Dewar M, Mackie M, Baird DT (1992) Mifepristone (RU 486) compared with high-dose estrogen and progesterone emergency postcoital contraception. N Engl J Med 327:1041-1044
10. Kekkonen R, Croxatto HB, Lähteenmäki P, Salvatierra AM, Tuominen J (1995) Effects of intermittent antiprogestin RU 486 combined with cyclic medroxyprogesterone acetate on folliculogenesis and ovulation. Hum Reprod 10:287-292
11. Li TC, Dockery P, Thomas P, Rogers AW, Lenton EA, Cooke ID (1988) The effects of progesterone blockade in the luteal phase of normal fertile women. Fertil Steril 50:732-742
12. Liu JH, Garzo G, Monis Strenkel C, Ulmann A, Yen SCC (1987) Disruption of follicular maturation and delay of ovulation after administration of the antiprogestin RU 486. J Clin Endocrinol Metab 65:1135-1140
13. Marions L, Gemzell Danielsson K, Bygdeman M (1998) The effect of antiprogestin in integrin expression in human endometrium. An immunohistochemical study. Hum Reprod 4:491-495
14. Mäentausta 0, Svalander P, Gemzell Danielsson K, Bygdeman M, Vikho R (1993) The effects of an antiprogesterone, mifepristone, and an antiestrogen, tamoxifen, on endometrial 17b-hydroxysteroid dehydrogenase and progestin and estrogen receptors during the luteal phase of the menstrual cycle. An immunohistochemical study. J Endocrinol Metab 77:913-918
15. Swahn ML, Bygdeman M, Xing S, Cekan S, Masironi B, Johannisson E (1990) The effect of RU 486 administered during the early luteal phase on bleeding pattern, hormonal parameters and endometrium. Hum Reprod 5:402-408
16. Swahn ML, Johannisson E, Daniore V, de la Torre B, Bygdeman M (1988) The effect of RU 486 administered during the proliferative and secretory phase of the cycle on the bleeding pattern, hormonal parameters and the endometrium. Hum Reprod 3:915-921
17. Ulmann A, Silvestre L, Chemama L, Rezvani Y, Renault M, Aquillaume CJ, Baulieu EE (1992) Medical termination of early pregnancy with mifepristone (RU 486) followed by a prostaglandin analogue. Acta Obstet Gynecol Scand 71:278-283
18. WHO task force on methods for the determination of the fertile period (1983) A prospective multicentre trial of the ovulation method of natural family planning. III. Characterization of the menstrual cycle and the fertile phase. Fertil Steril 40:773-778
19. Webb AMC, Russel J, Elstein M (1992) Comparison of Yuzpe regimen, danazol and mifepristone (RU 486) in oral postcoital contraception. Br Med J 305:927-931
20. Marions L, Gemzell Danielsson K, Swahn ML, Bygdeman M (1998) Contraceptive efficacy of low doses of mifepristone. Fertil Steril (in press)
21. Wilcox AJ, Weinberg CR, Baird DT (1995) Timing of sexual intercourse in relation to ovulation. N Engl J Med 333:1517-1521

12 Natural Methods in Family Planning

Günter Freundl

Introduction and General Considerations

The term Natural Family Planning is used for methods of contraception based on the biological fact that women are only fertile for a short time during the menstrual cycle. Accordingly, this method depends on the ability of the couple to identify the fertile phase in each menstrual cycle and the couple's motivation and discipline to practice abstinence when required [9].

A significant proportion of couples find it difficult to predict or identify accurately the onset and end of the fertile phase. They may also take chances when practising-periodic abstinence and break the rules. Accordingly, appropriate and relevant counselling, adequate teaching of the technique and supportive follow-up are essential for the effectiveness of this methods.

Periodic abstinence can be a very effective contraceptive method when both partners are highly motivated and able to practise abstinence strictly according to the rules applying to the technique. However, a significant proportion of couples take a chance and break the rules which may lead to a high failure rate. Two factors have been found to have a major influence on the effectiveness of the natural methods [32]. One is the standard of teaching given to a woman about how to use their chosen method. The second factor is the motivation of the couple. The influence of these two factors is apparent in the results acquired by various multi-centre effectiveness studies. The user failure rate (Pearl index), for example, for the sympto-thermal method varies among different countries from 2.5 to 15.5, with a method failure rate of 0.5 to 2.6, as did about 25% of those using the cervical-muous method, compared with less than 5% of those using oral contraceptives or intrauterine devices. While the sympto-thermal method is more effective than the cervical mucus method, both methods show wide and overlapping ranges of failure and discontinuation rates among different groups of women. These rates seem high when compared with other methods. However, cumulative pregnancy rates showed that although, in the short term, oral contraception produced a lower pregnancy rate after 1 year of use than the calendar method (28 vs 36), at the end of the third year, the calendar method was more effective than oral contraception [26, 29]. Also the results differ from couples who want to prevent a pregnancy and those who merely intend to space the children.

Periodic abstinence may be the only choice for individuals and couples who cannot or do not want to use other methods of fertility regulation for a variety of reasons. Family planning associations should include periodic abstinence methods in their contraceptive education and counselling activities. Service providers should familiarise themselves with these techniques and be prepared to teach them if requested or to refer clients to special centres where the methods are taught. Couples electing to use periodic abstinence should be clearly informed about the failure rates of the method, the need to adhere strictly to the abstinence rules and the risks involved in not doing so. Appropriate counselling and training should be provided to both partners until they feel confident in their ability to recognise the fertile phase and to modify their sexual behaviour. Follow-up may be required to support them over time and to provide counselling on other contraceptive alternatives if they experience problems with the periodic abstinence techniques selected [3, 4].

Family planning by periodic abstinence from sexual intercourse has a long and somewhat chequered history. For a long time, its use has been strongly promoted by certain religious groups. Recently, the desire of many modern women to liberate their bodies from the dictates of drugs and doctors has led some to take a close look at the natural methods of family planning (NFP). Natural methods of family planning rely on the following biological conditions:

- The ovum can only be fertilized during the 12-18 h after release (limited live-span of the ovum).
- The life of sperm is longer and more susceptible to variation and can reach 4-5 days, when cervical mucus is present.
- There is only one ovulation per cycle.
- The fertile days can be determined by the woman herself by self-observation of signs and symptoms of her body.

It is the aim of NFP to identify the fertile time in the cycle so that couples can choose to abstain from sexual intercourse if they wish to avoid a pregnancy or continue sexual activity if they wish to conceive.

The cycle is controlled by the complex interplay of hormones and the reproductive organs, which ensures that each month an ovum is released from the ovaries at just the right time for possible fertilization by a sperm. There are hormones involved: the pulsatile secretion of LHRH from the hypothalamus produces the excretion of FSH and LH by the pituitary gland. These hormones control the production of the ovarian hormones oestrogen and progesterone. Oestrogen is mainly active in the pre-ovulatory phase. It is produced by the ripening follicle. During the post-ovulatory phase of the cycle, the dominant influence is progesterone produced by the corpus luteum (resulting from the dominant follicle after having released the ovum). If an ovum is not fertilized and does not implant, the endometrium is shed, thus producing the menstrual bleeding [21].

Oestrogen and progesterone have a wide range of other effects, some of which can be readily observed. Oestrogen produces physico-chemical alterations in the cervical mucus, which changes from a thick, opaque sticky plug to a thin, clear, lubricant substance as ovulation approaches. When the cervical mucus gets more fluid it descends the vagina and can be observed at the vaginal entrance. Progesterone is thermogenic, producing a rise in basal body temperature (BBT) after ovulation. The reason for this effect can be a direct thermogenetic effect of the progesterone on the hypothalamus. It could also be that the constrictory effect of the progesterone on the peripheral vessels causes less energy loss from the body and so the central body temperature rises.

It is the observation and recording of these phenomena that provide the physiological basis for the modern approach to NFP. They provide markers as to the stage of development of the cycle under scrutiny. In this they differ fundamentally from the older approach based on predicting the time of ovulation solely on the basis of the length of previous cycles (calendar or rhythm method).

If sexual intercourse is to lead to conception, it must take place around the time of ovulation during the fertile phase of the cycle. Before and after that time are the infertile phases. Confining intercourse to the infertile phases, especially that after ovulation, greatly reduces the chance of conception. Periodic abstinence techniques include:

- The cervical mucus or ovulation method (Billings)
- The basal body-temperature method (Döring, Marshall)
- The sympto-thermal method (Rötzer, Thyma)

According to the definition of WHO, the calendar method / rhythm method (Ogino, Knaus) does not belong to the NFP methods as it does not allow determination of the fertile time by self-observation in the actual cycle. It is rather a probability calculation method.

It should be noted that the techniques used for periodic abstinence can also be used for contraceptive practice, whereby a couple choose to use barrier methods only on those days estimated to be fertile (F.A./Mix). Couples who wish to achieve pregnancy can improve their chances of conception if they can recognise the fertile phase of the reproductive cycle. Methods of ovulation prediction are valuable in the management of infertility as well.

The Methods

Cervical Mucus Method

Following the end of menstruation, there are a number of 'dry days'. During this time the cervical mucus consists of a thick plug at the cervix, with none flowing down the vagina. The woman experiences a positive sensation of dryness at the vaginal entrance.

Under the influence of the rising level of oestrogen, the mucus changes first to a thick, sticky, opaque substance which reaches the vaginal entrance and can be detected there, either by the sensation it produces or by visual observation. The change continues until the mucus is thin, clear and slippery, giving rise to a sensation of 'wetness' and 'lubrication'. The last day of this type of mucus marks the estimated day of ovulation, after which the mucus reverts to a thick dry state or disappears entirely. The last day on which the mucus is not necessarily most abundant, but most slippery and lubricative is known as 'peak' day, which can only be detected retrospectively, i.e., on the day after, when it no longer possesses these characteristics.

Practical Instructions

1. Observations should be made throughout the day at convenient times, for instance, when going to the toilet.

2. Observation includes both the sensation experienced and visual inspection of mucus which appears at the vulva.
3. Sensation will be positive dryness or nothing, then a feeling of moistness or wetness, followed again by dryness.
4. Inspection shows a change from a thick, sticky, opaque substance to a thin, clear, watery, slippery substance. In the latter state, the mucus can be stretched as an unbroken thread between the fingers or between folded leaves of toilet tissue.
5. The results of the observations throughout the day should be recorded each evening on a chart.
6. Intercourse can take place during the dry days following menstruation. It is recommended that intercourse only takes place on alternate dry days, to avoid the risk of residual semen masking the first appearance of mucus. Not every woman has dry days following menstruation; sometimes mucus appears immediately, in which case the fertile phase starts immediately.
7. Once mucus appears there must be abstinence from intercourse, if the intention is to avoid pregnancy.
8. The day of peak mucus – that is the last day when mucus is slippery and lubricative – is marked by a cross on the chart.
9. Intercourse can be resumed on the fourth day after peak.

Thus, if peak day is marked by a cross and the next three days numbered 1, 2, 3, intercourse begins on the first unmarked day. It can continue as often as desired until the next menstrual period.

Advantages and Disadvantages

It has the advantage of requiring nothing beyond a means of recording the observations. However, the frequency of unexpected pregnancies is higher than with BBT, and has ranged from 5 up to 35 pregnancies per 100 woman-years of use.

The Modified Mucus Method

A modified mucus method (MMM) is being used in some programmes [12]. The rules of the method are less conservative than the original mucus method. It is different from the original method on the following points:

- MMM allows sexual intercourse in the first month of use, while the original method does not.
- In women who have regular cycles, MMM allows sexual intercourse on pre-ovulatory days, when thick mucus is present, contrary to the original method.
- Sexual intercourse is permitted on the third day after the peak mucus day, in contrast to the fourth day in the original method.

Basal Body Temperature Method

This was the first scientific method based on periodic abstinence to be developed. Essentially, a woman records her temperature immediately on waking each morning to get a basal reading. Following menstruation during the early part of the cycle the BBT remains at a lower level. Around ovulation, it rises by about 0.2-0.4°C and then is maintained at a higher level or plateau until the onset of the next menstruation.

The shift of temperature from a lower to a higher level is the marker of ovulation. By waiting until three consecutive daily temperatures at the higher level have been recorded, the woman can then start intercourse with very little risk of conception. This is because of the short life of the ovum.

The post-ovulatory infertile phase continues until the next menstruation. The BBT gives no indication of the approach of ovulation, and since sperm may survive for 4-5 days, intercourse cannot take place during the first part of the cycle between menstruation and ovulation, if a pregnancy has definitely to be prevented. Ovulation mostly takes place 1 day or 2 days prior to the first or on the day of the first higher temperature reading itself. Taking into account the life span of the sperm, the 7-8 days before the temperature rise have to be considered as fertile. The infertile phase at the beginning of the cycle can be determined by taking the earliest temperature rise out of 10-12 cycles minus 8 days (=last infertile day pre-ovulatory).

Practical Instruction

1. The BBT must be recorded immediately on waking before undertaking any activity. It is advisable to use a mercury thermometer.
2. The temperature may be taken by various routes: rectally, vaginally or orally (underneath the tongue), the thermometer being left in position for 3-5 min (orally 6-8 min). The same route must be used throughout a menstrual cycle. Oral temperatures give the least satisfactory record, because they are more susceptible to minor irregularities.
3. The temperature should be recorded on a chart designed specially for the purpose of easy identification of the rise of temperature to the best advantage.
4. The post-ovulatory infertile phase starts after three consecutive daily temperatures, all of which are above the level of the immediately preceding six consecutive daily temperatures, have been recorded. The last one of these three readings should be 0.2°C higher than the previous six lower readings.
5. There must be abstinence from intercourse throughout the early part of the cycle, from the onset of menstruation to the day on which the third higher temperature reading has been recorded. Intercourse can take place from that point to the onset of the next menstruation.

Advantages and Disadvantages

The BBT method alone can only detect the end of the fertile phase. If sexual intercourse is restricted to this latter part of the cycle, it offers a high degree of reliability.

This clearly requires a long period of abstinence in each cycle. In this case, an unexpected pregnancy rate of less than one to four per 100 woman-years of use can be achieved, according to the standard of instruction and motivation of the couple. Since the BBT method requires the identification of ovulation before sexual intercourse can resume, it is not a very useful or appropriate method for women with very irregular cycles. Also, thermometer breaking and replacing can be a problem for some women.

Sympto-thermal Method

Combining BBT and mucus observations has the obvious advantage of using two markers of ovulation, which should increase the accurate identification of the fertile period. It is essential that always two indicators are used to determine the beginning and the end of the fertile phase [1-4]: mucus observation and some kind of calculation rule (first 5 days or earliest temperature rise out of 12 cycles minus 8) is used to determine the last infertile day according to the principle of whichever comes first. The end of the fertile phase is determined by mucus observation and temperature measurement according to the principle, whichever comes last.

The rule of resuming intercourse with the mucus method is the evening of the fourth day after peak and, for the BBT method, the evening of the third higher temperature reading. The two, however, frequently coincide because the peak tends to precede and the temperature shift to follow ovulation. When there is discrepancy, the later day should be followed, to make the sympto-thermal method as effective as possible. Some women using this approach also monitor one or more secondary signs or symptoms to help to determine the fertile phase of the cycle. These include intermenstrual pain ('Mittelschmerz'), intermenstrual bleeding, breast tenderness, oedema and mood changes. However, these are not often used on their own.

Practical Instructions

1. To diagnose the fertile/infertile stage of the cycle, it is necessary to use both indicators of fertility, the cervical mucus and the temperature. To detect the beginning of the fertile phase calendar calculation and the first mucus symptom, whether detected by sensation or appearance, has to be used. Whichever of these indicators comes first marks the beginning of the fertile phase. To detect the end of the fertile phase, the temperature shift and the peak mucus symptom has to be used. Whichever of these indicators comes last marks the end of the fertile phase.
2. Sensation will be positive dryness or nothing, then a feeling of moistness or wetness, followed again by dryness.
3. Appearance shows a change from a thick, sticky, opaque substance to a thin, clear, watery, slippery substance. In the latter state, the mucus can be stretched as an unbroken thread between the fingers or between folded leaves of toilet tissue.
4. The temperature has to be taken according to the rules of the temperature method.
5. Two additional rules will help to evaluate difficult charts: (a) if the third temperature reading is not 0.2°C higher than the basic values, you have to wait for another temperature reading on the next day. This must just be higher than the previous six

lower readings. If you have three higher readings, one between them can drop down then the third higher reading must be 0.2°C or more.

Advantages and Disadvantages

Studies of the sympto-thermal method show a method failure rate below 1 (Pearl-Index), the use-effectiveness rate varies between 2.0 and 16 pregnancies per 100 women-years [19]. Effectiveness depends very much on the standards and the quality control of the respective NFP teacher organisation [3, 4]. However, organisations that have fairly good use-effectiveness rates also concede, that the users frequently take risks and have intercourse during the fertile phase, mostly not in the highly fertile phase, but just at the beginning of the fertile phase, believing that nothing will happen at this time.

Cervical Palpation

Self-palpation of the cervix has attracted increasing interest. This is best done standing with a foot on a chair, while one or two fingers are inserted into the vagina. In the early part of the cycle after menstruation, the cervix is low in the vagina and can easily be felt. It is firm with a consistency rather like the tip of the nose. The cervical os is closed. As ovulation approaches, the cervix becomes soft; its consistency is that of the lips rather than the tip of the nose. The os begins to open and is felt as a dimple, and as the cervix is higher in the vagina it is more difficult to reach. After ovulation, the changes revert to give a low, firm cervix with a closed os.

A recent study has shown [28] that with 851 women practising NFP in 12470 cycles, cervical palpation was performed in only 2470 cycles (19.8%). Often it is used in combination with the symptothermal method.

Calendar or Rhythm Method

The calendar or rhythm method reportedly is the most widely used of all periodic abstinence techniques. Properly used, it involves numerical calculations based on previous menstrual cycles to estimate the fertile period. It has a high failure rate, since it relies on past information to predict length of future cycles, a prediction which has a limited accuracy. Women who have reasonably regular cycles may find it more convenient to use this method since it does not require daily monitoring of fertility signs.

Practical Instructions

1. The method is not advisable for women with irregular or very long cycles. Also women who are breast-feeding cannot use the method. In order to predict the lengths of future cycles, a record of at least the past six consecutive cycles (better twelve cy-

cles) is necessary. During this period, other methods of contraception can be used, provided that this is not a hormonal method.
2. Calculate the first fertile day, subtract 18 from the shortest cycle. First fertile day = shortest cycle – 18.
3. Calculate the last fertile day, subtract 11 from the longest cycle. Last fertile day = longest cycle – 11.
4. Avoid sexual intercourse during the fertile phase. For example, if the last six cycles were 28, 26, 29, 27, 29 and 27 days long, the first day of the fertile phase = 26-18=8. The last day of the fertile phase = 29-11=18. Avoid sexual intercourse from day 8 to day 18 of the cycle, inclusive.

Advantages and Disadvantages

1. The most severe disadvantage is the fact that the effectiveness of these methods is rather low.
2. Also, it is a method in which body signals, which have the best correlation to the cycle events, have to be detected from calculations
3. The abstinence requested may be rather long.
4. It is not useful for clients with very irregular cycles.

The Effectiveness of the NFP Methods

Estimates of NFP effectiveness in the literature vary widely [32]. Many reasons exist for these variations. First, investigators use different techniques to calculate pregnancy rates, making it difficult to interpret the results and compare estimates of effectiveness among studies. Second, NFP is not just one method. Different NFP methods use different indicators to identify the fertile time and they have different rules for abstinence, and, therefore, must be considered and evaluated separately. Third, many published reports omit important information, i.e. teaching situation of the couples, study population, the time that was necessary for the participants to reach autonomy. Also, many times, reports do not have the necessary information concerning perfect and imperfect use of a method [38].

Table 1 [19, 32] shows the results of well-designed prospective clinical studies concerning life table probabilities of pregnancy during typical use. Summarised, it is found that with the cervical mucus method, the theoretical Pearl-Index (method PI) is located between 1.2 and 2.9, the practical Pearl-Index (user effectiveness) between 15.5 and 34.9. The effectiveness of the temperature method is much higher than the one of the cervical mucus method: theoretical Pearl-Index between 0 and 1.2, practical Pearl-Index between 0.26 and 6.6.

With the sympto-thermal method, Rice [33] reported, in a prospective multinational study where established teacher organisations were involved, a theoretical Pearl-Index of 0.75 and a practical of 7.6. In this study, for the beginning of the fertile time, a calculation rule was used, whereas the end of the fertile time was detected using temperature. It is interesting that great international variations were found in the Rice study, i.e. use-effectiveness of 18.05 in Columbia and 4.85 in the States.

Table 1. NFP studies reporting 12-month single-decrement (gross) life table probabilities of pregnancy during typical use (modified according to V. Lamprecht and J. Trussell (1997) and Raith, Frank-Herrmann, Freundl (1994)

Reference (year)	Method tested	Pregnant (%)	Instructor	Financing
Johnston et al. (1978)	OM STM 1 STM 2	26.4 14.3 13.3	Married women with children	Goverment
Klaus et al. (1979)	OM	15.8	?	NFP-organisations, government
Medina et al. (1980)	OM STM 3	29.2 26.1	NFP-teachers	Foreign aid
Rice et al. (1981)	STM 4	8.3	Lay people: couple to couple	NFP-organisations, church, government
Wade et al. (1981)	OM STM 5	37.2 13.9	Lay people: couple tocouple	Government
WHO (1981)	OM	19.6	Lay people: couple to couple	WHO
Thapa et al. (1990)	OM MMM	2.5 10.3	NFP-teachers	Foreign aid
Frank-Herrmann et al. (1997)	STM 6 STM 7	2.5 7.8	NFP-teachers	NFP-organisation, church, government

OM, ovulation method or Billings method (1980); MMM modified mucus method according to Dorairaj (1991); STM sympto-thermal method; STM 1-7, different double-check methods.

Table References:

1. Billings JJ, Billings EL, Catarinich M (1980) Atlas of the ovulation method. 4th advocate, Melbourne
2. Dorairaj K (1991) The modified mucus method in India. Am J Obstet Gynecol 165:2066-2067
3. Frank-Herrmann P, Freundl G, Gnoth C, Godehardt E, Kunut J, Baur S, Sottong U (1997) Natural family planning with and without barrier method use in the fertile phase: efficacy in relation to sexual behaviour: A German prospective longterm study. Adv. Contraception 13: 179-89
4. Johnston JA, Roberts DB, Spencer RB (1978) NFP services and methods in Australia: a survey evaluation. Synopsis. IRNFP 2:143-154
5. Klaus H, Goebel J, Muraski B (1979) Use effectiveness and client satisfaction in six centers teaching the Billings Ovulation Method. Contraception 19:613-629
6. Lamprecht V, Trussell J (1997) Natural family planning effectiveness: evaluating published reports. Adv Contracept 13:155-165
7. Medina J, Cifuentes A, Abernathy J, Spieler J, Wade M (1980) Comparative evaluation of two methods of natural family planning in Columbia. Am J Obstet Gynecol 138:1142-1147
8. Raith E, Frank P, Freundl G (1994) Natürliche Familienplanung heute. Springer Verlag, Berlin Heidelberg New York
9. Rice FL, Lanctot CA, Garcia-Devesa C (1981) Biological effectiveness of the symptothermal method. An international study. Int J Fertil 26:222-230
10. Thapa S, Wonga M, Lampe P, Pretojo H, Soejoenoes A (1990) Effectiveness of three variations of periodic abstinence in Indonesia. Stud Fam Plann 21:327-334
11. Wade ME, McCarthy P, Braunstein GD (1981) A randomized prospective study of the use-effectiveness of two methods of natural family planning. Am J Obstet Gynecol 141:368-376
12. WHO (1981) A prospective multicenter trial of the ovulation method of natural family planning. II. The effectiveness phase. Fertil Steril 36:591-598

Wade [39] compared the STM with the OM and published in 1981 for the STM a theoretical Pearl-index of 0 and a practical of 16.6. The practical PI for the OM was 34.9. This project was a high cost project of the US government. Randomisation occurred between STM and OM. The teachers were trained during the study course. The participants were offered free medical care during the study. There was already a drop-out rate of 54% during the learning phase. At the end of the study, there were from 573 OM only 68 left, and from 590 STM only 139.

We have evaluated the results of our prospective use-effectiveness study of NFP in Germany, which we have performed since 1984 with the NFP-research project at the Heinrich-Heine-University of Düsseldorf [19]. Until summer 1997, we had 758 women NFP-beginners, aged 19-45 years, with 14.870 cycles, who wanted to avoid a pregnancy from the beginning. Twenty-eight unintended pregnancies were studied. Of the couples, 54.2% of the couples used NFP only or predominantly and 45.9% used mixed methods (additional barrier-method use in the fertile phase in 55.7% of the cycles). Also, 28 pregnancies were reported. There was no significant difference between NFP-only users and mixed-method users and, also, no significant effect of duration of use in the first 5 years. The overall pregnancy rate after 12 cycles of exposure (life table rate) was 2.2% according to the actuarial method. It was found that during the learning phase there was no increased risk of pregnancy. Of the 28 unplanned pregnancies, 24 occurred because unprotected intercourse took place during the fertile phase. One pregnancy followed condom-protected intercourse in the fertile phase, and three pregnancies occurred with perfect abstinence in the fertile phase.

In our trial, we divide the results into two groups: the group with typical use and the group with perfect use. So, during perfect use, the pregnancy rate at 12 months was 0.63% (method pregnancy rate). Table 2 shows the pregnancy rates in relation to perfect and imperfect use of the STM, which is used by the AG NFP Germany [4]. In a prospective European efficiency trial [20], we found a use-effectiveness of 2,4 P.I. for the sympto-thermal method.

The reports about the effectiveness of the rhythm method differ greatly: The theoretical Pearl-Index is said to be 3.3, the practical Pearl-Index lies between that and 47.

Table 2. Pregnancy rates in relation to perfect and imperfect use of the sympto-thermal method according to Frank-Herrmann et al. 1997 [19]

Sexual behaviour in the fertile phase	Cycles (%)	Unintended pregnancies (*n*)	Pregnancy rate (% per year *)	Confidence interval (x0.0001)
Abstinence	41.4	3	0.63	1.00-14.20
Abstinence most probable	11.5	0	0	0
Genital contact	5.7	4	4.54	7.37-103.45
Unprotected intercourse (ui)	15.9	17	8.96	42.16-15.98
Protected intercourse (pi)	19.6	1	0.45	0.09-19.10
ui and pi	5.9	3	4.33	7.02-98.68

*According to the formula: p = 100 ◊ (1-(1-P)), where P is the probability per cycle (pregnancies/cycle)

General Considerations

Motivation is essential for successful family planning of any kind. Nowhere is this more true than in the practice of natural family planning. Motivation is best secured through a thorough understanding of the method. Prescription of a set of rules to be followed blindly is unlikely to work. A couple must understand what they are doing and why. The background knowledge required for the practice of NFP promotes this understanding. The physiological principles need not be coached in highly technical terms; a simplified version of the phases of the cycle can be grasped by anyone.

Couples appreciate learning about phenomena that they have already observed, the significance of which they have not understood. They enjoy knowing more about their bodies and their fertility. The need to acquire this knowledge means that couples are making a positive choice to learn and use the methods which, in turn, strengthen their motivation. This knowledge is best conveyed by other successful users who have been specially trained for the task. Their personal experience combined with their training as teachers of the method make them credible. These methods, though inexpensive in terms of equipment, can be costly in terms of personnel. However, most organisations teaching the methods use trained volunteers.

In Germany during the last 16 years, a NFP organisation has been established to train teachers and to co-ordinate the activities of the NFP teachers, to promote high and international standards of NFP training and practice and to facilitate an exchange of updated information about research on fertility. Standardised teaching materials have been developed by the Working Group of NFP [1-4], which is located with its organisational part with the Malteserwerke in Cologne and with its research branch with the Heinrich-Heine-University of Düsseldorf. There is a marvellous co-operation with international NFP organisations worldwide.

Many of our studies have shown that most women who want to learn these methods are able to do so, regardless of their educational level. It appears that when the methods are taught and followed correctly, they can be very effective in preventing unplanned pregnancies. The methods can also be used to advantage in timing sexual intercourse, so as to improve the chances of conception when a pregnancy is desired.

Side Effects

Periods of abstinence may, when used positively, enhance rather than detract from a relationship. In strongly motivated couples, the bonds between them may be strengthened. However, in some instances, there may be psychological strain on the relationship, especially if one partner is more highly motivated than the other. Couples may, in these circumstances, use barrier methods during the fertile phase of the cycle, so that sexual intercourse can continue (F.A./Mix). It is essential if the method is to be effective that the woman observes her signs of fertility and infertility with the same care as she would if abstaining during the fertile phase.

There were discussions on the role of aged gametes in the fertilization process. However, the studies performed did not confirm the theory, that if fertilization involving ageing gametes does occur, there is a raised possibility of congenital abnormalities in the offspring. Simpson et al. [35] found that the overall rate of spontaneous abortions was not increased in NFP users, nor to date was the rate of anomalies. Of special interest was the lack of association between NFP and Down syndrome [11].

The suggestion has also been made that if fertilization takes place late in the menstrual cycle, there may be a higher than usual probability of ectopic pregnancy and placenta praevia, with their associated risks for the method and infant. This hypothesis, though supported by some observational data, has not been confirmed.

We conclude that knowledge of the most fertile, least fertile and infertile phases of the human menstrual cycle is important knowledge, which women should understand whether they wish to conceive, to use periodic abstinence for fertility regulation, or whether they wish to use coitus interruptus and/or barrier methods only during the fertile phase.

New Technologies to Detect Fertility in NFP

For some women, the identification of the subjective symptoms in the cycle to detect the fertile phase is inconvenient and, therefore, makes NFP methods unacceptable. The difficulties most often cited are the chore of making accurate daily observations and charts, their relative imprecision and subjectivity and the inability of the clinical indicators to cope with erratic or delayed fertility in a cycle. Another problem is the detection of the beginning of the fertile time by measurable cycle signals. Therefore, over the past decade, devices and tests have been developed particularly for the detection of ovulation and the fertile phase. They are called new technologies in NFP.

Electronic thermometers, such as "Evatherm" and "Roland" are able technically to measure temperature with an accuracy of 0.1°C. This accuracy is enough that this thermometers can be used in NFP. The advantage is that the time of measurements is minimised in relation to mercury-chrome thermometers.

At this time, the most advanced new technologies are computer thermometers, which have programs that use the rules of the temperature method (Babycomp/Ladycomp, Bioself, Cyclotest), and a hormonal computer system called Persona, which measures the hormones estriol-glucuronide (E3G) and LH in the urine and calculates fertile and infertile days with an inborn algorithm.

Temperature Computers

At this time, three temperature computers are marked in Germany: Babycomp/Ladycomp, Bioself Plus and Cyclotest 2 Plus. We carried out efficacy finding studies (EFS) with these devices. Unfortunately, with the exception of Bioself 110, no prospective effectiveness studies (pES) have been performed until now, as they are very expensive. I want to report briefly about our EFS results [22, 23]: points of reverence for this studies were: ultrasound/ LH in urine/ sympto-thermal method.

Babycomp/Ladycomp is a computer which is programmed according to the rules of the temperature method. We have tested 20 women in 204 cycles. The age of the women ranged between 18 years and 45 years, and they mostly had a cycle length of 25-35 days. In conclusion, we found that Babycomp safely determined the beginning as well as the end of the fertile phase. However, it does not shorten, but on the contrary it extends the length of the fertile phase.

In a retrospective clinical trial (rES) the effectiveness of Babycomp/Ladycomp was tested with more than 600 users [5]. The P.I. for the user efficacy rate was 4.2 [6], the method effectiveness was 0.7 P.I. Compared with the original temperature method, Babycomp takes clearly more than 30 s, often several minutes, until the measurement is completed. However Babycomp is suitable for women who do not want to record their temperature every morning. A problem of the design is the present high price.

Bioself 110 also uses the rules of the calendar method. Using these rules, it cannot be better than the calendar method itself. However, some of the women like this apparatus as it is very handy and easy to read. The Bioself 110 showed in a pES with 131 women and 1238 cycles a use effectiveness rate of 22.9 and a method effectiveness rate of 1.9 [13, 18]. The correct detection (no risk for an unwanted pregnancy) of the fertile phase was given in 86% of the cycles studied. No studies have been reported until now regarding the actual sold device Bioself plus. With Cyclotest D, we have tested in a prospective way the fertile time shown by the device compared with the fertile time detected by objective cycle parameters like sonography of the growing follicle and determination of the LH peak in urine [8, 23]. With 69 cycles in 57 ovulatory cycles, the temperature rise was detected at the day of ovulation or until 2 days after ovulation.

In summary, it has to be stated that for the actual temperature devices sold on the marked today, there are no actual data on effectiveness and acceptability. In our experience from earlier tests, we expect that these devices are rather safe, but we expect that the fertile phase, i. e. the requested time of abstinence, may be rather long, thus influencing the acceptability and efficacy of such devices.

Hormonal Computers

Home-based, self-test kits to measure cyclical hormone changes in urine are still being developed. Contraception detection of three hormones or their metabolites is interesting: estradiol, LH and progesterone. Estradiol should be able to mark the beginning, and LH or progesterone to detect the end of the fertile phase.

Now the personal system of hormone monitoring Persona has been put on the market, which allows the rapid assay of E3G and LH in urine to determine the fertile period. A first prospective European effectiveness trial (pES) has just been performed with women who were spacing their next pregnancy. The trial was carried out in UK, Ireland and Germany. The figures from Germany are published [25], the multicentre figures will follow. Seven hundred and ten volunteers (median age 30 years) were admitted to the study and contributed 7209 cycles of use. Using the prototype system, 67 method pregnancies were identified in 6833 cycles, giving a 13-cycle life-table method pregnancy rate of 12.1%. In addition, 92 user pregnancies and 3 unsure pregnancies were identified. With a revised algorithm generated for an extended fertile time, 33 of the method pregnancies would have been prevented giving a calculated method pregnancy rate of 6.2% (95% confidence interval 4.2-8.3%).

The Cyclotest 2 plus has also to be mentioned. In this device, in addition to a temperature program, a LH peak, determined by the users from an urine test, can be entered. This device has just been evaluated in a thesis in Düsseldorf [14].

The Safeplan, which is a urinary test, detects the pregnandiol-glucuronide rise in the urine after ovulation. It is a test, which should be able to detect the post-ovulatory infertile phase. Until today we saw problems with the sensitivity of the test or better with the exact calibration of the pregnandiol rise observed.

Electrical Resistance Gauges

We have tested devices for measuring the electrical resistance. Such devices are the CUE-Fertility Monitor, the ovulation controller or the dist-4. At the present stage, they are not yet fully recommendable, as the number of false negative results is still too high.

The CUE-Fertility-Monitor measures the salivary and vaginal fluid resistance. We have checked 45 cycles of eight women using the CUE-Fertility-Monitor [24]. We found that the CUE peak occurred 7±1.6 days prior to the first BBT rise. The vaginal low occurred 1.6±0.2 days prior to the first higher reading, the vaginal rise (VR) 0.6±1.9 days prior to BBT+1. From the standard deviation reported, you can see that there was not much difference in the individual values. In other papers [16, 30, 31], the efficiency was reported to be higher.

In summary, we found that it is possible, to use the CUE peak to predict the ovulation. In each normal and well-defined cycle, the CUE peak precedes the fertile phase of the cycle. We recommend to find a better algorithm than the one used in the CUE now to evaluate the single readings of each day in comparison with the day of ovulation and in comparison with biphasic and monophasic cycles.

Other Devices

There are available self tests for body fluids. With plastic vaginal aspirators (Rovumeter, Ovutrac), it is possible to measure the varying volumes of the cervico-vaginal fluid. In a prospective efficacy study (pES), Flynn et al. 1988 [17] found a use effectiveness of more than 95%. In Germany, this device is not on the market.

Methods that use enzyme reaction to detect the fertile time have to be mentioned. One of these devices is called Calgiswopä. It was tested in 57 cycles. The handling is rather easy, the result is shown clearly by a colour change, the reaction time is about 6 min. However, well-designed studies would be necessary to test the efficacy of the device and the individual variations [15].

Saliva microscopes, such as PC2000 and PG53 have been tested in small studies [6, 7]. With PC2000 in 300 cycles, fertility was detected only in 81.6% [38]. With PG 53, the fertility status could only be detected in 87.5% of the cycles. All the other devices have not been tested in prospective efficacy studies. Thus, figures concerning effectiveness are highly speculative.

There are other developments that rely on phenomenons in the menstrual cycle that are not generally recognized [10, 27]. A device was developed measuring fingertip electrical potentials, which are said to change during the cycle [36]. Another device detects the ratio of palminic acid and cholesterol in the skin of the face. A brazier originally developed to measure the temperature of the breast to detect tumours of the breast using built-in probes now measures the post-ovulatory temperature rise and the increase of circulation caused by oestrogens. An ovulation watch developed by Weiland and endowed with the Philipp-Moris-research award measures the skin temperature at the wrist.

It would be very interesting if a woman could predict her ovulation using direct measurements at home, for example, personal ultrasound at home. This is not possible at this time. Thus, she has to use signals that are as closely related to ovulation as possible. Finally, only well-designed effectiveness studies can prove the value of a new technical method.

Is There a Competition Between new Technologies and Natural Family Planning Methods?

The sympto-thermal method of NFP is a very effective method of family planning and can compete with the pill or the IUD in women who cannot or will not use these other modern methods for contraception. It is also suitable for women who wish to recognise the fertility of their own bodies, who want to live in accordance with their body and who feel responsible for their own contraception. If they are not willing or able to recognise or chart the signals of their body, then the new technologies offer an interesting alternative. However, the efficiency of the various devices must be known to the users for their decision. We think that the woman who uses the original NFP method is different from the woman who uses the new technologies. Therefore, there is no competition, but a completion.

References

1. AG NFP Köln, Brachi M, Tibaldeschi G (eds) (1989): Naturale e sicuro. vol 1. Edizioni Piemme S.p.A., Piemme
2. AG NFP Köln, Skupina PD (eds) (1992) Naravno in Zanesljio. vol 1. Mohorjeva Druzba, Celje
3. AG NFP Köln (ed) (1988) Natürlich und sicher: Arbeitsheft. vol 2. Ehrenwirth Verlag, München
4. AG NFP Bonn (1994) Natürlich und Sicher. Ehrenwirth Verlag, München
5. Bachhofer D (1997) Der Miniaturcomputer Babycomp/ Ladycomp in der Natürlichen Familienplanung. Promotion an der Medizinischen Fakultät der Heinrich-Heine-Universität, Düsseldorf
6. Barbato M, Bertolotti G (1988) Natural methods of fertility control: a prospective study. Int J Fertil Suppl :48-51
7. Barbato M, Pandolfi A, Guida M (1993) A new diagnostic aid for natural family planning. Adv Contracept 9:335-340
8. Bremme M, Freundl G, Frank-Herrmann P (1992) Analysis of the computer-thermometer "Cyclotest D" to be used for natural family planning. Adv Contracept 8:221-221
9. Brown JB, Blackwell LF, Billings JJ, Conway B, Cox RI, Garrett G, Holmes J, Smith MA (1987) Natural family planning. Am J Obstet Gynecol 157:1082-1089
10. Calamera JC, Vilar O, Nicholson R (1986) Changes in sialic acid concentration in human saliva during the menstrual cycle. Int J Fertil 31:43-45
11. Castilla EE, Lopez-Camelo JS, da Graca Dutra M, Queenan JT, Simpson JL, NFP-ECLAMP Group (1997) The frequency and spectrum of congenital anomalies in natural family planning users in South America: no increase in a case-control study. Adv Contracept 13:395-404
12. Dorairaj K (1991) The modified mucus method in India. Am J Obstet Gynecol 165:2066-2067
13. Drouin J, Guilbert EE, Desaulniers G (1994) An evaluation of the Bioself 110 electronic fertility Contrace indicator as a contraceptive aid. Contraception 50:229-238
14. Fatthagian (1997) Gebrauchssicherheit des Cyclotest 2 plus. Promotion an der Med. Fakultät der Heinrich-Heine-Universität, Düsseldorf

15. Fazleabas AT, Segraves MM, Khan-Dawood FS (1990) Evaluation of salivary and vaginal electrical resistance for determination of the time of ovulation. Int J Fertil 35:106-111
16. Fernando RS, Regas J, Betz G (1988) Ovulation prediction and detection with the CUE ovulation predictor. Hum Reprod 3:419-424
17. Flynn AM, McCarthy AM, Docker M, Royston JP (1988) The temporal relationship between vaginal fluid volumes obtained with Rovumeter vaginal aspirator and the fertile phase of the cycle. Hum Reprod 32:201-205
18. Flynn A, Pulcrano J, Royston P, Spieler J (1991) An evaluation of the Bioself 110 electronic fertility indicator as a contraceptive aid. Contraception 44:125-139
19. Frank-Herrmann P, Freundl G, Gnoth Ch, Godehardt E, Kunert J, Baur S, Sottong U (1997) Natural family planning with and without barrier method use in the fertile phase: efficacy in relation to sexual behaviour - a German prospective study. Adv Contracept 13:179-189
20. Freundl G (1993) Prospective European multi-center study of natural family planning (1989-1992): interim results. The European Natural Family Planning Study Groups. Adv Contracept 9:269-283
21. Freundl G, Tigges J (1995) Gynäkologische Endokrinologie für die Praxis. Fischer Verlag, Jena
22. Freundl G, Bremme M, Frank-Herrmann P, Baur S, Godehardt E (1992) Familienplanung: Was können Temperaturcomputer wirklich leisten?. Sexualmedizin 21:424-428
23. Freundl G, Baur S, Bremme M, Döring GK, Frank-Herrmann P, Godehardt E, Kunert J (1992) Temperaturcomputer zur Bestimmung der fertilen Zeit im Zyklus der Frau: Babycomp, Bioself 110, Cyclotest D. Fertilität 8:66-76
24. Freundl G, Bremme M, Frank-Herrmann P, Baur S, Godehardt E, Sottong U (1996) The CUE Fertility Monitor compared to ultrasound and LH peak measurements for fertile time ovulation detection. Adv Contracept 12:111-121
25. Freundl G, Bonnar J, Flynn AM, Frank-Herrmann P, Kirkman R, Snowden R (1998) Effektivität eines neuen Verhütungscomputers "PERSONA" - Bericht über Testergebnisse in Deutschland. Fortschr Med 116 Orig. I: 25-30
26. Gnoth C, Frank-Herrmann P, Freundl G, Kunert J, Godehardt E (1995) Sexual behavior of natural family planning users in Germany and its changes over time. Adv Contracept 11:173-185
27. Jordan V, Pilka L, Roztocil A (1992) The possibility of natural family planning by means of estrogen peak evaluation in saliva. Adv Contracept 8:223-224
28. Klose A (1992) Die Wertigkeit der Zervixveränderungen im Rahmen der Natürlichen Familienplanung. Med. Fakultät der Heinrich-Heine-Universität Düsseldorf, Düsseldorf
29. Laing JE (1984) Natural family planning in the Phillippines. Studies Family Planning 15:49-61
30. Loewit K, Hoppichler F, Ledermüller G (1990) Ovulation prediction from cyclic changes in salivary conductivity. Am J Obstet Gynecol 163:708-710
31. Moreno JE, Weitzmann GA, Doody MC, Gibbons WE, Besch P, Goldzieher JW (1988) Temporal relation of ovulation to salivary and vaginal electrical patterns: implications for natural family planning. Contraception 38:407-418
32. Raith E, Frank P, Freundl G (1994) Natürliche Familienplanung heute. Springer Verlag, Berlin Heidelberg New York
33. Rice FJ, Lanctot CA (1979) Fairfield international collaborative study on the sympto-thermal method. In: ed. NFP Research Workshop Linden Hill Hotel 1979. Bethesda, Maryland
34. Roumen FJ, Dieben TO (1988) Ovulation prediction by monitoring salivary electrical resistance with the Cue Fertility Monitor. Obstet Gynecol 71:49-52
35. Simpson JL, Gray RH, Perez A, Mena P, Barbato M, Castilla EE, Kambic RT (1997) Pregnancy outcome in natural family planning users: cohort and case control studies evaluating safety. Adv Contracept 13:201-214
36. Stoller KP, Brooks PG (1986) Detection of ovulation via fingertip electrical potentials: a preliminary report. Mt Sinai J Med 53:506-509
37. Treves C, Vincenzini MT, Vanni P, Bardazzi F, Cattaneo A, Ogier E (1986) Changes in enzyme levels in human cervical mucus during the menstrual cycle. Int J Fertil 31:59-66
38. Trussel J (1990) Contraceptive Failure of the ovulation method of periodic abstinence: Results from the WHO multi-country study. Family Planning Perspect 3:
39. Wade ME, McCarthy P, Braunstein GD (1981) A randomized prospective study of the use-effectiveness of two methods of natural family planning. Am J Obstet Gynecol 141:368-376
40. WHO (1981) A prospective multicenter trial of the ovulation method of natural family planning. II. The effectiveness phase. Fertil Steril 36:591-598

13 Female and Male Sterilisation

Marcus Filshie

Introduction

Current information on the world use of contraception remains elusive, not least because of the logistic difficulties involved in amassing such data. However, the United Nations, when they assessed global levels and trends in contraceptive use in 1998, suggested that the number of couples at that time who had already opted for a surgical end to childbearing was of the order of 180,000 million [1]. Spira [2], who re-analysed data from the late 1980s, implied that a little over one half (53%) of couples in the world then used a contraceptive method; well over one-third of these users had undergone a surgical procedure. At the global level, the data suggest female sterilisation to have been used four times as frequently as male surgery. Marked variations could be seen between the various regions of the world, with the more-developed regions having - as a whole - a lower resort to surgery. Correspondingly, the less-developed regions - despite problems of access to services - had a higher use of surgical contraception. Indeed, by the late 1980s, it would appear that approximately one-half the contraceptive users in China and Asia had been sterilised [2].

Data cited by the US Collaborative Review of Sterilisation indicate that, by 1988, tubal sterilisation had become the most prevalent method of contraception among ever married women in the USA and that, by 1990, more women had undergone sterilisation surgery than were using any other single method of fertility control - including oral contraception [3]. In the UK, data on contraceptive use are routinely collected, usually biennially, via the General Household Survey [4]. Figures for the period 1986-1995 show that around one in four women of reproductive age or their partners rely on sterilisation. By 1995, for women aged 40 years or over, this figure approached one in two, with slightly more than half of the cases involving tubal surgery rather than vasectomy (24% female sterilisation versus 20% vasectomy among 40-44 year olds, and 26% against 20% among the 45-49 years age group). Over the same time period, the proportion of younger women who had been sterilised fell from 25% to 18% for women aged 30-34 years and from 42% to 32% for the 35 to 39-year-old group between 1986 and 1995; oral contraceptive use correspondingly increased in these age groups. These changes in contraceptive practice are consistent with a substantial proportion of women in the UK delaying the start of childbearing until they reach their early or mid-thirties [5].

Female Sterilisation

Historical Review

The first reported case of female sterilisation appeared in a text book over 160 years ago by Blundell, who recommended removing part of the fallopian tube at the time of caesarean section in patients with a contracted pelvis. Fifty years later, in Ohio, USA, in 1880, Lungren ligated the fallopian tube, also at caesarean section, in a woman with a similar problem. Since then, a multitude of different methods of occlusion of the fallopian tubes have been developed, the most notable being the Madlena procedure of 1910 and techniques of Irving 1924, Pomeroy 1930, Aldridge 1934, Kroener 1935 and Uchida 1946. These have been ably summed up by Rioux [6].

The main indications were for medical reasons or for grand multiparity. The procedures were performed at the time of caesarean section or immediately post-partum. Female sterilisation was not performed frequently until the advent of laparoscopy, which enabled the patient to have the procedure performed safely on a day-care basis. Although crude laparoscopy was originally performed in 1910 by Kelling, in dogs, Jacobeus from Sweden first introduced a laparoscope into humans in 1911, and it was he who coined the phrase 'laparoscopy'. The use of the laparoscope to perform female sterilisation was first recorded by Ruddock in 1934. Anderson (1937) from the USA first designed a purpose-built electrode for tubal fulguration. Powers & Barnes, in 1941, wrote an article on laparoscopic tubal fulguration techniques. It was not until 20 years later, in 1960, when Palmer of France gave a huge impetus to laparoscopic tubal fulguration and popularised the method in France. Later, in 1964, Frangenheim from Germany and, in 1965, Steptoe from the UK popularised these methods in their respective countries. The laparoscope was substantially improved by the addition of the Hopkins-Ron Lens system, together with the advent of the cold light source. Laparoscopic tubal ligation was later adopted by Cohen & Wheeless in the USA.

Laparoscopic tubal ligation became so popular that it was used for sterilising women for social reasons as well as medical reasons. As large numbers of patients had the operation, so complications and fatalities relating to bowel burns came to light from unipolar diathermy, and these burns were often at a site distant from the operating field. To reduce these complications, bipolar cautery was introduced by Rioux (Canada), Kleppinger (USA) and Hirsch (Germany). Despite bipolar cautery, thermal injuries still continued and, so, a number of mechanical methods of tubal occlusion emerged (Fig. 1). These included the Fallope ring in 1975 [7], the Hulka clip in 1973 [8] and the Filshie clip in 1981 [9]. Tupler and Bleier plastic clips also emerged. Today, only the Fallope ring, Hulka and Filshie clips are being used on a regular basis.

Surgical Routes

The laparoscopic technique is widely used and is preferred. Its use is popular both in the developed and in the developing countries. The procedure may be performed under local [10] or general anaesthesia. The patient is placed on the operating table, usually in the lithotomy position, and following catheterisation, a pneumoperitoneum is created by instilling, through a Veress needle just below the umbilicus, 2-3 l

Fig. 1

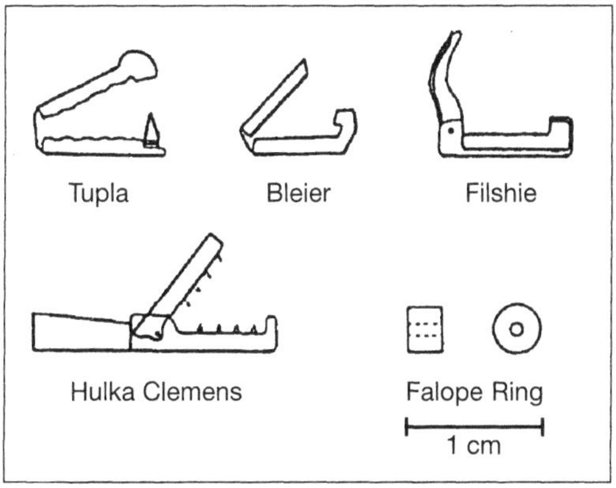

C02 or N20 if local anaesthetic is employed. A trocar and cannula is inserted just below the umbilicus to allow the insertion of a standard laparoscope. The patient is placed in the Trendelenberg position and the pelvic organs, including the fallopian tubes, are visualised. Using a supra-pubic second puncture, a further trocar and cannula is inserted to allow the introduction of the appropriate operating instrument, e.g. a clip applicator, ring applicator or cautery forceps. The tubes may be anaesthetised by dropping local anaesthetic, e.g. 2 ml 4% lignocaine or 10 ml 0.5% bupivocaine to reduce the per- and post-operative discomfort [11], whether the procedure is performed by local or general anaesthesia. There are single puncture techniques for all these methods and their use depends on the surgeons preference. As a rule, single-puncture technique is more difficult to perform, but may be more acceptable in certain patients.

Mini Laparoscopy

In countries where laparoscopy is not available, mini laparoscopy, performed under either local or general anaesthetic, is available. This method is perfectly acceptable and has minimal extra morbidity when performed by skilled surgeons.

Culdescopically or Culdotomy

This route is feasible and well tried, but its reputation for increasing pelvic infection has made the route less popular.

Methods and Efficacy

Although female sterilisation has been adopted by over 140 million women throughout the world, there have been remarkably few pivotal studies comparing the most popular methods of tubal occlusion; most studies are single and not comparative studies. The results, therefore, demonstrate a wide scatter of effectiveness, making two comparisons impossible. Pivotal studies are when patients are randomised to methods where the surgeon is competent at each method and follow-up data are obtained without the knowledge of the method employed. The popular methods to consider are:

1. Partial salpingectomy (Pomeroy or Parkland)
2. Bipolar cautery
3. Fallope Rings
4. Filshie clips
5. Hulka clips

Partial Salpingectomy

This method [12] is commonly performed in the post-partum period or at the time of caesarean section. It is also employed for interval tubal occlusion in the developing world, when laparoscopic facilities are not available. The Pomeroy technique is popular and has a failure rate of 3.3 per thousand. The Parkland technique, which involves the excision of a portion of the fallopian tube and each end, is then ligated separately. This involves slightly more surgery, but it has a low failure rate [13].

Unipolar Cautery

Unipolar cautery is of interest from a historic point of view, as it is considered to have a complication rate which is unacceptable by today's standards.

Bipolar Cautery

Bipolar cautery is usually performed laparoscopically. Unipolar diathermy, which is very efficient, has been largely replaced by bipolar diathermy because of the rare, but serious, consequences of inappropriate bowel burns. When diathermy is used, the tube is desiccated in two to three places, which usually involves a substantial portion of the fallopian tube. The temperature at the point of contact may reach over 300°C. Cutting the tube following the procedure has been used, but has been associated with a higher failure rate. The short-term failure rate is reportedly below two per thousand [14], but long-term results are much higher [13].

Cold Coagulation

A low-voltage, low-temperature technique has been developed to decrease yet further complications of heat. The temperature between the jaws of the forceps reaches approximately 120-140°C; when the forceps have become heated to the pre-operative temperature, they are kept in place for 20 secs at each place of burning.

The Fallope Ring

The Fallope ring is the most commonly used mechanical device throughout the developing world. It is an ingenious technique and can be made relatively cheaply for developing countries. The ring is made of silicone rubber 1x2.2x3.6 mm, which is expanded onto the end of a cannula. The forceps grasp the isthmic portion of the fallopian tube and pull the tube into the lumen of the operating cannula. The expanded ring is then pushed off the cannula to contract around a knuckle of approximately 3 cm of the fallopian tube, resulting in a Madlener type of technique.

The failure rate is less than four per thousand [15, 16]. This method is not recommended for post-partum use as the tubes are hypertrophied.

Hulka Clemens Clip

The Hulka Clemens clip is a spring-loaded clip, first described in 1972. The clip is made of lexan plastic and has interdigitating teeth on the jaws to prevent expulsion of the tube during closure of the clip. The clip is kept closed by a spring that is made of gold-plated stainless steel. This clip maintains pressure between the jaws of the clip holding the enclosed tube so that a vascular necrosis occurs within the jaws. The clip is 3 mm wide 15 mm long.

The short-term failure rate is less than five per thousand and this is higher when associated with pregnancy [15, 16].

Filshie Clip

The Filshie clip is made of titanium with an inner cushioned lining of silicone rubber. It has a front-locking mechanism to reduce the chance of the tube slipping out of the jaws when correctly applied. It is the most widely used method in Scotland [17] and the UK, Canada and Australia, and has been available in the US since the end of September 1996. The clip is 4 mm wide and 13 mm long.

The failure rate is less than three per thousand, but is higher in the post-partum period [18].

Operative Risk

All operations have a risk, particularly of sepsis and haemorrhage. The laparoscopic approach, when correctly performed, has remarkably few immediate complications, particularly of sepsis. In one of the largest mortality survey series published involving 29 deaths [19], 38% were related to anaesthetic problems and 24% due to sepsis - most of which related to bowel injury including bowel burns. Haemorrhage was associated with 14% of cases. The remainder were due to a miscellaneous group, including myocardial infarction, pulmonary embolus and gas embolus. The present estimated mortality from female sterilisation is 3.6% per 100.000 [20], which is considerably lower than the mortality of childbearing, which is 5.5% per 100.000 [21]; this benefit is particularly important in developing countries where the maternal mortality can be in excess of 100 per 100.000.

Long-Term Effects of Tubal Ligation

The long-term effects of tubal ligation include long-term failures, ectopic pregnancies and menstrual effects.

Long-Term Failures (8-14 years)

A long-term follow-up of female sterilisation has only recently been made available by the Crest study, conducted by the Centre for Disease Control [13]. As this is an American study, the Filshie clip data were not included. However, a long-term study is presently being conducted. The long-term follow-up for unipolar coagulation by polar coagulation, Fallope rings and Hulka clips is now available. In the Crest collaborative study, 10,863 patients were enrolled and 10,685 were followed up. Data were collected at 1, 3, 5, 8 and 14 years following the procedure. Cumulative 10-year morbidities were highest using the Hulka-clip method (36.5 per thousand cases) and was lowest using the unipolar coagulation (7.5 per hundred thousand). Young women have the highest failure rate and this included 53.3 per thousand with bipolar coagulation and 51.2 per thousand with Hulka-clip application. Pregnancies occurred fairly evenly throughout the successive years following the operation.

Ectopic Pregnancy Following Sterilisation

Ectopic pregnancies are potentially life-threatening complications, particularly in the third world, where access to surgery may be limited. Stock has described three types of fistulae leading to ectopic pregnancies:
a) A direct tubo-peritoneal fistula derived from the stump of the tube following any method of tubal ligation
b) As a result of endosalpingeosis following tubal ligation
c) A tubo-tubal fistula causing an ectopic pregnancy to lodge in the site of the fistulous connection

Electrocoagulation methods have the highest rate of ectopic pregnancy with regard to failures, whereas mechanical failures have the lowest in recent studies [18]. Filshie-clip failures have a 4% ectopic pregnancy rate following failure and this compares with 20% for the tubal ring and 67% for electro cautery. In this study, the Hulka clip demonstrated no ectopic pregnancies.

Menstrual Problems

A long-term effect on menstrual function has been conflicting. Increased loss and spotting has been reported, as has an increased reporting of pelvic pain, whereas absence of pain and no menstrual dysfunction have also been reported [22]. Some studies have involved over 10,000 subjects. In a prospective study of 5000 patients, followed up for 5 years, it was found that an increased number of menstrual disturbances, including pain, bleeding and spotting, occurred [23]. Also these problems were not related to the degree of tissue destruction at the time of the original operation. The disturbances increase with time following the procedure.

Hysterectomy has been reported to involve an increased number of women following sterilisation. It has also been concluded that women who have been sterilised will more readily accept a hysterectomy in the future.

Pelvic abscesses have been recorded with the Filshie clip in one patient [24]. Expulsion of Hulka clips have also been reported [25]. In a study of 6000 patients [18], three patients have been observed to have a clip pass per urethra, per rectum and per vaginum. All three patients were subsequently examined and no cause or morbidity was found. Migration is a common problem of clips but it is only rarely associated with morbidity.

Pre-operative Counselling

Counselling is a process of information gathering carried out by the couple so that they can understand the nature of the operation and its consequences sufficiently well to be able to give informed consent. Prior to the procedure, counselling both partners is ideal, although exceptions can be made. The principal of counselling is the same for both female and male sterilisation. A medical history of both partners is important, and concomitant pathology should be noted for each, e.g. menstrual problems relating to fibroids or the presence of ovarian cysts may make gynaecological surgery imminent or, as far as a man is concerned, he may have a hernia or a scrotal tumour. If related surgical procedures are contemplated, then, the sterilisation could be performed at that particular time. If a woman is to come off the pill after many years, her periods may become heavier, whereas if she has an IUD prior to the sterilisation her periods may become lighter. If both patients are fit and well then either may be sterilised. There are a number of special circumstances that need extra time when formulating a decision:

- *Age.* When a patient is under 25 years of age, a couple should understand fully that regret is more likely as there is a longer time to have a change in terms of life events, e.g. marital breakdown or death of a child or spouse.
- *Low parity.* As with younger patients, low-parity patients should be certain that they understand the permanency of the procedure and accept the consequences, even in the face of a loss of a child or spouse.
- *Performing a sterilisation in association with pregnancy.* Regret of the procedure following birth, termination of pregnancy or miscarriage is higher. This fact must be clearly understood by the patient and accepted. There is some evidence that there is a higher failure rate with some methods at this time. If the method is associated with a higher failure rate then the patient should be aware of this.
- *Financial considerations.* Poor financial circumstances can be highly motivating towards sterilisation. Patients should be aware of improved financial circumstances in the future.
- *Illness of a spouse or child.* These circumstances are difficult to respond to, as the condition could be genetically transmitted, familial or sporadic. On balance it would be preferred if the ill spouse be sterilised providing that it would not com-

promise their health. Ultimately, however, it is the couple's decision as to who should be sterilised.

- *Psychosexual problems or marital disharmony.* A sterilisation only rarely improves a marital relationship or psychosexual problems. If such problems are identified, then the issue should be addressed by Relate or psychosexual counselling prior to sterilisation.
- *Peri-menopause.* The cost effectiveness of a sterilisation operation is much less as the menopause becomes nearer, particularly as fertility declines substantially at this time. However, there are some couples who would not accept an abortion under any circumstances and would prefer to have a method with the best efficacy.
- *Reversibility of sterilisation.* This should not be a serious consideration. Although methods with minimal tissue destruction, e.g. clips, have a higher success rate when reversed [26].
- *Medico-legal aspects.* A failure of a sterilisation procedure is the most common cause of medico-legal complaints in the UK. The Medical Protection Society reports that this is responsible for 29% of claims in obstetrics and gynaecology [27]. The three areas of litigation involve:
  1. Failure to warn patients that there is a failure or complication rate
  2. Negligence in performing the sterilisation
  3. Inadvertently causing injury during the course of the procedure

Careful, and meticulous, attention to surgical techniques should reduce items 2 and 3. To reduce the incidence of item 1, careful counselling should be adopted by the general practitioner, the counsellor and also the surgeon. It is helpful if full documentation of the counselling can be made. This should include the following: the patient should be aware of other methods of family planning available, including vasectomy; the patient should be aware of the main complications of a sterilisation procedure and this should include the failure rate, which is usually given as 2-3 per thousand (anything less than 1% should be acceptable); the patient should accept the responsibility of not becoming pregnant at the time of tubal ligation and to continue family-planning methods until the next menstrual period has arrived. Ideally, the operation should be performed in the follicular phase of the cycle. If the operation is performed in the luteal phase, then it is possible that a sperm could have already entered the reproductive tract and this could result in an intra-uterine pregnancy, or indeed an ectopic pregnancy; the patient should accept the permanency of the operation; if the patient is obese or has medical problems, then this could increase the risk and this fact should be discussed and documented.

A dedicated Consent Form for sterilisation should be signed. Although a spouse is also often requested to sign, this is not a legal necessity.

Future Possible Methods

Most new methods of tubal ligation are related to the transcervical route as this would be less intrusive than the abdominal route.

Transcervical Obliteration of the Interstitial Portion of the Fallopian Tube

Cryocautery, diathermy, NG Yag lasers have all been used to destroy the interstitial portion of the fallopian tube. The power of regeneration of the endosalpinx is substantial and patency has been recorded in up to 50% of cases.

Transcervical Insertion of Tubal-Blocking Devices

There have been a number of intra-uterine plugs of titanium and silicone rubber, ceramics and nylon plus hydrogel. The latter is called P-block, which is designed by Brundin [28] and has had a number of studies carried out on it. Recent studies have demonstrated a Pearl index of 0.3.

Transcervical Application of Chemical Agents that Flow Down the Fallopian Tubes

Silver nitrate, zinc chloride, copper sulphate, formeldahyde, methyl cyanoacrilate and quinacrine pellets have all been described. The most promising of these has been quinacrine pellets. This technique involves the introduction 0f 7x36 mg pellets through a modified CuT intra-uterine device introducer into the uterine cavity. A single application, or two applications separated by 1 month is satisfactory. In one study [29] of over 31,000, there were no deaths and the pregnancy rate varied between 2.63 after 1 year to 4.3 at 2 years [3].

Male Sterilisation

Vasectomy

Introduction

Vasectomy was only rarely performed prior to 1970. However, following a publication from the Margaret Pyke Centre of 1000 vasectomies [30] followed up for 1 year, the operation gained wide-spread support. When family-planning services became freely available in 1974, many local authorities included vasectomy amongst their services, and when vasectomy became an item of service for family planning, vasectomy became totally accepted.

Prevelance

Vasectomy is becoming increasingly popular. Whereas it was estimated that some 50,000 procedures were performed annually in the UK in 1975, some 100,000 procedures are now thought to take place annually in the UK. In the developed world, there are approximately equal numbers of vasectomies and female sterilisations. However, vasectomy is less popular or illegal in developing countries.

Methods

A vasectomy may be performed under general or local anaesthesia. At present, most patients have a local anaesthetic procedure, as it is quicker and safer. Traditionally the local anaesthetic is administered to the skin and vas either in the mid-line or in preparation for a lateral incision. An incision is made through the skin down to the spermatic sheath. The sheath and vas is then grasped through the incision by special forceps, e.g. Soonerwalla. The sheath is incised until the vas is encountered. The vas is picked out from the sheath (a no.-1 needle is helpful here) and the vas is freed from the surrounding tissue. A portion of the vas is removed and both ends of the vas are ligated. Ideally, a needle-point diathermy is then inserted down each vas to cauterise the lumen. The testicular end is sometimes tied back on itself. This helps to keep the end out of the sheath, whilst the other end falls into the sheath. Bleeding points are cauterised and the procedure is repeated on the other side. A dissolvable skin suture is usually placed in the skin incision.

The No-Scalpel Technique. This procedure was developed in China by Dr Li [31] and involves the use of two special instruments. The first is ring-grasping forceps and the second is a sharp pair of pointed dissecting forceps. A local anaesthetic is injected 2-3 cm cordally around the vas to affect a proximal block (Fig. 2). Both vasa are anaesthetised. The oedema generated by the local anaesthetic is therefore 2-3 cm away from the operating site, so that the vas can be palpated easily. The vas, and anaesthetised overlying skin, is grasped by the ring forceps (Fig. 3). The skin is punctured by one blade of the sharp dissecting forceps and, through this puncture site, both blades are inserted down to the vas (Fig. 4). The forcep blades are then opened to spread the

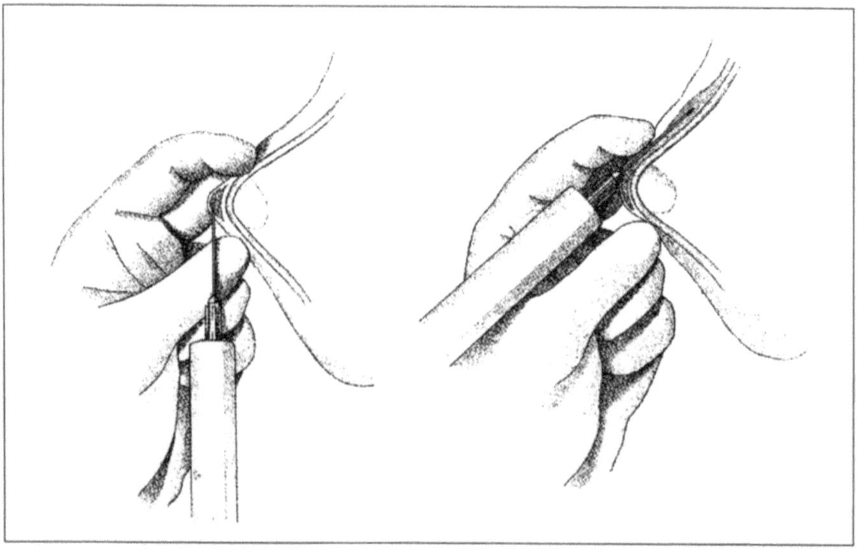

Fig. 2

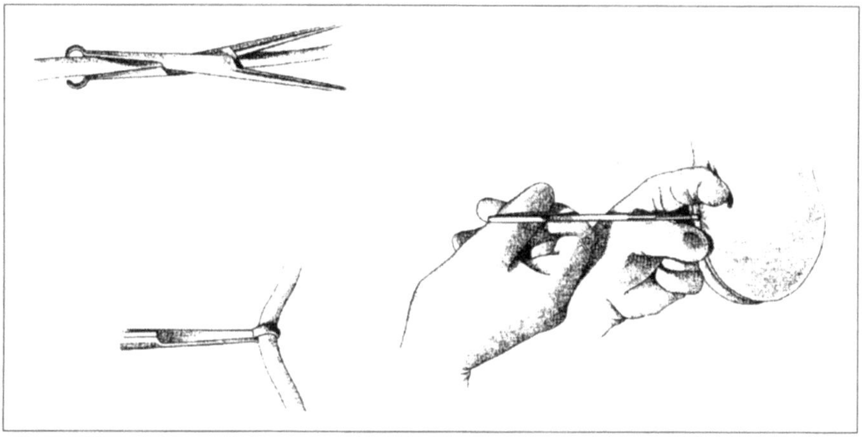

Fig. 3

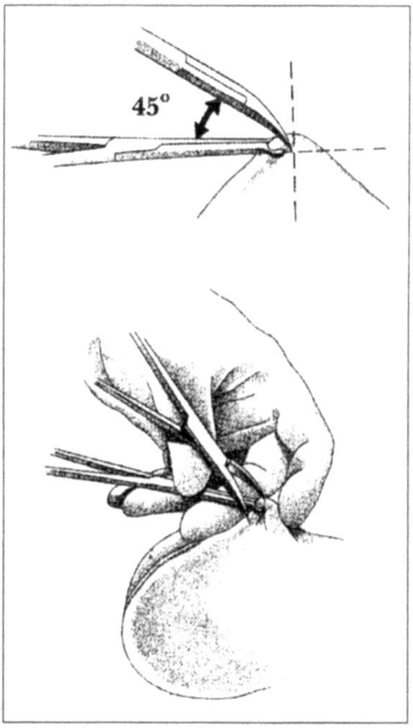

Fig. 4

tissue and the vas can, therefore, be seen immediately (Fig. 5) and exteriorised by the dissecting forceps (Fig. 6). The vas is stripped clear of any tissue and ligated as before (Fig. 7). The placing of fascia between the two ends has been advocated to reduce the failure rate, although this stage has been regarded as optional. No suture is usually required.

In a study from Thailand, Bangkok, at the King's Birthday Festival on 5 December 1987, when 1203 patients were operated on [32], a comparison was made between a standard vasectomy technique and the no-scalpel technique. The following results were recorded:

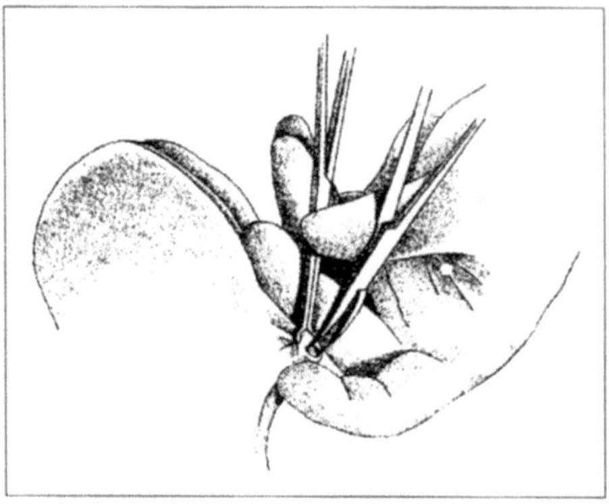

Fig. 5

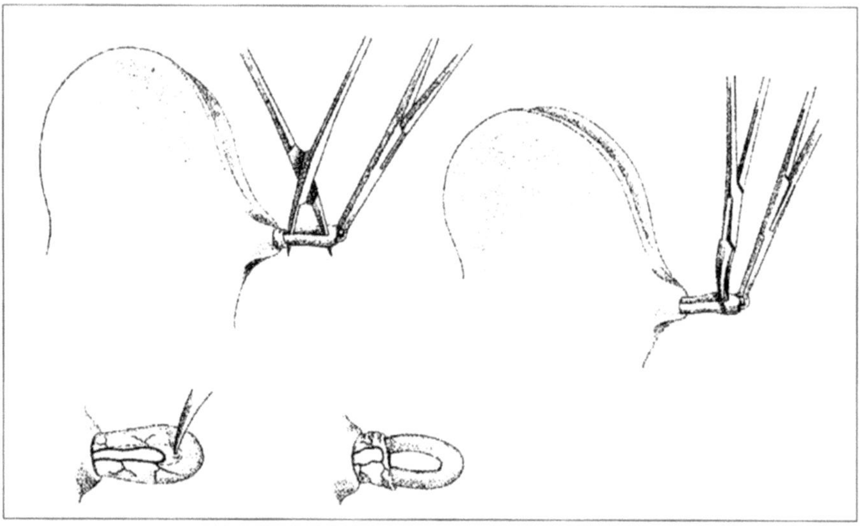

Fig. 6

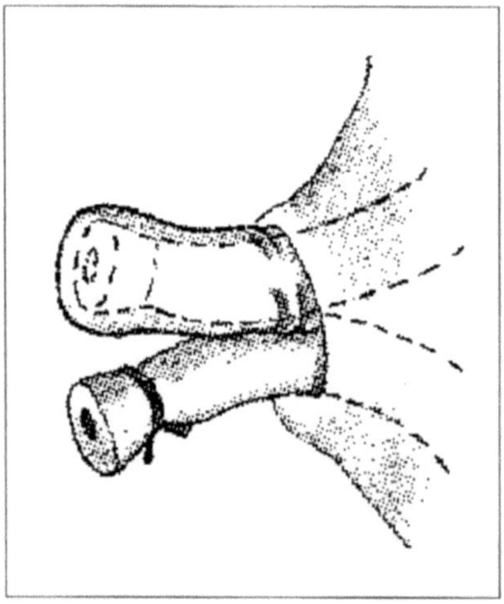

Fig. 7

Twenty-eight physicians operated on 1203 patients. Twelve physicians utilised the no-scalpel technique, whereas 16 physicians used a standard technique. The mean number of procedures was 57 (SD=12) for the no-scalpel technique and 33 (SD=13) for the standard procedure. Nineteen complications were reported during the 2 weeks following the operations: 16 occurred during the standard technique (3.1 per 100 procedures) and 3 occurred following the no-scalpel technique (0.4 per 100 procedures). Haemorrhage was the most common complication and two patients required surgical drainage. Nine of 11 haemorrhages (including those requiring drainage) were from the standard procedure. Eight patients had an infection diagnosed; seven of those had undergone the standard technique and one occurred following the no-scalpel technique.

Morbidity

Vasectomy has a very low mortality, but it has a relatively high morbidity. Approximately 4%-5% of cases will develop a small haematoma or experience sepsis. Large haematomas may need evacuation, as would an abscess. However, such interventions are required only one or two times per thousand cases. Long-term problems are rare: sperm granulomas and neuromas have been noted. There is no evidence that testicular cancer is increased with vasectomy, as is cardiovascular disease. However, there may be a very small increase in prostatic cancers, but it is regarded as so small to be insignificant when comparing a vasectomy with its benefits [33].

Counselling

The principals for counselling are the same as those adopted for female sterilisation. However, there are extra facts to be understood and accepted by the patient. There is a short-term failure rate of 3-5 per thousand. These can be identified by performing two sperm counts following the procedure. This may vary between 10 weeks and 20 weeks post-operatively. Patients are therefore advised to continue other forms of contraception until these two counts have proved negative. There is evidence of long-term intermittent presence of sperm in the ejaculate which could, very rarely, result in a pregnancy [34]. Complications of the procedure should be mentioned and also accepted by the patient. It is wise to ensure that the patient should seek immediate advice should any complications occur. A leaflet describing the procedure and its complications should be available for the couple to read.

Future Methods Being Considered

Intravasal chemicals and silicone plugs are being evaluated. The object would be to have a simple, reversible method. The techniques are more cumbersome and prolonged than existing methods and the results of the efficacy and reversibility are being evaluated. Percutaneous diathermy of the vas has also been investigated. The procedure appears simple and safe, but the efficacy appears to be less than normal. However, should the operation fail, a repeat procedure is easy to perform.

References

1. United Nations (1992) Levels and trends of contraceptive use as assessed in 1988. United Nations, New York
2. Spira A (1994) Contraception by the end of the 20th Century. Hum Reprod 9[Suppl 2]:125-128
3. Peterson HB, Xia Z, Hughes JM, Wilcox LS, Taylor LR, Trussell J (1996) The risk of pregnancy after tubal sterilisation: findings from the US collaborative review of sterilization. Am J Obstet Gynecol 174:1161-1168
4. Rowlands O, Singleton N, Maher J, Higgins V (1997) Living in Britain: results from the 1995 General Household Survey. The Stationery Office, London
5. Office of National Statistics (1997) 1995 Birth Statistics. Series FM1, No.24. The Stationery Office, London:
6. Rioux JE (1991) Female sterilisation. In: Filshie GM, Guillebaud J (eds) Contraception, science & practice. Butterworths, Chap. 12
7. Yoon I, King TM (1975) A preliminary and immediate report on a new laparoscopic tubal ring procedure. J Reprod Med 15:54
8. Hulka JF, Fishbourne J, Mercer JP et al. (1973) Laparoscopic sterilisation with a spring clip. A report of the first fifty cases. Am J Obstet Gynaecol 116:715
9. Filshie GM, Casey D, Pogmore JR et al. (1981) The titanium/silicone rubber clip for female sterilisation. Br J Obstet Gynaecol 88:655-662z
10. MacKenzie IZ, Turner E, O'Sullivan GM, Guillebaud J (1987) Two hundred outpatient laparoscopic clip sterilization's using local anaesthesia. Br J Obstet Gynaecol 94:449-453
11. Wheatley SA, Millar JM, Jadad AR (1994) Reduction of pain after laparoscopic sterilisation with local bupivacaine: a randomised, parallel, double-blind trial. Br J Obstet Gynaecol 101:443-446
12. Population Report (1990) Female sterilisation. No.10. p. 11. Nov
13. Peterson HB, Zhisen X Hughes JM et al. (1996) The risk of pregnancy after tubal sterilisation: findings from the US Collaborative Review of Sterilisation. Am J Obstet Gynecol 174:1161-1170
14. Hirsch HA, Nesser E (1983) Bipolar high frequency coagulation. In: van Lith DAF, Keith LG, van Hall EV (eds) New trends in female sterilisation. Year Book Medical, Chicago, pp 83-90
15. Chi I-C, Laufe LE, Gardner SD et al. (1980) An epidemiological study of risk factors associated with pregnancy following female sterilisation. Am J Obstet Gynecol 136:768-771
16. Chick PH, Frances M, Paterson PJ (1985) A comprehensive review of female sterilisation - tubal occlusion methods. Reprod Fertil 3:81-87
17. Penney GC, Soutar V, Glasier A, Templeton AA (1997) Laparoscopic sterilisation: opinion and practice among gynaecologists in Scotland. Br J Obstet Gynaecol 104:71-77
18. FDA Advisory Panel Meeting. 26 February, 1996
19. Peterson HB, De Stefano F, Rubin GL et al. (1983) Deaths attributable to tubal sterilisation in the United States: 1977-1981. Am J Obstet Gynecol 164:131-136
20. Kawachi, Ichiro, Colditz GA, Hankinson S (1994) Long term benefits and risks of alternative methods of fertility control in the United States. Contraception. 50:1-16
21. Report on confidential enquiries into maternal deaths in the United Kingdom. 1991-1993. HMS
22. Bhiwandiwala PP, Mumford SD, Feldblum PJ (1982) A comparison of different laparoscopic sterilisation occlusion techniques in 24, 439 procedures. Am J Obstet Gynecol 144:3
23. Wilcox L, Martinez-Schnell B, Peterson HB, Ware JH, Hughes JM (1992) Menstrual function after sterilisation. Am J Epidemiol 135:1368-1381
24. Robson S, Kerin J (1993) Recurrence of pelvic abscess associated with a detached Filshie Clip. Australia, N Z J Obstet Gynaecol 33:446
25. Gooden MD, Jaroslav F, Hulka MD, Cristman GM (1993) Spontaneous vaginal expulsion of Hulka clips. Obstet Gynaecol 81:884-886
26. Hulka JF, Noble AD, Letchworth AJ, Lieberman B, Owen E, Gomel V, Taft RC, Haney A, Wheeless CR, Imrie AH, Winston RCS, Loefler FE (1982) Reversibility of clip sterilisation. Lancet 2:927
27. Orr CJB (1985) Female sterilisation - the medico-legal aspects. In: Chamberlain GVP, Orr CJB, Sharp F (eds) Litigation: obstetrics & gynaecology vol. 163. Royal College of Obstetrics & Gynaecology, London, pp 76
28. Brundin J (1982) Hysteroscopy for sterilisation. In: Hafez ESE, Os WAA van (eds). Contraceptive delivery systems vol. 3. Elsevier, Amsterdam, pp 63-74
29. Mumford SD, Kessel E (1992) Sterilization needs in the 1990's: the case for quinacrine nonsurgical female sterilisation. Am J Obstet Gynecol 167:1203-1207

30. Margaret Pyke Centre (1973) One thousand vasectomies. BMJ 4:216-221
31. Li S, Goldstein M, Zhu J, Huber D (1991) The no-scalpel vasectomy. J Urol 145:341-344
32. Niraphpongporn A, Huber D, Krieger JN (1990) No-scalpel vasectomy at the Kings birthday vasectomy festival. Lancet 335:894-895
33. Scwingl PJ, Guess HA (1996) Vasectomy and cancer: an update. Gynaecol Forum 1:24-28
34. Philip T, Guillebaud J, Budd D (1984) Late failure of vasectomy after two documented analysis showing azoospermic semen. BMJ 289:77-79

14 Male Contraception: Promising New Approaches

Sigrid von Eckardstein, Eberhard Nieschlag

Background of the Development of a Reversible Male Contraceptive

Unlike women, who have a large variety of choices for contraception, men are presently restricted to a limited number of contraceptive choices, such as condom use, vasectomy or coitus interruptus. In Germany approximately 25% women of reproductive age report that they rely on one of these male methods in their sexual relationships (Oddens et al. 1994).

The last World Conference on Population and Development in Cairo (1994) recommended the development of a reversible male contraceptive for two principal considerations. First, especially in industrialized countries, there is an increasing demand from both men and women to share the responsibility and burden of family planning. Furthermore, continued growth of the world population, estimated to reach at least 8 billion people by the year 2020, makes it incumbent upon us to develop and make available reliable contraceptive choices to men and women. For similar reasons, scientists involved in research of male contraception recently formulated the "Weimar Manifesto" (see insert), which urgently requests the community and industry to support efforts on behalf of the development of a reversible male contraceptive.

The present article outlines the current status of male contraception with special respect to methods that have reached an advanced stage of development (hormonal suppression of spermatogenesis), as well as approaches that are currently still at a more experimental stage (Table 1).

Table 1. Approaches to a reversible male contraceptive

Principle	Approaches under clinical investigation	Approaches under experimental investigation
Prevention of sperm migration	Reversible occlusion of the vas deferens	
Suppression of spermatogenesis	Hormonal inhibition of gonadotropin secretion	
Prevention of sperm maturation/ function		Immunization against GnRH, FSH or FSH receptor Nitroimidazole derivatives, tripterigyium wilfordii, immunization against sperm antigens

The Weimar Manifesto on Male Contraception

Leading researchers from all over the world met in Weimar (Germany) on June 29, 1997, for a Summit Meeting to discuss the current status and prospects for male hormonal contraception. The researchers represented academic institutions as well as international organisations such as the Population Council (New York) and the World Health Organisation (Geneva).

All agreed that contraception is an essential component of reproductive health for men and women. Without contraception, all socioeconomic progress and the future of this planet are endangered. Apart from vasectomy and condoms, no contraceptives are available for men. New forms of male contraception are required to involve men more actively in family planning to share the benefits and burdens of contraception more equitably.

The researchers agreed that clinical research had shown that a reversible male hormonal contraceptive is feasible and effective. However, it has not yet been possible to show wide acceptability due the inadequate funding for large scale clinical trials.

There is a pressing need for product development and clinical trials of new, long-acting testosterone preparations and combinations with other agents. With adequate funding, a male hormonal contraceptive could be available in the near future.

Since any contraceptive method can only be brought to practical usage by pharmaceutical companies, the researchers urged the pharmaceutical industry to become actively involved in the development of novel male contraceptives. They also appealed in the spirit of the UN Cairo Declaration to politicians and research foundations to commit themselves to the development of male contraception for the sake of future generations.

Prof. E. Nieschlag (Chair)
University of Münster, Germany

Dr. H. M. Behre
University of Münster, Germany

Prof. M. T. Mbizvo
WHO, Geneva, Switzerland

Prof. W. Bremner
University of Washington, Seattle, USA

Dr. C. Meriggiola
University of Bologna, Italy

Prof. E. Diczfalusy
Karolinska Hospital, Stockholm, Sweden

Dr. K. Sundaram
Population Council, New York, USA

Prof. D. J. Handelsman
University of Sydney, Australia

Prof. R. Swerdloff
University of California, Los Angeles, USA

Prof. I. Huhtaniemi
University of Turku, Finland

Prof. C. Wang
University of California, Los Angeles, USA

Dr. E. Johansson
Population Council, New York, USA

Dr. F. Wu
University of Manchester, UK

Traditional Methods of Male Contraception

Barrier Methods

Traditional methods of male contraception, such as periodic abstinence or coitus interruptus, have the disadvantage of disturbed sexual activity and a relatively high rate of undesired pregnancies. Condoms are the oldest barrier method available. Unintended conception rates with condom use are relatively high with 12 of 100 couples conceiving during the first year of use (Trussell et al. 1990). However, safety of condom use may increase with the experience of the couple (Messiah et al. 1997). Worldwide acceptance of condoms varies with different sociocultural backgrounds. Recently, considerable financial effort and manpower was spent on educational programs for condom use as a potential protection from HIV infection (de Vincenzi 1994). Demonstration of long-term efficacy of these campaigns is still outstanding. National surveys in developed countries noted that the frequency of condom use has increased since the beginning of the AIDS epidemic, but preferentially among couples using an additional safer method of contraception (Larsson et al. 1996; Douglas et al. 1997).

Vasectomy

Vasectomy is a safe method for male contraception and has the advantage that it is technically easy to perform. Besides classical surgical vasectomy, minimal invasive procedures (Xiaozhang & Shunqiang 1993, Reynolds 1994) based on percutaneous electrocoagulation or chemical denaturation of the vas have diminished post-operative patients' complaints even further (Skriver et al. 1997). Unwanted pregnancies after vasectomy occur in less than 1% (Trussell et al., 1990). Possible reasons for failure are recanalization or intercourse before follow-up examinations are carried out. Less than two-thirds of patients undergo the two consecutive semen analyses recommended as a minimum to assure azoospermia (Maatmann et al. 1997).

In industrialized countries, vasectomy, like tubal ligation in women, is chosen preferentially with advancing age (Edouard 1997). This is mainly due to the fact that both procedures can be considered irreversible. Vasectomy reversal is requested in 2% - 7% of men (Engelmann & Hertle 1996), mainly due to changes in life circumstances. Refertilization can be successfully performed by means of microsurgical techniques, but the high incidence of sperm antibodies after vasectomy (Heidenreich et al. 1994) can be an obstacle to achieving a spontaneous pregnancy. In these cases, in vitro fertilization in combination with intracytoplasmatic sperm injection (ICSI) may be required to induce a pregnancy.

To make vasectomy a more widely chosen male contraceptive, Djerassi came up with the idea of sperm cryopreservation prior to vasectomy performed early in male reproductive life (Djerassis and Leibo 1994). This concept implies that a large human population, including both men and women, would be willing to relegate personal reproduction to medical techniques, divorced from sexual activity, which possibly prevents this approach from becoming a well-accepted procedure. Curiously, this idea converges with Crow´s suggestion that young men should cryopreserve their sperm early for paternity later in life, and undergo vasectomy to avoid mutational hazard to germ cells and reduce genetic diseases in their offspring that might otherwise increase with advanced age (Crow 1997).

New Approaches Towards Reversible Male Contraception

Posttesticular Contraception

Posttesticular contraception may act as classical male contraception at the site of the vas deferens or by interfering pharmacologically or immunologically with the process of sperm maturation in the epididymis (Fig. 1a, b). During epididymal transit, sperm undergo several maturation steps which are prerequisites for the acquisition of sperm motility and the ability to interact with the oocyte during fertilization (Cooper 1995). Theoretically, these may be disrupted at different sites; altering the process of fluid secretion and absorption could interfere with the optimal transit time and acquisition of sperm viscosity. Modifying the pattern of epididymally secreted proteins may change the optimal environment for maturation and storage of sperm (Cooper 1992). In practical terms, the search for effective and safe substances turned out to be difficult because of imbalances between effectivity and toxicity.

Non-surgical Vasectomy

Chinese investigators suggested a non-surgical vas occlusion by injection with a polyurethrane elastomer (Zhao 1990). Azoospermia was achieved in 95-98% of men within an interval of 18 months after the procedure. Full reversibility of the method by surgical extraction of the plug was reported for a limited number of patients. Histological examinations of the vas more than 4 years after the procedure are available, and showed a high rate of obstruction proximal and distal to the plug (Chen et al.

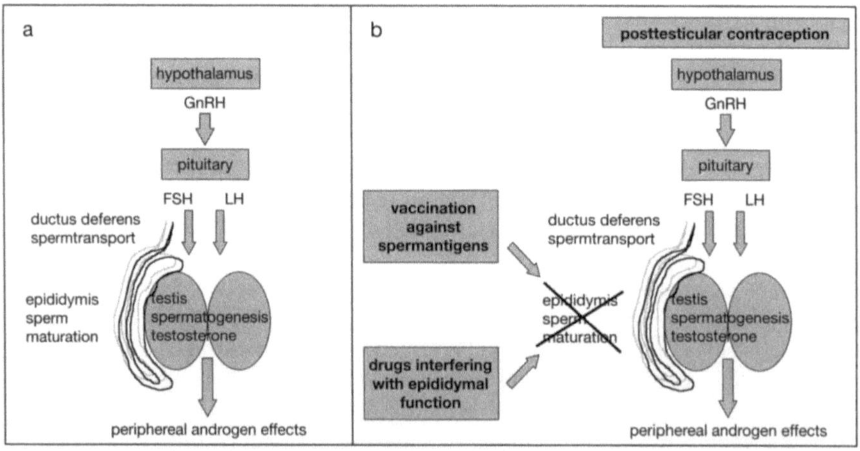

Fig. 1a, b. Possible sites for posttesticular interference with male reproductive capacity: *a* = normal situation, *b* = contraceptive approach

1996), casting some doubt on the reported success rates for refertilization. There is no confirmational data on non-surgical vasectomy from outside of China.

Inhibition of Sperm Maturation

A variety of substances is known to interfere with sperm maturation and exert anti-fertility effects in the presence of normal sperm numbers. Until now, none of these could be used for contraceptive purposes because the early appearance of toxic side effects prohibited long-term use. Gossypol, the substance best evaluated in humans, had to be eliminated because, at higher doses, it leads to severe potassium deficiency and irreversible damage of spermatogenesis (Prasad & Diczfalusy 1982, Waites & Wang 1998).

Trypterigium wilfordii is a plant product containing at least six components used in traditional Chinese medicine against fever, edema and localized infections. Given orally, it decreases fertility in animal models and some of its components were shown to reduce sperm motility and sperm counts in humans as well. The exact mechanism of action is not fully understood, probably because most data available refer to single components. Besides a post-testicular effect, a direct effect on spermatogenesis was proposed. At least in the rat model trypterigium wilfordii affected in vitro the human chorionic gonadotrophin (hCG)- stimulated testosterone secretion of Leydig cells, although in vivo the effective treatment dose did not alter serum levels of testosterone or gonadotropins. Upon histological examination (rat), an impairment of all spermatogenic stages was found. The degree of reversibility was not reported. At high doses, irreversible damage to the seminiferous epithelium, along with reduced serum testosterone concentrations were observed. Preliminary analysis of toxicity in animal models are suggestive of immunosuppressive side effects (for review Zhen et al. 1995). This agrees with the fact that, in men, the anti-fertility effects of trypterigium wilfordii were first observed when the plant was evaluated for treatment of rheumatoid arthritis because of its hypothesized immuno-modulatory functions.

On oral intake, ornidazole, a nitromimidazole-derived antimycoticum, effectively and reversibly inhibits fertility in the rat model at a dose of 400 mg/kg body mass. Impaired fertility is found in the presence of normal sperm counts and, as in vitro and in vivo studies suggest, results from an impairment of sperm energy production and changes in sperm velocity, leading to a failure in capacitation and oocyte fertilization (Yeung et al. 1995). Though animals tolerated treatment well and showed normal mating behavior during the period of drug feeding, they gained less body weight than controls. Whether this observation is suggestive of toxic side effects has not been investigated further and clinical trials for contraceptive purposes are still outstanding.

Although to date the reported studies did not succeed in finding a safe product interfering with sperm function, they show that this approach can be effective and deserves further exploration.

Immunization Against Spermantigens

From patients, it has long been known that the presence of sperm autoantibodies in the male or female partner is connected with impaired fertility. Anti-sperm antibodies may interfere with sperm transport in the female genital tract or inhibit sperm–egg interaction (Peters and Coulam 1992). Vaccination against sperm antigens has been successfully performed in female non-primate animal models (guinea pig), mainly targeting antigens such as PH-20 (Primakoff et al. 1990) and SP-10 localized on the acrosomal membrane. Using bovine in vitro fertilization, SP-10 antibodies were found to inhibit binding of capacitated spermatozoa to the zona pellucida (Coonrod et al. 1996). In the female non-human primate (baboon), vaccination with a synthetic peptide based on the immunoactive epitope of LDH-C4, a testis-specific isoenzyme of lactate dehydrogenase, reversibly decreased fertility over a 1-year period to 75% compared with control animals (O´Hern et al. 1995).

So far a variety of concerns has prevented studies on vaccination in male subjects beyond the preclinical level. Because of the blood-testis barrier, the testis is normally an immunologically privileged site. Immunization against sperm antigens present in the testis may be accompanied by irreversible testicular damage. Antibodies raised against antigens presented exclusively on post-testicular sperm may be less likely to induce autoimmune orchitis (Jones 1994), but presently only limited data from animal studies are available. To a certain extent, progress has been impaired by technical limitations, as identification of antigens was restricted to SDS-page analysis. Recent progress in molecular technology, including the availability of specific cDNA libraries, now allows improved identification and characterization of a variety of possible target antigens on sperm (Diekman & Herr 1997), implying the possibility of further advances in this field. PH-20 and PH-30 (fertilin), as antigens present on acrosome-reacted sperm, have been used for immunization of male guinea pigs and cynomolgous monkeys, respectively, leading to a marked reversible inhibition of fertility (Primakoff et al. 1990; Ramarao et al. 1996). In contrast to other reported immunization targets, no signs of testicular damage were observed in these experiments. Passive immunization, e.g. against prostatic inhibin peptide, though being an antigen only expressed in the prostate and the epididymis, was followed by an elevation of serum FSH levels, suggesting the induction of testicular damage (Vanage et al., 1992).

Suppression of Spermatogenesis

For female contraception, it is basically sufficient to interfere with the process of ovulation mediated through the midcycle LH peak to prevent pregnancies. For male contraception, it is essential to inhibit the whole process of spermatogenesis, which is, as in the female, regulated by a complex system of endocrine, paracrine and autocrine factors. Approaches currently being tested are based on preventing pituitary hormones from maintaining an intact process of spermatogenesis (Fig. 2a, b).

Immunization

Vaccination against gonadotropins as the major component involved in the hormonal feedback system controlling testicular function is one of oldest approaches to reversible male contraception (Nieschlag 1975; Wickings et al. 1980; Srinath et al. 1983). Theoretical advances claimed in favor of contraceptive vaccines are:

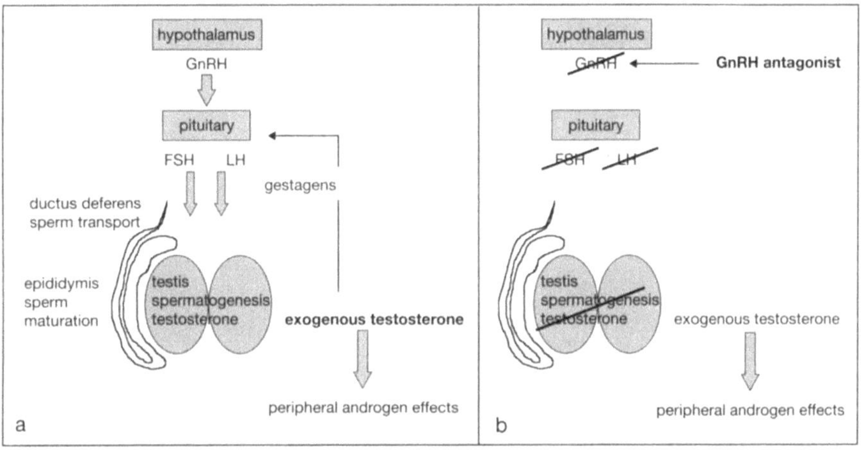

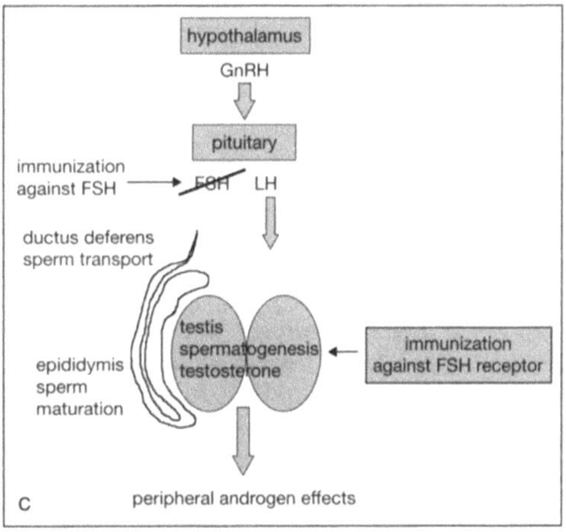

Fig. 2a-c. Hormonal and immunological approaches to the suppression of spermatogenesis: *a* Testosterone with or without gestagens. *b* GnRH antagonist with testosterone supplementation. *c* Immunological approaches

1. a potentially long-lasting effect
2. the possibility of large-scale production on a reasonable cost-effectiveness basis, and
3. the fact that in developing countries vaccination is a long-established medical principle (Jones 1994).

In women, immunization against hCG is at an advanced stage of research, with recently completed clinical trials (Talwar et al. 1997a). The effect of anti-hCG antibodies was found in the presence of regular menstrual cycles, suggesting that the anti-fertility effect is, as intended, prior to implantation. The HSD-hCG vaccine was highly effective with only one pregnancy occurring in more than 1200 cycles, observed as soon as antibody titers of more than 50 ng/ml were reached. Endocrine side-effects were absent, an especially important effect considering the high homology between hCG and other pituitary hormones.

Vaccination approaches in men are more difficult as there is no hormonal target which is as exclusively involved in regulation of reproductive function as hCG is in establishment and maintenance of early pregnancy in women. To better understand problems which were seen targeting FSH for immunocontraception, it is essential to look briefly at the current concepts on the regulation of spermatogenesis.

The classical concept of hormonal regulation of human spermatogenesis attributes LH primarily to the regulation of Leydig cell function and FSH to that of Sertoli cell function. Several lines of evidence from the human and non-human primate support the concept that the action of both hormones is needed to sustain quantitatively and qualitatively intact spermatogenesis (Weinbauer & Nieschlag 1996). Active immunization against FSH markedly reduces sperm output in monkeys (Srinath et al. 1983). When monkeys depleted of gonadotropins by treatment with GnRH antagonists were treated with FSH, it turned out that spermatogonia were present in the testis to a normal extent, but further stages of spermatogenic development (spermatocytes and spermatids) were numerically decreased (Weinbauer et al. 1991). These data suggest that FSH is critically involved in the induction of spermatogenesis, but quantitative maintenance of the complete spermatogenic cycle probably requires further cofactors. In the human, administration of FSH after testosterone-induced inhibition of spermatogenesis restores sperm counts to a certain extent, but complete restoration can only be achieved by co-treatment with hCG, substituting LH (Matsumoto & Bremner 1983, 1986). From patients with idiopathic hypogonadotropic hypogonadism, it is also known that normally administration of hCG plus hMG (substituting FSH) is necessary to produce sperm in the ejaculate (Kliesch et al. 1994). Normally hCG cannot be substituted by testosterone (Schaison et al. 1993), though occasionally hCG alone can be sufficient to induce spermatogenesis to some extent (Burris et al. 1987). Recent clinical observations are suggestive of a more central role for FSH and the FSH receptor in preserving fertility. Gromoll et al. (1995) described a hypophysectomized man who had undisturbed semen parameters and fathered three children during periods of testosterone substitution. He was shown to have an activating mutation of the FSH receptor. Therefore vaccination targeting the FSH receptor itself may lead to a considerably different outcome than FSH immunization.

In monkey studies, vaccination against endogenous FSH has the potential to disturb fertility severely in the presence of oligozoospermia, but constantly high antibody titers are required to overcome the testicular/ pituitary feedback system (Mougdal et al. 1992). Comparable to anti-hCG vaccines, cross-reactivity arising from structural homologies of glycoproteins (LH, TSH) may limit the use of antisera against whole FSH. Anti-FSH antisera were shown to have a high amount of anti-LH activity (Westhoff et al., 1996), raising the possibility that with long-term use, symptoms of testosterone deficiency such as impairment of sexual function, bone density and erythropoesis may be induced. On the other hand, residual anti-LH activity may have contributed to the contraceptive effect as the intratesticular testosterone content, as outlined in the chapter on hormonal male contraception, is discussed as one factor limiting spermatogenic suppression (Anderson et al. 1996). To overcome these problems, recently antisera against specific peptides (FSH sequence ß33-53 and ß81-95) were raised, addressing those antigenic sites that were previously found not to cross-react with LH (Westhoff et al. 1997). In rabbits, antibodies against a tandem form of the FSH ß33-53 subunit suppressed FSH bioactivity without altering LH-activity, as would be desirable for contraceptive purposes. Effects on fertility have not been investigated so far.

With increasing knowledge of molecular genetic techniques, further interesting immunization strategies became feasible. Recently, Mougdal et al. (1997) used antibodies raised against the extracellular domain of the FSH receptor for contraceptive vaccination in male bonnet monkeys. Sperm count and fertility results were comparable to those seen in immunization studies against FSH, with one animal of three impregnating a female during a 4-month mating episode. All animals had reduced fertility indices calculated from sperm count and motility and showed a significant impairment of spermatogenic development indicated by a decrease in the ratio of tetraploid to diploid cells on flow-cytometric analysis of testicular biopsies. FSH-receptor expression is restricted to gonadal tissue and is probably regulated by a number of factors not fully understood to date (Simoni et al. 1997). For these reasons, approaching the FSH-receptor rather than FSH may be of advantage and deserves further exploration. Currently available data may also be different in primates which do not have a seasonal breeding pattern.

From investigations on hormonal male contraception, it is known that pharmacological suppression of GnRH in combination with substitution of testosterone is an effective way to induce azoospermia in men. In the rat, immunization against GnRH has been used in models of spermatogenic physiology (McLachlan et al. 1994) and has also been proposed as a contraceptive approach (Awoniyi et al. 1992). When GnRH is linked to a carrier protein, it seems to have sufficient immunogenic properites. Three different conjugates have been created so far. Preliminary evaluations of toxicity are available for two of them. One was approved for clinical trials in India and Austria for the treatment of four patients with advanced stage prostate carcinoma. A decline in testosterone and PSA levels occurred in a dose-dependent fashion (Talwar 1997b). These preliminary results raise the possibility of a useful approach to contraception in men and women.

Hormonal Male Contraception

At the present state of research, hormonal male contraception is the most advanced and promising approach (Nieschlag & Waites 1996). Cessation of spermatogenesis is achieved via suppression of gonadtropins in combination with testosterone substitution to maintain the extratesticular effects of testosterone (Nieschlag & Behre 1996b).

Testosterone

The earliest approach to suppression of spermatogenesis via inhibition of the hormonal pituitary / testicular feedback mechanism is the systemic application of testosterone itself, which at the same time guarantees the maintenance of peripheral testosterone effects. Testosterone enanthate (TE), which is injected intramuscularly in an oily solution, is the substance on which the largest amount of data is available. In WHO-guided trials (WHO 1990, 1996), it turned out to be an effective but inconsistent inducer of azoospermia (Table 2). The second multicenter study was especially aimed at

Table 2. Efficacy of different regimens for hormonal male contraception

Study	Medication	Number of volunteers	Rate of azoospermia	Rate of oligo-zoospermia	Sperm count above
				($<3 \times 10^6$/ml)	($>3 \times 10^6$/ml)
Nieschlag et al., 1977)	Testosterone undecanoate (3x80 mg per day orally)	7	1/7 (14%)	0/7	6/7 (86%)
WHO 1990, WHO 1996 (Caucasian and Asian men)	Testosterone enananthate 200 mg/week	670	425/670 (63%)	not azoospermia 45/670 (37%)	
Handelman et al. 1995	Testosterone implants (1200 mg)	9	5/9 (56%)	4/9 (44%)	0/9
Knuth et al. 1985	19 - Nortestosterone	12	8/12 (67%)	2/12 (16.5%)	2/12 (16.5%)
Behre et al. 1995	Testosterone buciclate (1800 ng single injection)	8	3/8 (38%)	0/8	5/8 (62%)
For review Nieschlag et al. 1992	GnRH agonist (5-500 µg+ testosterone enanthate	106 (12 studies)	21/106 (20%)	32/106 (30%)	53/106 (50%)
For review Nieschlag & Behre, 1995	GnRH antagonist (7.5 to 20 mg/d) + testosterone enanthate or 19 - Nortestosterone	40 (5 studies)	35/ 40 (88%)	5/40 (12%)	0/40
Merigiolla et al. 996	Testosterone enanthate (100 mg/week) + Cyproteroneacetate (50 or 100 mg/d)	5	5/5 (100%)	0/5	0/5
Merigiolla et al. 1997	Testosterone undecanoate (80 mg twice a day) + Cypoteronacetate (12.5 mg twice a day)	8	1/8 (12%)	5/8 (62%)	2/8 (26%)
Knuth et al. 1989 (Germany) WHO, 1993 (Indonesia)	Testosterone enanthate (200 mg/month) or 19 - Nortestosterone + depot-medroxyprogesteron acatate (100-150 mg/month)	12 90	9/12 (75%) 87/90 (98%)	3/12 (25%) 3/90 (2%)	0/12
Bebb et al. 1996	Testosterone enanthate (100 mg/week) + Levonorgestrel (500µg/d)	18	12/18 (67%)	5/18 (28%)	1/18(5%)

studying contraceptive efficacy in azoospermic and non-azoospermic men (WHO 1996). Over an observation period of 12 months, all men who developed continuous azoospermia induced no pregnancy. In the oligozoospermic group, five pregnancies occurred, giving a pregnancy rate of 15.9% per 100 person years comparable to the Pearl Index found in condom users. Sperm function seems to be unaltered in the remaining sperm of oligozoospermic volunteers when tested for induction of acrosome reaction or oocyte penetration in the zona-free-hamster test (Wang et al. 1997), giving additional evidence that upcoming contraceptive trials should aim for azoospermia. In both WHO trials (1990, 1996) and local smaller studies (Aribarg et al. 1996), men from Asian centers more often suppressed to azoospermia than Causcasian volunteers. Whether this non-uniform response is attributable to ethnicity is still not clarified, though the only study addressing this aspect of non-uniform response argues against anthropometic or ethnic differences (Handelsman 1995). These findings suggest individually different thresholds for effective suppression of the pituitary axis, because responders showed a more pronounced rebound of FSH and LH after the suppression phase than non-responders.

Another problem limiting the use of testosterone enanthate for male contraception arises from the necessity of weekly injections. The search for longer-lasting testosterone preparations goes back to 19-nortestosterone hexoxyphenylpropionate (Anadur), which was the first long-acting preparation investigated (Knuth et al. 1985). Azoospermia rates were comparable to those for testosterone enanthate, but application intervals could be extended to 3 weeks.

Subcutaneous testosterone implants have a comparable potency in suppressing spermatogenesis over an interval of 5-6 months (Handelsman et al. 1992). The minor surgery required for implantation and occasional problems with infection and extrusion (Jockenhövel et al. 1996) to date prevented implants from more extensive investigations, except for some Anglo-Saxon countries.

Testosterone buciclate, developed under the guidance of WHO, is a substance with a very favorable pharmacokinetic profile resulting in normal testosterone levels over at least 3 months (Nieschlag & Behre 1996). A single injection of a low dose (1200 mg) is sufficient to suppress sperm counts (Behre & Nieschlag 1995). Data on higher doses or repeated injections are still outstanding but are expected to be promising.

Whether a newly developed testosterone preparation (injectable testosterone undecanoate) has a potential for male contraception is not clear to date. Currently it is under clinical investigation for substitution therapy in male hypogonadism (Abshagen et al. 1997).

Furthermore, in in vitro studies of a synthetic androgen, 7α-methyl-19-nortestosterone (MENT) had a high androgenic effect on muscles and on the pituitary. As it does not undergo 5α-reduction, it is supposed to have lesser effects on the prostate (Agarwal & Monder 1988). It has been evaluated for its potency to suppress gonadotropins in vivo in men. A single dose of 4 mg injected intramuscularly resulted in a short-term reduction of LH and FSH levels to 70% and 57%, respectively, after 5 days (Suvisaari et al. 1997). From these results, it appears that MENT may become another candidate substance as the androgenic component in a hormonal male contraceptive.

GnRH Analogues and Testosterone

As azoospermia rates resulting from suppression with testosterone alone are not completely satisfying and frequent testosterone administrations are inconvenient, interest focused further on combination therapies consisting of testosterone and other drugs enhancing gonadotropic supression.

From treatment of advanced-stage prostate carcinoma GnRH agonists are known to effectively suppress serum testosterone levels via inhibition of gonadotropins, which make them an attractive tool to enhance the suppressive effect of testosterone alone. GnRH agonists specifically bind to GnRH receptors in the pituitary gland and, after initial activation of the receptor, lead to suppression of LH and FSH secretion via down-regulation of GnRH receptors. For unexplained reasons the combination of different GnRH agonists with testosterone very insufficiently inhibited spermatogenesis (Table 2). From monkey and rat studies it has been suggested that this problem is due to coadministration with testosterone, which prevents adequate FSH suppression (Akhtar et al. 1983). Recent availability of newer long-acting GnRH agonist preparations did not result in reevaluation of this approach to hormonal male contraception.

GnRH antagonists competitively block GnRH receptors and immediately lead to a drop in LH and FSH secretion. In a sequence of studies in non-human primates it could be shown that GnRH antagonist treatment combined with a delayed onset of testosterone supplementation most effectively suppressed spermatogenesis (Weinbauer et al. 1988, Weinbauer et al. 1989). In the clinical studies performed so far (for review Nieschlag & Behre 1996a) GnRH antagonist turned out to induce azoospermia very efficiently independently of whether testosterone coadministration was delayed or not. The onset of suppression varied between a very early onset of 4 weeks and 16 weeks, depending on the dose of the GnRH antagonist administered. Unfortunately administration of GnRH antagonists remains inconvenient because of the necessity of daily subcutaneous injections. An improvement is offered by administration schemes which, after an initial loading of 5 days with GnRH antagonist, maintains gonadotropic suppression for at least 30 days on a diminished dose (Behre et al. 1997). Whether this is also effective for contraception still has to be shown. In our own study attempts to maintain spermatogenic suppression after initial administration of GnRH antagonist with 19-nortestosterone hexoxyphenylpropionate showed a slight rebound in gonadotropins and reappearance of sperm after the antagonist was withdrawn (Nieschlag & Behre 1996a).

Gestagens and Testosterone

The high efficacy of GnRH antagonist cotreatment underlines the fact that complete inhibition of the pituitary axis is an important prerequisite in achieving optimal suppression of the spermatogenic process in all men. Interest currently focuses on other drugs acting on the gonadotropic axis but less expensive and less inconvenient to apply. Female contraception has shown gestagens to be effective suppressors of FSH and LH. For male contraception gestagens have been used with different results. In German volunteers 19-nortestosterone hexoxyphenylpropionate (Anadur) together with depot-medroxyprogesteroneacetate (DMPA) was only slightly more efficient than

19-nortestosterone hexoxyphenylpropionate given alone (Knuth et al. 1989), while it leads to nearly complete azoospermia in Indonesian men (WHO 1993).

Recently, Bebb et al. (1996) reported very satisfying results combining testosterone enanthate administered intramuscularly with the oral gestagen levonorgestrel at a dose of 0.5 mg daily (Table 2). By this mode of administration the dose of testosterone enanthate could be reduced to half (100 mg), but weekly injections were still required.

Cyproterone acetate is a synthetic steroid with antiandrogenic and gestagenic actions. In men it has been traditionally used for testosterone suppression in cases of hypersexuality and sexual delinquency. Its property of suppressing spermatogenesis was first evaluated in studies conducted around 1980 (Fogh et al. 1979; Moltz et al. 1980; Wang & Yeung 1980). Doses between 5 and 20 mg considerably impaired sperm counts in the ejaculate. However, because of symptoms of androgen deficiency, i.e., decreased libido and general activity patterns, it was neglected for male contraception until recently. In a preliminary small study the combination of cyproterone acetate at comparably high doses of 100 or 50 mg/day with testosterone enanthate (Merigiolla et al. 1996) partly overcame this problem and turned out to be very effective in terms of reduced sperm output (Table 2). Though overt symptoms of androgen deficiency were lacking, mild manifestations such as slight anemia and reduction in body weight occurred. The mechanism of action for the effect of cyproterone acetate on spermatogenesis still needs to be elucidated. It has been claimed that the degree of inhibition of spermatogenesis depends on intratesticular conversion of testosterone to DHT, at least in testosterone enanthate trials (Anderson et al. 1996). Whether antiandrogens are capable of diminishing intratesticular testosterone action remains a matter of speculation.

Coadministration of lower doses of cyproterone acetate with an oral androgen preparation turned out to be far less effective in suppression of spermatogenesis (Merigiolla et al. 1997), probably underlining the necessity of constantly high levels of testosterone, which at the moment are best achieved by injectable preparations or implants. It further demonstrates the problem of developing a self-administered male contraceptive, which we also faced in a clinical trial combining transdermal testosterone patches with levonorgestrel. Azoospermia rates were comparably low and therefore this approach deserves optimization (Büchter et al. 1998).

Outlook

At present, the status of research of hormonal male contraception is most advanced in clinical trials and probably nearer to wide range application than immunization protocols or posttesticular approaches. In the coming years interest will focus on further increasing efficacy and practical applicability. The development of long-acting testosterone preparations may be an important step forward in this regard. Presently the results of ongoing clinical trials on the efficacy of different testosterone preparations with different gestagens are awaited. Here, too, when establishing the minimally effective dose of components, possible side-effects must not be overlooked.

Besides FSH, LH and testosterone, a variety of other intratesticular factors such as growth factors, stem cell factors and estrogens are possibly involved in the regulation of intact spermatogenesis (Schlatt et al. 1997). Further research in this field may reveal additional targets for male contraception. For example, in monkeys it was reported that inhibition of aromatization of testosterone to estrogens is accompanied by a decrease in sperm production (Shetty et al. 1997). However, with regard to the human, such appoaches are presently limited by our sparse knowledge on estrogen actions in men.

Acknowledgement. The work on male contraception at the Institute of Reproductive Medicine, University of Münster has been supported by grants from WHO, BMG and DFG.

References

Abshagen K, Behre HM, Oette W, Hübler D, Nieschlag E (1997) Intramuscular injection of testosterone undecanoate for the treatment of male hypogonadism: phase I-studies. Experim. Clin. Endocrinol. Diab. 105 (Suppl.1): 21 (Abstract)

Agarwal AK and Monder C (1988) In-vitro metabolism of 7α-methyl-19-nortestosterone by rat liver, prostate and epididymis. Endocrinology 123: 2187-2193

Akhtar FB, Marshall GR, Nieschlag E (1983) Testosterone supplementation attenuates the antifertility effects of an LHRH agonist in male monkeys. Int. J. Androl. 6: 461-468

Anderson RA, Wallace AM, Wu FC (1996) Comparison between testosterone-enanthate induced azoospermia and ologozoospermia in a male contraceptive study. III. Higher 5α-reductase activity in oligozoospermic men administered supraphysiological doses of testosterone. J. Clin. Endocrinol. Metabol. 81: 902-908

Aribarg A, Sukcharoen N, Chanprasit Y, Ngeamvijawat J, Kriangsinyos R (1996)Suppression of spermatogenesis by testosterone enanthate in Thai men. J. Med. Assoc. Thai. 79: 624-629

Awoniyi CA, Kim WK, Hurst BS, Schlaff WD Immunoneutralization of gonadotropin-releasing hormone and subsequent treatment with testosterone silastic implants in rats: an approach toward developing a male contraceptive. Fertil. Steril. 58: 403-408

Bebb RA, Anawalt BD, Christensen RB, Paulsen CA, Bremner WJ, Matsumoto AM (1996) Combined administration of levonorgestrel and testosterone induces more rapid and effective suppression of spermatogenesis than testosterone alone: a promising male contraceptive approach. J. Clin. Endocr. Metab. 81: 757-762

Behre HM, Baus S, Kliesch S, Keck C, Simoni M, Nieschlag E (1995) Potential of testosterone buciclate for male contraception: endocrine differences between responders and nonresponders. J. Clin. Endocr. Metab.; 80: 2394-2403

Behre HM, Kliesch S, Pühse G, Reissmann T, Nieschlag E (1997) High loading and low maintainance dose of a GnRH antagonist suppress serum LH, FSH and testosterone effectively in normal men. J. Clin. Endocrinol. Metab. 82: 1403-1408

Büchter D, v. Eckardstein S, Behre HM, Nieschlag E (1998) Hormonal male contraception with transdermal testosterone patches and levonorgestrel. Abstract Europ. Soc. Endocrinol.

Burris AS, Rodbard HW, Winters S, Sherins RJ (1987) Gonadotropin therapy in men with isolated hypogonadotropic hypogonadism: the response to human chorionic gonadotropin is predicted by initial testicular size. J. Clin. Endocrinol. Metabol. 66: 1144-1151

Chen ZW, Gu Y, Liang X, Shen L, Zou WZ (1996) Morphological observations of vas deferens occlusion by the percutaneous injection of medical polyurethane. Contraception 53: 275-279

Coonrod SA, Westusin ME, Herr JC (1996) Inhibition of bovine fertilization in vitro by antibodies to SP-10. J. Reprod. Fertil. 107: 287-297

Cooper TG (1992) The epididymis as a site of contraceptive attack. In. Nieschlag, E., Habenicht, U.F. (eds): Spermatogenesis, fertilization, contraception. Springer: 419-460

Cooper TG (1995) Functions of the human epididymis. In: Hamamah, S., Mieusset, R., Dacheux, J.L. (eds.): Frontiers in endocrinology. Epididymis: role and importance in male infertility treatment. Ares Serono Symposia: 1-12

Crow JF (1997) The high spontaneous mutation rate: Is it a health risk? Proc. Nat. Acad. Sci. 94: 8380-8386

de Vincenzi I (1994) A longitudinal study of human immunodeficiency virus transmission by heterosexual partners. N. Engl. J. Med. 331: 341-346

Diekmann AB, Herr JC (1997) Sperm antigens and their use in the development of an immunocontraceptive. Am. J. Reprod. Immunol. 37: 111-117

Djerassi C, Leibo SP (1994) A new look at male contraception. Nature 370:11-12

Douglas JM, Hoxworth T, Rogers J, Malotte CK, Bolan GA, Zenilman J, Lenz A (1997) Contraceptive practices before and after an intervention promoting condom use to prevent HIV infection and other sexually transmitted disease among women - selected US sites, 1993-1995. JAMA 277:1752-1753

Edouard L (1997) On the determination of contraceptive prevalence using health care utilization data. J. Clin. Epidemiol. 50: 481-484

Engelmann U & Hertle L (1997) Vaectomy and refertilization. In In: Nieschlag, E. & Behre, H.M. (eds): Andrology: Male reproductive health and dysfunction. Springer, Heidelberg: 380-386

Fogh M, Corker CS, Hunter WM, McLean H, Philip J, Schon G, Skakkebaek NE (1979) The effects of low doses of cyproterone acetate on some functions of the reproductive system in normal men. Acta Endocrinol. 91: 545

Gromoll J, Simoni M, Nieschlag E (1996) An activating mutation of the follicle-stimulating hormone receptor (FSHR) autonomously sustains spermatogenesis in a hypophysectomized man. J. Clin. Endocr. Metab. 81: 1367-1370

Handelsman DJ, Conway J, Boylan LM (1992) Suppression of human spermatogenesis by testosterone implants. J. Clin. Endocr. Metab. 75: 1326-1332

Handelsman DJ, Farley TM, Peregoudov A, Waites GM (1995) Factors in nonuniform induction of azoospermia by testosterone enanthate in normal men. Fertil. Steril. 63: 125-133

Heidenreich A, Bonfig R, Wilbert DM, Strohmaier WL, Engelmann UH (1994) Risk factors for antisperm antibodies in infertile men. Am. J. Reprod. Immunol. 31: 69-76

Jockenhövel F, Vogel E, Kreutzer M, Reinhardt W, Lederbogen S, Reinwein D (1996)Pharmacokinetics and pharmacodynamics of subcutaneous testosterone implants in hypogonadal men. Clin. Endocrinol. 45: 61-71

Jones WR (1994) Gamete immunology. Hum. Reprod. 9, Suppl. 2: 107-124

Kliesch S, Behre HM, Nieschlag E (1994) High efficacy of gonadotropin or pulsatile gonadotropin-releasing hormone treatment in hypogonadotropic hypogonadal men. Eur. J. Endocrinol. 131: 347-354

Knuth UA, Behre HM, Belkien L, Bents H, Nieschlag E (1985) Clinical trial of 19-nortestosterone hexyloxyphenylpropionate (Anadur) for male fertility regulation. Fertil. Steril. 44: 814-821

Knuth UA, Yeung CH, Nieschlag E (1989) Combination of 19-nortestosterone hexyloxyphenylpropionate (Anadur) and depot-medroxyprogesterone acetate (Clinovir) for male contraception. Fertil. Steril. 51: 1011-1018

Larsson G, Milsom I, Andersch B, Blohm F (1996) A comparison of contraceptive habits and pregnancy outcome at 19 years of age in two cohorts of Swedish women born 1962 and 1972. Contraception. 53: 259-265

Maatman TJ, Aldrin L, Carothers GG (1997) Patient noncompliance after vasectomy. Fertil. Steril. 68: 552-555

Matsumoto AM, Karpas E, Paulsen CA, Bremner WJ (1983) Reinitiation of sperm production in gonadotropin-suppressed normal men by adminstration of follicle-stimulating hormone. J. Clin. Invest. 72: 10051015

Matsumoto AM, Karpas E, Bremner WJ (1986) Chronic human chorionic gonadotropin administration in normal men: evidence that follicle-stimulating hormone is necessary for the maintainance of quantitatively normal spermatogenesis in man. J. Clin. Endocrinol. Metab. 62: 1184-1192

McLachlan RI, Wreford NG, Tsonis C, De Kretser DM, Robertson DM (1994) Testosterone effects on spermatogenesis in the gonadotropin-releasing hormone-immunized rat. Biol-Reprod.; 50: 271-280

Merigiolla MC, Bremner WJ, Paulsen A, Valdiserri A, Incorvaia L, Motta R, Pavani A, Capelli M, Flamigni C (1996) A combined regimen of cyproterone acetate and testosterone enanthate as a potentially highly effective male contraceptive. J. Clin. Endocrinol. Metabol. 81: 3018-3023

Merigiolla MC, Bremner, Constantino A, Pavani A, Capelli M, Flamigni C (1997) An oral regimen of cyproterone acetate and testosterone undecanoate for spermatogenic suppression in men. Fertil. Steril. 68: 844-850

Messiah A, Dart T, Spencer BE, Warszawski J (1997) Condom breakage and slippage during heterosexual intercourse: a French national survey. French National Survey on Sexual Behavior Group (ACSF). Am. J. Public. Health. 87: 421-424

Moltz L, Römmler A, Post K, Schwartz, Hammerstein J (1980) Medium dose cyproterone acetate (CPA): effects on hormone secretion and on spermatogenesis in man. Contraception 21: 393-413

Mougdal NR, Ravindranath N, Murthy GS, Dighe RR, Aravindan GR, Martin F (1992) Long term contraceptive efficacy of vaccine of ovine follicle stimulating homone in male bonnet monkeys (Macaca radiata). J. Reprod. Fertil. 96: 91-102

Mougdal NR, Sairam MR, Krishnamurthy HN, Sridhar S, Krishnamurthy H, Khan H (1997) Immunization of male bonnet monkeys (M. radiata) with a recombinant FSH receptor preparation affects testicular function and fertility. Endocrinol. 138: 3065-3068

Nieschlag E (ed) (1975) Immunization with hormones in reproduction research. Proceedings of the International Symposium on Immunization with Hormones in Reproduction research. North-Holland/American Elesevier, Amsterdam and New York

Nieschlag E, Hoogen H, Bölk M, Schuster H, Wickings EJ (1978) Clinical trial with testosterone undecanoate for male fertility control. Contraception 18: 607-614

Nieschlag E, Behre HM, Weinbauer GF (1992) Hormonal male contraception: a real chance? In. Nieschlag E, Habenicht UF (eds): Spermatogenesis, fertilization, contraception. Springer: 477-501

Nieschlag E & Behre HM (1996a) Hormonal male contraception: Suppression of spermatogenesis with GnRH antagonists and testosterone. In Filicori M, Flamigni C (eds.): Treatment with GnRH analogs: controversies and perspectives. Parthenon Press, London: 243-248

Nieschlag E & Behre HM (1996b) Männlicher Beitrag zur Kontrazeption: Experimentelle Ansätze. In: Nieschlag E & Behre HM (eds): Andrologie: Grundlagen und Klinik der reproduktiven Gesundheit des Mannes. Springer, Heidelberg: 409-416

Nieschlag E & Behre HM (1997) Testosterone therapy. In Nieschlag E, Behre HM (eds) Andrology: Male reproductive health and dysfunction. Springer, 298-309

Nieschlag E & Waites GMH (1996) The myth of a male pill. Nature Medicine 7: 722 (letter)

Oddens BJ, Visser AP, Vemer HM, Everaerd WTAM (1994) Contraceptive use and attitudes in reunified Germany. Eur. J. Obstet. Gynecol. 57: 201-208

O´Hern PA, Bambra CS, Ishakia M Goldberg E (1995) Reversible contraception in female baboons immunized with a synthetic epitope of sperm-specific lactate dehydrogenase. Biol. Reprod. 52: 331-339

Peters AJ, Coulam CB (1992) Sperm antibodies. Am. J. Reprod. Immunol. 27: 157-162

Prasad MR, Diczfalusy NE (1982) Gossypol. Int. J. Androl. (Suppl.) 28: 53

Primakoff P, Lathrop W, Woolman L, Cowan A, Myles D (1988) Fully effective contraception in male and female guinea pigs immunized with the sperm protein PH-20. Nature 335: 543-546

Ramarao CS, Myles DG, White JM, Primakoff P (1996) Initial evaluation of fertilin as an immunocontraceptive antigen and molecular cloning of the cynomolgous monkey fertilin ß subunit. Mol. Reprod. Dev. 43: 70-75

Reynolds RD (1994) Vas deferns occlusion during non-scalpel vasectomy. J. Fam. Pract. 39: 577-582

Schaison G, Young J, Pholsena M, Nahoul K, Couzinet B (1993) Failure of combined follicle-stimulating hormone-testosterone administration to initiate and/or maintain spermatogenesis in men with hypogonadotropic hypogonadism. J. Clin. Endocrinol. Metabol. 77: 1545-1549

Schlatt S, Meinhardt A, Nieschlag E (1997) Paracrine regulation of cellular interactions in the testis: factors in search of a function. Eur. J. Endocrinol. 137: 107-117

Shetty G, Krishnamurthy H, Krishnamurthy N, Bhatnagar S, Mougdal RN (1997) Effect of estrogen depriviation on the reproductive physiology of male and female primates. J. Steroid. Biochem. Molec. Biol. 61: 157-166

Simoni M, Gromoll J, Nieschlag E (1997) The follicle-stimulating hormone receptor: biochemistry, molecular biology, physiology, and pathophysiology. Endocr. Rev. 18: 739-773

Skriver M, Skovsgaard F, Miskowiak J (1997) Conventional or Li vasectomy: a questionnaire study. Br.J.Urol. 79: 596-598

Srinath BR, Wickings EJ, Witting C, Nieschlag E (1983) Active immunization with follicle-stimulating hormone for fertility control: a 4,5-year study in male rhesus monkeys. Fertil. Steril. 40: 110-117

Suvisaari J, Sundaram K, Noe G, Kumar N, Aguillaume C, Tsong YY, Lähteenmäki P, Bardin CW (1997) Pharmacokinetics and pharmacodynamics of 7 alpha-methyl-19-nortestosterone after intramuscular administration in healthy men. Hum. Reprod. 12: 967-973

Talwar GP, Singh OM, Gapta SK, Hasnain SE, Pal R, Majumbar SS, Vrati S, Mukhopaday A, Srinivasan J, Deshmakh U, Gauga S, Maudokhot A, Gupta A (1997a) The HSD-hCG vaccine prevents pregnancy in women: feasibility study of a reversible safe contraceptive vaccine. Am. J. Reprod. Immunol. 37: 153-160

Talwar GP (1997b) Fertility regulating and immunotherapeutic vaccines reaching human trials stage. Hum. Reprod. Update 3: 301-310

Trussell J, Hatcher RA, Cates W, Stewart FH, Kost K (1990) Contraceptive failure in the United States: an update. Stud. Fam. Plan. 21: 51-54

Vanage GR, Garde SV, Sheth AR (1992) Passive immunization against prostatic inhibin peptide as a male contraceptive. Intern. J. Androl. 15: 114-126

Waites JGM & Wang C (1998) Gossypol. Int. J. Androl. in press

Wang C, Yeung KK (1980) Use of a low dosage of cyproterone acetate as a male contraceptive. Contraception 21: 245-272

Wang C, Leung A, Superlano L, Steiner B, Swerdloff R (1997) Oligozoospermia induced by exogenous testosterone is associated with normal functioning residual spermatozoa. Fertil. Steril. 68: 149-153

Weinbauer GF, Göckeler E, Nieschlag E (1988) Testosterone prevents complete suppression of spermatogenesis in the gonadotropin-releasing hormone (GnRH) antagonist-treated nonhuman primate (macaca fascicularis). J. Clin. Endocrinol. Metabol. 67: 284-290

Weinbauer GF, Kurshid S, Fingscheidt U, Nieschlag E (1989) Sustained inhibition of sperm production and inhibin secretion induced by a gonadotropin-releasing hormone antagonist and delayed testosterone substitution in the nonhuman primate (macaca fascicularis). J. Endocrinol. 123: 303-310

Weinbauer GF, Behre HM, Fingscheidt U, Nieschlag E (1991) Human follicle-stimulating hormone exerts a stimulatory effect on spermatogenesis, testicular size and serum inhibin levels in the gonadotropin-releasing hormone antagonist-treated non human primate. Endocrinology 129:1831-1839

Weinbauer GF & Nieschlag E (1996) The Leydig cell and male contraception. In Payne AH, Hardy MP, Russell CD: The Leydig Cell. Cache River Press: 630-662

Westhoff WE, Slootstra JW, Puijk WC, Kuperus D, Flinterman JF, Schaaper WMM, Oonk HB, Meloen RH (1996) Detection of epitopes on follicle stimulating hormone and FSH-antiserum-induced suppression of bioactivity of follicle-stimulating hormone and luteinizing hormone. J. Reprod. Immunol. 30: 133-149

Westhoff WE, Slootstra JW, Puijk WC, van Leeuwen L, Schaaper WMM, Oonk HB, Meloen RH (1997)In vitro inhibition of the biological activity of follicle-stimulating hormone by anti-peptide antisera representing the follicle-stimulating hormone beta subunit sequence 33-53. Biol. Reprod. 56: 460-468

WHO Task Force on Methods for the Regulation of Male Fertility (1990) Contraceptive efficacy of testosterone-induced azoospermia in normal men. Lancet 336: 955-959

WHO Task Force on Methods for the Regulation of Male Fertility (1993) Comparison of two androgens plus depot-medroxyprogesterone acetate for suppression to azoospermia in Indonesian men. Fertil. Steril. 60:1062-1068

WHO Task Force on Methods for the Regulation of Male Fertility (1996) Contraceptive efficacy of testosterone induced azoospermia and oligozoospermia in normal men. Fertil. Steril. 65: 821-829

Wickings EJ, Usadel KH, Dathe G, Nieschlag E (1980) The role of follicle-stimulating hormone in testicular function of the mature rhesus monkey. Acta Endocrinol. 95: 117-128

Xiaozhang L, Shunqiang L (1993) Vasal sterilization in China. Contraception 48: 255-265

Yeung CH, Oberländer G, Cooper TG (1995) Effects of the male antifertility agent ornidazole on sperm function in vitro and in the female genital tract. J. Reprod.Fertil 103: 257-264

Zhao SC (1990) Vas deferens occlusion by percutaneous injection of polyurethrane elastomer plugs: Clinical experience and reversibility. Contraception 41: 453-459

Zhen QS, Ye X, Wie ZJ (1995) Recent progress in research on Tripterygium: a male antifertility plant. Contraception 51: 121-129

MIX
Papier aus verantwortungsvollen Quellen
Paper from responsible sources
FSC® C105338

If you have any concerns about our products,
you can contact us on
ProductSafety@springernature.com

In case Publisher is established outside the EU,
the EU authorized representative is:
Springer Nature Customer Service Center GmbH
Europaplatz 3, 69115 Heidelberg, Germany

Printed by Libri Plureos GmbH
in Hamburg, Germany